Health Studies
An Introduction

Second edition

Edited by
Jennie Naidoo and Jane Wills

palgrave
macmillan

First edition 2001
Reprinted 8 times
Second edition 2008

Published by
PALGRAVE MACMILLAN
Houndmills, Basingstoke, Hampshire RG21 6XS and
175 Fifth Avenue, New York, N.Y. 10010
Companies and representatives throughout the world

PALGRAVE MACMILLAN is the global academic imprint of the Palgrave
Macmillan division of St. Martin's Press, LLC and of Palgrave Macmillan Ltd.
Macmillan® is a registered trademark in the United States, United
Kingdom and other countries. Palgrave is a registered trademark in the
European Union and other countries.

ISBN-13: 978–0–230–54520–5 paperback
ISBN-10: 0–230–54520–3 paperback

This book is printed on paper suitable for recycling and made from fully
managed and sustained forest sources. Logging, pulping and manufacturing
processes are expected to conform to the environmental regulations of the
country of origin.

A catalogue record for this book is available from the British Library.

10   9   8   7   6   5   4   3   2   1
17 16 15 14 13 12 11 10 09 08

Printed and bound in Great Britain by
Cromwell Press Ltd, Trowbridge, Wiltshire

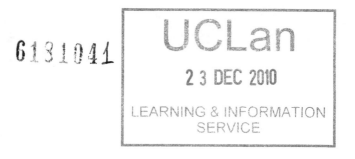

Contents

List of figures

List of tables

List of examples

List of abbreviations

ADP	adenosine diphosphate
AIDS	acquired immune deficiency syndrome
ASA	Advertising Standards Authority
ASH	Action on Smoking and Health
ATP	adenosine triphosphate
BMI	body mass index
BSE	bovine spongiform encephalopathy
CCTV	closed circuit television
CEO	chief executive officer
CHD	coronary heart disease
CHI	Commission for Health Improvement
CHRE	Council for Healthcare Regulatory Excellence
CLBP	chronic lower back pain
CPS	Crown Prosecution Service
CT	computed tomography
DCMS	Department of Culture, Media and Sport
DfES	Department for Education and Skills
DHA	district health authority
DHSS	Department of Health and Social Services
DNA	deoxyribonucleic acid
DoH	Department of Health
ECHR	European Court of Human Rights
ESC	embryonic stem cells
GDP	gross domestic product
GI	glycaemic index
GMC	General Medical Council
GNP	gross national product
GP	general practitioner
HDI	human development index
HDL	high density lipoprotein
HIV	human immunodeficiency virus
HPA	hypothalamic-pituitary-adrenal
HPC	Health Professions Council
HRT	hormone replacement therapy
HRV	heart rate variability
HSE	Health Survey for England
ICD	International Classification of Diseases
IT	information technology

(2007, Manchester University Press) and she is currently completing *The Care of Brute Beasts: A Social and Cultural Study of Veterinary Medicine in Early Modern England*, due for publication in 2008.

Norma Daykin is Professor of Arts in Health at the University of the West of England, Bristol. A sociologist with multidisciplinary interests, she has spent over 15 years researching and writing about health, focusing on the impact of illness and patients' and professionals' experiences of health services. She is co-author of *Improving Cancer Services through Patient Involvement* (2004, Radcliffe Medical Press) and *Health and Work: Critical Perspectives* (1999, Macmillan). She is an executive editor of *Arts & Health: An International Journal of Research, Policy and Practice*. Her current research examines the role and impact of arts and music in healthcare.

Peter Duncan is Senior Lecturer in Health Promotion, Centre for Public Policy Research, King's College London. He is the author of *Critical Perspectives on Health* (2007, Palgrave Macmillan) and (with Alan Cribb) *Health Promotion and Professional Ethics* (2002, Blackwell).

Mat Jones is Senior Lecturer in Health and Social Science at the University of the West of England, Bristol. He combines a lecturing role in the fields of social science, health studies and public health with a wide range of externally commissioned research, specializing in mixed-method studies of complex community health initiatives. Much of this work has centred on young people's perspectives on drugs, alcohol and food-related issues. It also encompasses wider agendas on health inequalities, wellbeing and social inclusion. His current academic interests include the relationship between gardening, cultural spaces and the public sphere in late modernity.

Lynne Kennedy is Lecturer in Public Health Nutrition at the University of Liverpool. She has over 15 years' experience in health promotion, with special interests in food and health policy, and the politics of food.

Liz Lloyd is Senior Lecturer in Social Gerontology at the School for Policy Studies, University of Bristol. Her research interests are in health and social care policies and practices related to ageing, particularly in relation to the end of life in old age. From her recent research, Liz has developed theoretical ideas concerning the role of care in promoting health in the context of chronic and degenerative disease and about the need for an ethics of care. Liz has an ongoing interest in multidisciplinary and multiagency practice, including the contribution of housing to the promotion of health.

Anne Mulhall is an independent research consultant. Her previous posts include Senior Scientific Officer at Queen Charlotte's Hospital, London, and Deputy Director of the Nursing Practice Research Unit, University of Surrey. Her particular interests are evidence-based practice, the dissemination and implementation of research, ethnography, epidemiology and infection control. She has written three books on nursing research.

Jennie Naidoo is Principal Lecturer in Public Health and Health Promotion at the University of the West of England, where she is a member of an interdisciplinary team delivering the MSc Public Health programme. Her background is in sociology and health promotion practice. She has co-authored several bestselling textbooks on health promotion and public health with Jane Wills. Her research interests focus on women's health and ethnic minority groups' access to services.

Jane Ogden is Professor of Health Psychology at the University of Surrey and is involved in research in a number of health-related areas including eating behaviour and obesity, communication in healthcare and aspects of women's health. She is author of over 100 research papers and five books, including two books on eating behaviour and one entitled *Health Psychology: A Textbook* (2nd edn, 2000, OUP).

Bob Pitt is Senior Lecturer in the School of Health, Community and Policy Studies at the University of the West of England. He has experience teaching social policy to a diverse range of students including youth and community workers, social workers and health professionals. His background is in community work and community education, where he has worked on oral history and reminiscence projects with older people in Bristol. His current research interest is on the educational journeys of adults returning to learn in further and higher education.

Hilary Scott is an independent consultant, supporting individuals, teams and organizations in their work to develop public services. She has more than 20 years' experience of working in the healthcare and voluntary sectors, at local, regional and national levels. Her career in healthcare included 10 years as a health authority and then trust Chief Executive, a period as Deputy Health Service Ombudsman and a senior level secondment to the Department of Health. Hilary chairs the board of trustees for the UK charity, Action on Elder Abuse. She is Associate Professor at Middlesex University Business School and an independent governor at the University of Westminster.

Katherine Smith is Research Fellow at Durham University. Her current research examines the interface between health inequalities research, policy and politics in Scotland and England.

Martin Walter was employed in the NHS in laboratory work, computing, management and staff training for some 33 years. From 1988, he was Senior Lecturer at London South Bank University, teaching health services management studies to both UK and international students. He is now a freelance lecturer and consultant.

Jane Wills is Reader in Public Health and Health Promotion at London South Bank University. She has written extensively on health promotion and has co-authored several texts with Jennie Naidoo. Her research interests have been pedagogical and on the development of practitioners. She is co-editor of

JENNIE NAIDOO and JANE WILLS

Introducing health studies

Health studies has the virtue of being a broad and interdisciplinary subject area that allows students to focus on the central topic of health without being confined to any one discipline. This book demonstrates how different disciplines construct health in different ways and have different ways of studying what health is and how it may be understood. This second edition of *Health Studies* has been extensively revised and updated to ensure its continuing relevance and two new chapters, on politics and history, have been included.

This introductory book will help the reader to:

- Become familiar with a variety of perspectives on health issues

- Explore different constructions of health and its management for individuals and populations

- Relate these perspectives to the ways in which health and social care services could and should be organized

- Use these different perspectives to explore key health issues and contemporary challenges

- Understand the different research methodologies and methods that may be used to study health

- Be guided to areas that merit further study

What is health studies?

Health studies is a relatively new field of enquiry that draws on theoretical perspectives from a wide range of disciplines or branches of knowledge. In some cases, it encompasses a study of health through a relatively traditional foundation course in social sciences. Elsewhere, interdisciplinary health studies courses emphasize, through a focus on specific topics, the many ways in which health may be understood and studied through the use of different academic disciplines. The concept of 'health' is studied in many different programmes and curricula, ranging from health studies, health sciences and health and wellbeing, to more vocational programmes such as health promotion and nursing. Some programmes select a combination of subject disciplines. It is the breadth of analysis and evidence that distinguishes health studies from being simply the application of any particular subject discipline to health.

Health studies as a unifying concept to facilitate **interdisciplinary** understanding has several unique strengths. First, health studies focuses on health but without any a priori ranking of different disciplines. Health studies therefore allows for creative exploration and collaboration around health needs and healthcare. Second, health studies encourages interventions to take place in different disciplines, professions and organizations simultaneously. This achieves a synergistic effect – the whole effect being greater than the sum total of the different component parts. Third, health studies allows creativity and exploration to flourish. Creativity is fostered when the accepted truths or ways of working are challenged by different perspectives within an overall attitude of mutual knowledge and respect.

A focus on health

This book is about the study of health. Most students probably have a clear idea what they will be studying when they look at health. Yet as individuals, groups and societies, our understanding of health differs and varies according to the context and situation. For example, a young female nursing student might tap into very different meanings of health according to whether she is conducting experiments in the laboratory with her tutor group (biology), discussing dieting with her friends (cultural), trying to persuade a patient to quit smoking (psychology and health promotion) or lobbying for better transport to and from university (social policy and environmental science). All these different meanings of health are valid within their own context. However, some definitions are more popular and more widely used than others. Historically and culturally, an objective, biological construction of health, derived from science and medicine, has dominated Western developed countries' concepts of health. However, this dominant definition of health is increasingly being challenged on many fronts, as will be demonstrated in this book.

Health can be defined as both an objective and a subjective phenomenon. In objective terms, health is the normal functioning of biological entities. Normal functioning is assessed via the measurement of physical bodies, organs or systems, for example body mass index (BMI) measurements and blood pressure rates. Health may also be defined in relation to populations, for example disease prevalence rates. Health is also defined in subjective terms, which in turn are affected by one's age, gender and social class. For example, most children see health as 'eating the right things' and 'being fit', whereas older people define health more in terms of 'being able to cope' and being able to continue to do daily tasks and activities.

Health can also refer to a number of different categories or entities, ranging from the cellular or organ focused (for example healthy hearts), the individually focused (for example healthy body and healthy mind), the socially focused (for example healthy societies with high levels of social capital and wellbeing) to the environmentally focused (for example sustainable housing and renewable energy sources). This diversity of meaning ensures that the concept of health is relevant to a wide range of disciplines and practitioners. However, it may also lead to confusion and misunderstandings if people attempt to use their definition of health in different contexts and situations.

One solution would be to have an overarching definition of health that encompasses all the different disciplinary and contextual meanings of health. Attempts have been made to do this. A holistic view of health was encapsulated in the World Health Organization's (WHO, 1946) definition:

> Health is a state of complete physical, mental and social wellbeing, not merely the absence of disease or infirmity.

In this definition, health may seem idealistic and unattainable but its frequent quotation reflects its symbolic significance in highlighting the importance of a multidimensional positive view of health. Other definitions suggest that health can be viewed in terms of resilience and the capacity of individuals, families and communities to cope successfully with risk or adversity. The following pronouncement from the WHO emphasizes the dynamic and aspirational nature of health and its many social and environmental correlates:

> To reach a state of complete physical, mental and social well-being, an individual or group must be able to identify and to realize aspirations, to satisfy needs, and to change or cope with the environment. Health is, therefore, seen as a resource for everyday life, not the objective of living. Health is a positive concept emphasizing social and personal resources, as well as physical capacities. (WHO, 1986, p. 1)

A consequence of the diversity of definitions of health is that the scope of health studies is vast, and although there is no consensus on what disciplines should be included or excluded in its study, it will certainly include far more than a study of illness or diseases or training in the care of the sick. Inevitably, this book presents a selection of disciplines that contribute to health studies. In the absence of a commonly accepted syllabus, the rationale for inclusion was to demonstrate the breadth of health studies and include what we perceive to be key contributory disciplines. A brief synopsis of the disciplines included in this book follows.

Outline of the book

In Western societies, health is frequently associated with the presence or absence of disease or illness. This derives from the dominance of medicine that offers a framework of scientific knowledge and understanding of the body. The body is understood to be an objective biological structure composed of different component parts and connecting pathways. Health and disease are objective states that are capable of being scientifically proven. Health is the normal functioning of the biological components of the body, whereas disease is manifested through signs and symptoms in parts of the body indicating a pathological abnormality. Someone has a disease if tests can verify the presence of a disease process such as a compromised immune system. The scientific biological concept of health is explored by S.H. Cedar in Chapter 1.

The scientific view of health has not always been the case. Health has been defined differently in different historical epochs. In ancient times, the Greeks defined *hygieia* (health) and *euexia* (soundness) as the ideal balance between the four bodily 'humours' of blood, phlegm, yellow bile and black bile. In the sixteenth and seventeenth centuries, scientists began increasingly to view the body as a machine that could be reduced to its component parts. This paradigm shift was underwritten by Descartes' (1596–1650) famous treatise, which proposed that the body and the soul are separate. Cartesian dualism, as this is called, allowed the corporeal body to be freed up for exploration through the methods of scientific study, which legitimized the exploration of the human body through dissection, something that had already been described by Vesalius in 1543. There followed a general trend towards empiricism (the idea that knowledge derives from observation or experiments rather than from theory). Historical concepts of health are discussed in Chapter 2 by Louise Hill Curth.

Epidemiology, the study of patterns of disease within populations, is particularly linked to public health. Epidemiological data contribute to the health agenda by identifying and prioritizing particular health problems according to their contribution to mortality and morbidity. Analysing patterns of disease and correlating these with the distribution of risk factors in populations can help to identify the causes of ill health and disease. Once causes and risk factors have been identified, strategies to address these factors and thereby improve the health of populations can be planned and implemented. Epidemiology uses the techniques of scientific enquiry and quantitative study designs to identify relationships between risk factors and resulting diseases, and this is the subject of Chapter 3 by Nicola Crichton and Anne Mulhall.

Epidemiological data confirm a link between socioeconomic status and health and the existence of social inequalities in health. While the impact of social class on health has been extensively researched and documented, there is increasing recognition and documentation of the effect on health of other structural factors such as gender, sexuality and ethnicity. Social factors are not just important predictors of health status, they can also be powerful agents of health improvements. McKeown's (1976) historical analysis showed that socioeconomic factors such as improved sanitation, nutrition and general improvements in living conditions were more significant in improving health than medical advances or health services. Supranational economic policies, globalization and the commodification of influences on health also impact on health (www.who.int/social_determinants). Sociology is concerned not just with objective phenomena, but also with the social construction of meaning. This branch of sociology has investigated topics such as the social construction of the body and the meanings we give to medical surveillance. In Chapter 4, Norma Daykin and Mat Jones discuss the contribution of sociology to health studies, focusing particularly on the evidence and debates concerning health inequalities in modern society.

However, knowing someone's socioeconomic status cannot predict either their objective state of health or their subjective perception of health. Subjective perceptions are affected by people's knowledge, attitudes and behaviour, and this field of enquiry is studied in psychology. Psychological explanations for health acknowledge that mental functioning affects behaviour and both may be influenced by wider social factors. Health psychology aims to understand and explain the role of psychological factors in the cause, progression and consequence of health and illness. Many health promotion and disease prevention programmes focus on trying to persuade people to change their behaviour and make healthier choices. These programmes are informed by theoretical models of behaviour change and personality traits drawn from the discipline of psychology. In Chapter 5, Jane Ogden explores what contributes to people's behaviour and how the views of patients may differ from those of health professionals.

It is common nowadays to think of health and ill health as an individual experience – as personal and unique. However, these individual perceptions and experiences are in turn shaped and moulded by cultural norms, concepts and meanings that are evident in language and popular media representations. Individual perceptions and experiences draw upon those shared meanings that are current in the common culture of our social group or wider society. For example, a disease like cancer is often seen as an uncontrolled invasion of our body and self by an alien entity (Sontag, 1989). Wellness is frequently expressed through independence and control. The growing interest in the body reflects our emphasis on the individual and it is through our bodies that we express and shape our identity. In Chapter 6, Sarah Burch examines the language and visual signs with which we describe health.

The protection and promotion of health, and the detection and treatment of illness, are key functions of modern democratic governments. Governmental responsibility in this area is reflected in legislation and policy-making to protect and promote people's health, and the provision of health and social care services. Social policies can promote health in diverse ways, ranging from protecting individual incomes and access to personal health and welfare services, to promoting sustainability and regeneration in neighbourhoods. However, health has to compete against other priorities (such as economic growth) in the policy-making arena. The need to rationalize the rising costs of healthcare has been a major feature of most health policy throughout the developed world. In Chapter 7, Bob Pitt and Liz Lloyd discuss different views on service provision and the emergence of the welfare state in the UK. Recent challenges to the welfare state, from both the Left and Right boundaries may involve exchanging the role of expert for one of novice. This can be challenging for the student, as it means being able and willing to go beyond one's 'home' discipline and accept other disciplines' constructions of health as valid, meaningful and helpful. As such, it is also a creative and productive endeavour.

Different disciplines may be thought of as different pathways leading to their chosen destination, hedged in by their own concepts, theories, concerns and methodologies. Most further and higher education is provided in terms of different disciplines – economics, psychology, politics and so on. The academic disciplines are discrete areas of knowledge characterized by specific theoretical concerns and allegiance to particular types of methodology. An academic discipline centres on a particular definition of what is deemed worthy of knowing and what constitutes truth or reality. This is referred to as 'ontology'. Each discipline also has accepted ways of knowing or finding out about truth or reality, referred to as 'epistemology'. This book shows that other explanations exist and that 'health' is far too complex to be interpreted in a single, all-embracing explanation.

Relationships between different disciplines are frequently strained and hostile. For example, biologists and sociologists have long misunderstood each other. Biology has led to the discovery of many cures and treatments for illnesses. Unfortunately, recourse to the biological in society has occasionally served inhumane or immoral ends, as in justifying eugenics as a means to bring about desirable genetic traits in individuals or societies. Recently, there has been a move to bring together sociology and biology. Stansfield (1999) asks whether a lack of social support (a psychologically perceived and socially produced process) can influence bodily physiology and contribute to illnesses such as cardiovascular disease. The evidence from epidemiological studies suggests that there is a relationship between the two variables but the causal mechanism is not known. This thesis has led to calls for more social support (or social capital) strategies, such as Sure Start, to be introduced on health grounds.

Conrad and Jacobson (2003) offer a fascinating and complex discussion of the overlap and links between the biological and social using the example of cosmetic surgery. Cosmetic surgery may be used by women to enhance their social position as well as to conform to media-created examples of beauty. The area of biogenetics raises fundamental questions about the practicalities and realistic expectations of genetically tailored cures for diseases, the ethics of ownership of, and access to, such knowledge and the funding and management of the global project. While biogenetics is firmly embedded within the disciplines of biology and physiology, its impact and usefulness will depend on many factors that are addressed by different disciplines, such as social policy, economics, organizational studies and ethics. These examples of projects that span biology and social sciences demonstrate how in real life health issues are interdisciplinary. In order to understand and engage with these issues, and achieve results, people need to be able to transcend disciplinary boundaries and become familiar with using interdisciplinary perspectives.

Each of the disciplines presented in this book is located within different paradigms or ways of seeing the world. Each, therefore, poses different sorts of questions and requires different methods for answering them. The second part of each chapter of the book discusses theoretical and methodological perspectives and you will find extended discussions of different **methodologies** ranging from scientific methods (Chapter 3) to social constructionism (Chapter 4).

Traditionally, a scientific approach tries to identify the cause of the phenomenon being studied, for example an illness, and aims to produce predictive models that can say that, in certain circumstances, X will happen. It does this through the observation and measurement of variables, ideally in the context of a randomized controlled investigation. Epidemiology, physiology, economics and psychology all use this kind of approach and use scientific methodologies. This approach is associated with the philosophy of positivism. Positivism assumes there are objective, external realities that can be known and understood, using appropriate scientific methodologies. The social and natural sciences have a common logical framework, which tries to understand the relationship or association between different variables. The quest to understand why something happens varies according to different disciplinary values. For example, a physiologist may be interested in the physical reactions that take place under stress. A psychologist might be interested in why certain situations are perceived as stressful.

At the opposite end of the spectrum lies the social constructionist epistemology or theory of knowledge. According to this perspective, there is no single, fixed reality but people have many different descriptions and accounts of health. We all try to interpret our experiences and learn to understand 'what health is' (for us). Thus we can begin to understand health as a social product, influenced and formed by class, political processes and values, historical antecedents, gender, family life and so on. People's 'worlds of meaning' are also shaped by and reflected in all the customs and practices of the culture and society in which they live. We can begin to understand this by looking at accounts of health and illness in discourse and narratives and in media representations. The chapters on sociology, cultural studies, social policy, history and politics explore this different approach to understanding.

In between the two extremes lie a range of epistemologies and methodologies that subscribe to elements of both science and social constructionism. Sociology and social policy use a scientific approach and quantitative data, while simultaneously advocating a critical stance towards such data. For example, the mortality rates of different social classes tell us that mortality is linked to employment status, but do not reveal the mechanisms linking the two. Such data may also obscure the impact of other factors that may be equally important, such as gender or ethnicity. This may lead us to further questions: Why are data on social class more widely available than data on had economic costs with lower productivity and lost output of £2 billion. The Department of Health's *Health Survey for England 2003* showed increasing obesity in children aged 2–15. The prevalence of obesity in children under 11 has risen from 9.9% in 1995 to 13.7% in 2003. The proportion of women classified as obese rose by 8% between 1993 and 2003, while for men the increase was nearly 10% (DoH, 2004a).

In 2004, the government set a target on tackling obesity in England. A public service agreement (PSA) target was agreed to halt the year-on-year rise in obesity among children aged under 11 by 2010. The PSA target was shared by the Department of Health, the Department of Culture, Media and Sport, and the Department for Education and Skills. A raft of policies has followed, including healthy school food initiatives, exercise initiatives and further action on food labelling and marketing.

Addressing the issue of food and nutrition demands answers to a range of questions:

- What is a healthy diet and is this culturally or historically relative?

- Do people know what constitutes a healthy diet?

- How is obesity defined and measured?

- How easy is it to access foods for a healthy diet?

- What influences individual food choices?

- Is what people eat an entirely individual matter or should governments be concerned?

- What accounts for the rise in overweight and obesity? Is this confined to the UK?

- What interventions are effective in promoting healthy eating and addressing obesity?

- What are the economic costs of the rise in overweight and obesity?

Each chapter illustrates the perspective that discipline offers on the issue. In Figure 0.1 below, we show how the questions that need to be answered in order to tackle a complex issue such as obesity or nutrition sit within different disciplinary paradigms. These may range from a risk factor analysis of individual lifestyles that give rise to obesity, an economic cost–benefit analysis for the health service, to organizational change analyses suggesting how organizations and workplaces can be more health promoting. It is important that readers understand how and why different explanations and interpretations are offered and that these build on, and reinforce, each other. A biomedical perspective is concerned with classification and measurement and the relationship between food and health. The classification of obesity as a disease, although not all people who are obese or overweight are ill, and disputes over the use of BMI measurements to identify obesity reflect both the dominance and limitations of this paradigm (Gard and Wright, 2005). On the other hand, social constructionist perspectives are concerned with the meanings and values attached to food and the ways these are reproduced and represented. We also know that the ability to choose, access and purchase a healthy diet is not the same for all groups, and a social science perspective shows how food and dietary behaviour are affected by socioeconomic status. To arrive at a comprehensive overview of a topic like obesity requires inputs from many different disciplines.

Interdisciplinary health studies is more than just a mixing of different disciplines. The bringing together of insights, knowledge and skills drawn from different disciplines has led to the creation of new areas of knowledge and practice that seek to protect and promote health in innovative and effective ways. Health promotion is a good example of this fertile merging of disciplinary knowledge and draws upon epidemiology, psychology, sociology, cultural studies and politics (among other disciplines) to understand and promote the health of populations. The next section discusses health promotion in greater depth in order to illustrate the power and productivity of interdisciplinary health studies.

Health promotion: an example of interdisciplinary practice

Many different professions use interdisciplinary definitions of health. For example, health visitors typically use a combination of physical, psychological and social perspectives to promote the health and wellbeing of children and families. Health promotion is a good example of interdisciplinary practice because it is built on several different academic disciplines and taps into many varied perspectives on health (Bunton and Macdonald, 2002). This brief discussion of health promotion will use healthy eating as an example of a health issue.

A focus on the ways in which health can be enhanced or promoted illustrates the contribution of many of the different disciplines outlined in this book. The term 'prevention', for example, suggests that it is possible to intervene in a causal process and implies that there are particular risks to health that we can detect and manage. The identification of risk in preventive health tends to derive from epidemiological data referring to large populations showing that exposure to a particular factor is associated with an increased probability of the relevant disease occurring. For example, obesity is a risk factor for type 2 diabetes, hypertension and coronary artery disease (WHO, 2003). Risk factors such as eating a high-fat or high-salt diet are then translated into health programmes and become the targets for intervention. Protective factors may also be identified through epidemiological analysis, leading to strategies designed to implement such factors throughout the

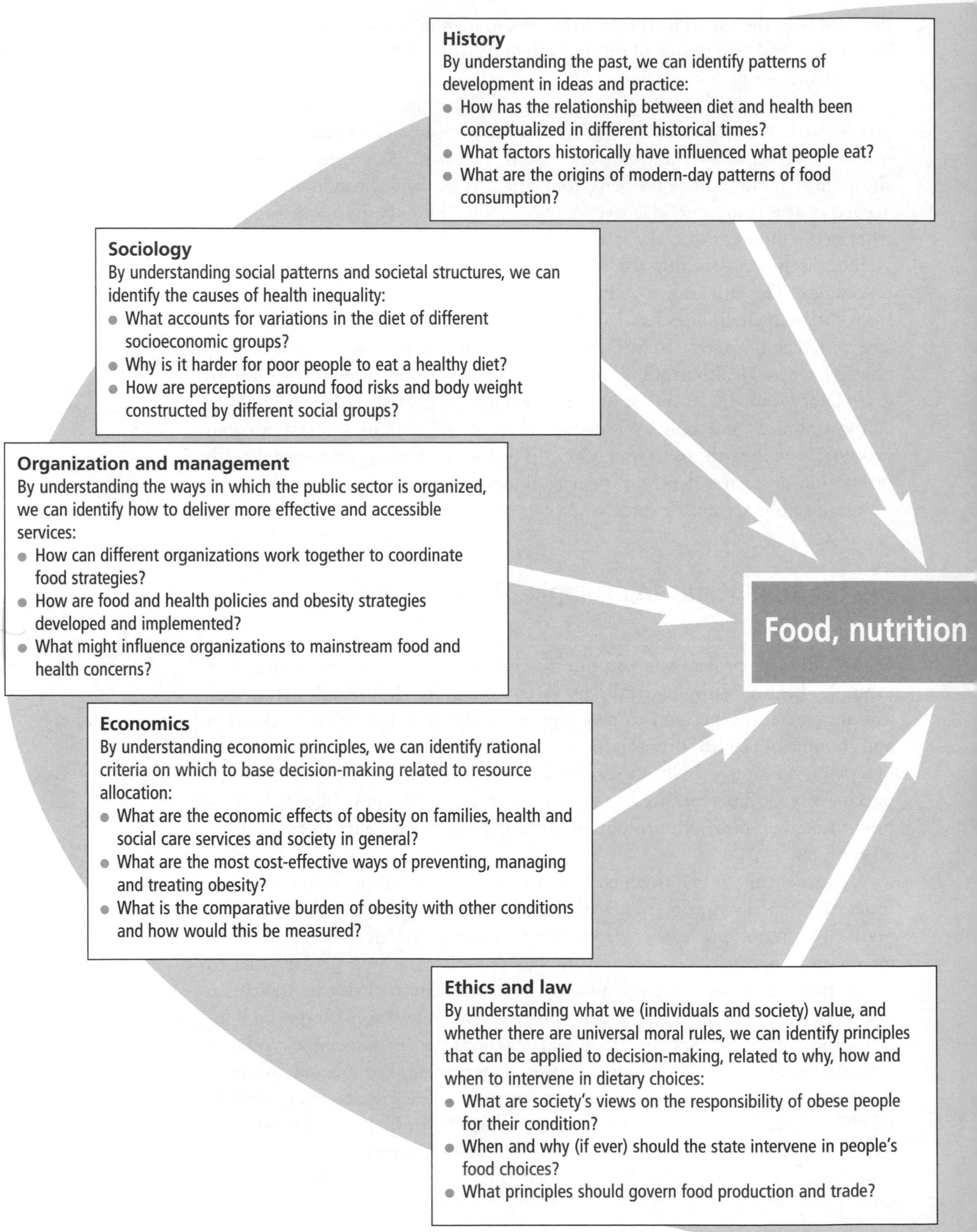

History
By understanding the past, we can identify patterns of development in ideas and practice:
- How has the relationship between diet and health been conceptualized in different historical times?
- What factors historically have influenced what people eat?
- What are the origins of modern-day patterns of food consumption?

Sociology
By understanding social patterns and societal structures, we can identify the causes of health inequality:
- What accounts for variations in the diet of different socioeconomic groups?
- Why is it harder for poor people to eat a healthy diet?
- How are perceptions around food risks and body weight constructed by different social groups?

Organization and management
By understanding the ways in which the public sector is organized, we can identify how to deliver more effective and accessible services:
- How can different organizations work together to coordinate food strategies?
- How are food and health policies and obesity strategies developed and implemented?
- What might influence organizations to mainstream food and health concerns?

Economics
By understanding economic principles, we can identify rational criteria on which to base decision-making related to resource allocation:
- What are the economic effects of obesity on families, health and social care services and society in general?
- What are the most cost-effective ways of preventing, managing and treating obesity?
- What is the comparative burden of obesity with other conditions and how would this be measured?

Ethics and law
By understanding what we (individuals and society) value, and whether there are universal moral rules, we can identify principles that can be applied to decision-making, related to why, how and when to intervene in dietary choices:
- What are society's views on the responsibility of obese people for their condition?
- When and why (if ever) should the state intervene in people's food choices?
- What principles should govern food production and trade?

Food, nutrition

Figure 0.1 Disciplinary perspectives on food, nutrition and obesity

esity Epidemic: Science, Morality and

nalism: A Sociological Analysis. San
ess.

ine: Dream, Mirage or Nemesis.
s Trust.

ckling Obesity in England. London:

social structure, in Parsons, T., Essays in
e Press, pp. 34–49.

01) 'The meanings of "culture" in health
mbined Trust in Somerset'. Journal of

trition and Food Poverty Toolkit.
lic Health, www.heartforum.org.uk.

rs. London: Penguin.

social cohesion, in M. Marmot and R.G.
f Health. Oxford: OUP, pp. 155–78.

al. (2003) Children and Healthy Eating:
Facilitators. London: EPPI Centre, Social
ucation, University of London.

46) Preamble of the Constitution of the
WHO.

86) Ottowa Charter for Health
nal Office for Europe.

00) Obesity: Preventing and Managing
l Report Series 894. Geneva: WHO.

03) Diet, Nutrition and the Prevention
t WHO/FAO Expert Consultation.

users' needs. The basic premise of this book is that working together across disciplinary and professional boundaries has a positive impact on health. Working in partnership with service users and other service providers means health needs can be met in a more holistic and sustainable manner. By engaging in truly interdisciplinary perspectives and action, the health and wellbeing of people will be maximized.

This hierarchy of professions presents yet another barrier to interdisciplinary study and practice. However, in order to aspire towards the provision for service users of seamless care that spans medical and social services, it is important to appreciate the contributions that different professions and disciplines can make towards the promotion of health.

Although health studies has no direct link to a single profession and does not offer training for a specific role, many students will go on to pursue a career in health and social care, some as frontline practitioners, some in an increasing range of 'lifestyle adviser' posts and some as managers. The value of a broad and fluid approach is recognized in the recent emergence of generic posts that cross specialist and professional boundaries such as 'children's worker'. By studying health in an interdisciplinary way, through health studies, students who wish to embark on a related career will find themselves better equipped to work with other professionals, patients, managers and the general public. Acknowledging and understanding the diversity of perspectives that people bring to the concept of health is the first step in successful partnership working.

The QAA subject benchmark statement for health studies includes the following employability skills that can be gained by studying health studies:

- The ability to analyse health and health issues, and health information and data that may be drawn from a wide range of disciplines

- The ability to synthesize coherent arguments from a range of contesting theories relating to health and health issues

- The ability to draw upon the personal and lived experience of health and illness through the skill of reflection and to make links between individual experience of health and health issues and the wider structural elements relevant to health.

Using this book

This book presents each discipline separately, showing what it can contribute to the understanding of 'health'. The chapters all follow a similar layout with certain features (see below). The 'connections' boxes make links to other chapters, flagging up shared concepts or methodologies. The complex health issue of food, health and obesity is addressed by each discipline in a case study at the end of the chapter. This discussion of a common issue

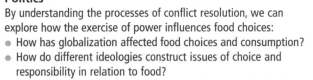

Politics
By understanding the processes of conflict resolution, we can explore how the exercise of power influences food choices:
- How has globalization affected food choices and consumption?
- How do different ideologies construct issues of choice and responsibility in relation to food?
- How much influence do food companies have over food policies?

Epidemiology
By understanding what factors are associated with obesity, we can identify which groups of people are more likely to become obese:
- What are the trends in obesity?
- What proportion of children are overweight or obese?
- What is the incidence of obesity-related health problems, such as type 2 diabetes?

Social policy
By understanding the links between ideology, policy process and service provision, we can identify how a range of pressing social concerns may be addressed by government:
- Why is obesity on the current policy agenda?
- How are concerns about obesity framed in current policy?
- How has the role of the state in promoting and protecting the nation's diet changed?

and obesity

Biology
By understanding the relationships between structure and function in the living world, we can identify how the human body works:
- How is obesity defined and measured?
- What accounts for the health risks from obesity?
- What constitutes a healthy diet?

Psychology
By understanding people's health beliefs, we can identify what might influence their diet-related decisions:
- What factors influence food preferences?
- Why do people overeat?
- What beliefs do people have about food?

Cultural and anthropology studies
By understanding how concepts of health are produced and represented, we are more able to read and decode everyday cultural experiences:
- What contemporary meanings are attached to fatness and thinness?
- What is the popular representation of obesity in the media?
- How do different groups understand a healthy diet?

sionals are allied to particular disciplines. For example, sociology underpins social work practice, whereas biology underpins medical practice. Professions are defined in part by their disciplinary knowledge and expertise. The traditional consensual functionalist definition of a profession is of an occupation possessing desirable traits including a body of theoretical knowledge (Parsons, 1954). More recent critical perspectives on professions retain disciplinary expertise as part of the definition of a professional. For example, Larson (1977) uses the term 'professional project' to refer to members of an occupation working collectively to improve their status and economic position. A key plank in this enterprise is the professional claim to knowledge, ratified through training and registration. Different professions use training and registration to create their own boundaries, reinforcing disciplinary boundaries and thereby magnifying them.

In addition to professional barriers, there are also professional hierarchies. The traditional three professions (medicine, law and the clergy) tend to retain the highest status and position in society. Health is commonly interpreted as healthcare, and healthcare and service delivery have historically been 'owned' by medicine, medical practitioners and nurses. Medicine, informed by biology and science, has dominated the health arena. By contrast, social care, 'owned' by sociology and social workers, has been a relatively subservient and invisible aspect of health.

There are many benefits, both academic and practical, to appreciating the concepts, methodologies and insights that different practitioners and professionals bring to bear on health-related issues. Many different practitioners focus on protecting, enhancing and promoting the health of their service users, each in their own unique way. For example, occupational therapists focus on service users regaining the skills and functions that enable independent living, whereas health visitors focus on parenting and the healthy development of children. Multiprofessional or interprofessional ways of working, where different professions work together across professional and organizational boundaries, is commonly cited as a goal for healthcare. However, it is not clear what this goal involves. Does it mean all professionals adopting a single new culture, or mutual understanding and respect between existing professional and organizational cultures (Peck et al., 2001)? If we replace culture with academic discipline, the answer is clearly the second interpretation. Unfortunately, what is often cited as interprofessional education is nothing more than shared learning, in which professional groups (for example social workers, health visitors and mental health nurses) may learn together on common core programmes, specialist elements being presented separately for each professional group. The intention of such programmes is to increase mutual professional knowledge, promote teamwork and encourage multiskilled professionals who can look beyond their particular specialism.

In practical terms, understanding the focus and approach of different practitioners enables and enhances multiprofessional working centred on service

---

throughout the book suggests that one level of explanation or s knowledge is inadequate and encourages the reader towards a interpretation. By comparing the different disciplines' approach gies to issues regarding food, nutrition and obesity, it is hoped th will appreciate the value of interdisciplinary and multiprofessi working. The book is clearly signposted and structured for ea and study. Each chapter starts with an overview of its contents a a bullet point summary of the main points. Key terms are highl text (in bold) and the complete glossary of highlighted terms is the book. Interspersed in the text are interactive features:

- *Questions* for discussion, reading and exploration

- *Thinking about* to enable the reader to use his or her experie understand and apply concepts

- *Examples* to illustrate concepts or methodologies or explore contemporary issues.

We hope this book will provide a tool to encourage students t meaning and promotion of health across different academic di professions, and thereby contribute to the promotion of health a

References

Bunton, R. and Macdonald, G. (eds) (2002) *Health Promotion Dis Diversity and Developments* (2nd edn). London: Routledge.

Conrad, P. and Jacobson, H.T. (2003) Enhancing biology? Cosmeti breast augmentation, in S. Williams, L. Birke and G. Bendelow (*Bilology: Sociological Reflections on Health, Medicine, and Soci* Routledge, pp. 223–35.

Crawford, R. (1984) A cultural account of health: control, release a body, in J. McKinlay (ed.) *Issues in the Political Economy of He* Tavistock: London, pp. 60–103.

DoH (Department of Health) (1998) *Saving Lives: Our Healthier N* London: Stationery Office.

DoH (Department of Health) (2000) *The National Service Framew Coronary Heart Disease*. London: Stationery Office.

DoH (Department of Health) (2004a) *Health Survey for England 2* Stationery Office.

DoH (Department of Health) (2004b) *Choosing Health: Making H Choices Easier*. London: Stationery Office.

Duncan, P. (2007) *Critical Perspectives on Health*. Basingstoke: Pal Macmillan.

Chapter

S.H. CEDAR

1

Human biology an

Outline of chapter

This chapter will enable readers to:

- Gain an appreciation of the scope of hu framework of homeostasis and health a examine ill health and disease

- Be aware of the scientific methods use bioscientists and biomedical scientists

- Understand how biology can contribute physical aspects of human health

Overview

The natural sciences seek to explain the natural world and the social sciences seek to explain human behaviour and societies. This book is largely made up of social science disciplines, but because its focus is health, the natural sciences and, in particular, biology offer a useful perspective. Natural science is limited in what it investigates: it investigates natural phenomena in the universe, but does not investigate human feelings, morals or beliefs. Biology contributes to the study of health by providing knowledge of the body's functions and how these are interlinked. These issues are illustrated later in the chapter using a biological analysis of nutrition and obesity. Human biology concerns how the body functions in terms of its cells, tissues and body systems. This chapter will briefly explain some biological theories such as the function of cells in all organisms; how each body system contributes to the maintenance of a constant internal environment (homeostasis) for its cells; and gene theory. Most importantly, biology is a science and science is an experimental, evidence-based pursuit. The discipline of science dates back about 2,500 years to ancient Greece (Wolpert, 2000). It is derived from the Greek *episteme*, which distinguishes science as knowing not only that something is so, an act of experience, but also why it is so, an act of the 'knowledge of first causes' as Aristotle would say in his *Metaphysics* (Finley, 1963). It uses scientific methods variously described as induction, deduction, falsification and hypothetico-deduction. This chapter will explain the principles and processes of the scientific method.

Introduction

Biology is the science of life (from the Greek words *bios* meaning life and *logos* meaning reasoned account). It is the study of living organisms, what they are made of and how they function and how they interact with each other and the environment. In biology, humans are seen as just one type of organism, one species or race. Species are defined as one kind when they can breed together and have viable offspring. As all humans can do this, all humans, biologically, are one race or species. In this chapter, while biology applies to all living organisms, it is the human species that interests students of health. Biology encompasses a broad spectrum of academic fields that are often viewed as independent disciplines, including zoology, botany and physiology. Physiology aims to unravel how the body functions, for example what are the mechanisms by which a person feels pain, pumps blood round the body, breathes in and out, absorbs food.

Science can be divided into 'basic' and 'applied'. Basic or pure science is the description and understanding of phenomena and can be applied to many areas. Applied science is the application of scientific principles to meet a specific, recognized need, for example **biomedical** sciences may apply scientific

Proof and falsification

How do we know when a law or theory is true or proven? Induction and deduction have their place, but can it ever be said that enough observations have been made to prove a law, or that enough predictions based on that law have been tested? Scientists are not naive observers – they make sense of observations through pre-existing theory, building on previous scientific information.

Falsification, as propounded by Karl Popper in the 1950s, acknowledged that scientists have some preconceptions about how phenomena happen. Popper also argued that is never possible to prove that something is true. The next observation might disprove the theory. Popper (1959) suggested that good science starts with a hypothetical explanation that is falsifiable – the **null hypothesis**.

Logically, deductions can be made from the hypothesis, and these can be tested. If the hypothesis does not stand up to testing, it is rejected; if it does, the hypothesis is not rejected, instead it is subjected to even more rigorous testing. This description of science, the hypothetico-deductive method, is still accepted today. This process builds evidence supporting a hypothesis, but at the same time acknowledges that the hypothesis is not an absolute truth, but a conditional truth. Science is therefore evidence based and its findings are in a constant state of flux, unlike absolute beliefs or morals that are held to be fixed and inviolable.

Kuhn (1962) suggested that science progresses by a series of revolutions. A number of contrary findings may challenge the existing explanatory framework. This leads to an alternative paradigm or framework being proposed that explains existing incompatible findings. A **paradigm shift** then occurs, whereby scientists adopt a new explanatory system. Einstein's law of relativity is an example of a paradigm shift from Newtonian physics.

Experimentation

The relationship between cause and effect is tested by experiment. Science is a systematic discipline involving the recording of observations made under carefully controlled conditions. The observations are a way of testing an idea. The results of scientific research are publicized and opened up for testing, that is, the same piece of work could be repeated by another person and identical results obtained. The equipment used must be accurate and must reliably measure whatever data are being recorded. The methods are clearly described in papers so that they can be repeated by others.

The unravelling of a biological pathway usually requires some intervention or interference whereby the changes can be noted and inferences drawn, for example if it is suspected that a gland in one part of the body controls another by hormones, the removal of that gland will result in physiological changes in the effector. If the hypothesis is that one part of the body controls another by nerves, cutting or inactivating the nerves will prevent the control system working and there will be clear differences between the observations recorded in the control (uncut) group and in the experimental (cut) group.

The important point to experimentation is, however, that if an experiment disproves a hypothesis, then the hypothesis is incorrect and a new one must be proposed. Hypotheses that are consistently confirmed can be considered acceptable 'theories' or 'laws' of nature. A key aspect of the scientific method is that, regardless of how many times a theory has been confirmed or rejected, it is always subject to the addition of new data. This explains why science continually finds new explanations to understand the universe and is not about protecting the status quo. It also explains why many subjects of interest cannot be 'scientifically' investigated because no rigorous experiment can be undertaken where just one variable is tested. When observing phenomena, explanations for the observed effect need to be tested before causation can be established. Just because two things happen together doesn't mean that one causes the other. To establish this means controlling for various influences that may contribute to the relationships between things. Biology, as a natural science, is able to test for causality by undertaking a controlled experiment.

CONNECTIONS

Chapter 3 further defines the concepts of causation and association.

Example 1.5

AN EXAMPLE OF THE LINK BETWEEN BIOLOGY AND HEALTH

Biology seeks to make a direct link between cause and effect rather than an indirect link or a correlation. Consider, for example, the link between scurvy (a disease suffered particularly by sailors in the seventeenth and eighteenth centuries when they were at sea for long periods of time) and a lack of vitamin C. Americans may still describe British people as 'Limeys', a reference to the sailors who carried fresh fruit, particularly lemons and limes, on voyages, because these fruits contain vitamin C. The link between lack of vitamin C and scurvy is a direct scientific finding, which also presents a direct solution.

Contemporary explanations for scurvy might look to a lack of access to fresh fruit, to a lack of education on nutrition, to the relatively high cost of fresh fruit or possibly to cultural reasons for not eating fresh fruit. All these indirect reasons do not deny that the cause is a lack of vitamin C, a scientific finding. The cure is known only because of scientific investigations into normal physiology and biochemistry. Therefore biology, albeit not a medical science, still has a direct impact on our health.

CONNECTIONS

The nature and process of 'social' experiments in randomized controlled trials are discussed in Chapter 3.

- Water – for osmotic balance, maintenance of normal blood pressure, transport and diffusion of chemicals around the body

Energy (calories) comes from food such as carbohydrates and fats, which can be converted by the cell into a chemical called adenosine triphosphate (ATP). When energy is needed, for example during physical exercise, ATP is converted into adenosine diphosphate (ADP). This conversion process releases energy. Fats are macromolecules composed of long chains of fatty acids. Fat, or adipose tissue, is used to store energy, provide insulation and protect the organs. When necessary, fat can be converted into energy. When food containing more calories than are used is consumed, the excess is stored as fat. If an individual is habitually eating more than their body uses, and is storing a large amount of excess fat, this condition is known as obesity.

There are several different ways of calculating obesity:

1. Using the body mass index (BMI). BMI is calculated as weight in kilograms divided by the square of height in metres. A person with a BMI of above 30 is considered to be obese. An increased BMI above the optimum score (23–24 for men, 22–23 for women) is linked to increased mortality from a variety of causes including heart disease and cancer, as outlined in Chapter 3.
2. Waist to hip circumference ratios are used to assess how much body weight is carried around the stomach (which is thought to pose a greater health risk) as opposed to around the hips and thighs. In addition to obesity, abdominal adipose tissue distribution, measured as the waist to hip circumference ratio, is a risk factor for the development of type 2 diabetes. Several studies have found that increased central adiposity is a risk factor for

mortality in women (Folsom et al., 1993; Simpson et al., 2007; Zhang et al., 2007). Compared to BMI, increased central adiposity has a stronger association with coronary vascular disease (Yusuf et al., 2004), but this is still under debate.
3. Obesity can also be defined using measures of body fat. Men with over 25% body weight as fat and women with over 30% body weight as fat are considered to be obese. The best means of measuring body fat is underwater weighing, but skin fold testing (to measure the subcutaneous fat layer) and bioelectrical impedance analysis may also be used. All these measures require specialist facilities and personnel, so are not as readily accessible as BMI or waist to hip circumference ratios.

There are many biological explanations for obesity. It may be associated with specific medical conditions or treatments. For example, some medical conditions, such as hypothyroidism, Cushing's syndrome and growth hormone deficiency, increase the risk of obesity. Some mental illnesses are defined as eating disorders and may lead to obesity, for example bulimia nervosa and binge eating disorder. Smoking cessation is often linked to weight gain, as nicotine is an appetite suppressant. Some medicines may also cause weight gain, for example steroids and some fertility medication.

Whether there is a genetic propensity towards fatness, which is the explanation of choice for those who become seriously obese, has long fascinated scientists. Those who have argued for a genetic explanation point to the genes that affect calorie consumption and feelings of hunger and satiation. Genes produce proteins and there is evidence that some peptides (small proteins) produced by the stomach and gastrointestinal (GI) tract may affect calorie intake. The discovery of leptin in 1994 triggered research into the many hormonal mechanisms that are implicated in appetite control, food intake, storage patterns of adipose tissue and the development of insulin resistance (Flier, 2004). Cholecys-tokinin (CKK), neuromedin B, enterostatin, somatostatin, glucagon-like peptide-1 (GLP-1) and apolipoprotein A-1V have all been identified as having possible involvement in feelings of satiety. Another peptide, grehlin, increases in fasting and is reduced in response to a meal. Grehlin and leptin are thought to be complementary in their influence on appetite, with grehlin affecting short-term appetite, and leptin affecting long-term appetite. Insulin and leptin hormones are secreted in proportion to the amount of adipose tissue (fat) in the body, stimulating receptors in the brain to reduce food intake. If the genes involved in the production of these peptides, insulin or hormones are functioning abnormally, or are absent, normal feelings of satiety would be affected, which could cause habitual overeating, resulting in obesity. A small percentage of obese people are leptin deficient, and many more obese people are leptin resistant.

The mediators mentioned above affect appetite by acting on the hypothalamus, the part of the brain that processes signals related to metabolic state and energy storage. One theory is that one region of the hypothalamus, the lateral hypothalamus, affects feelings of hunger, while another region, the ventromedial hypothalamus, affects feelings of satiety; however, this theory has been challenged by more recent research (Flier, 2004).

Isolating any individual gene(s) responsible for obesity has proved elusive until recently. However, in 2007, the results were published from a large Wellcome Trust study originally set up to identify suscepti-bility for type 2 diabetes (Frayling et al., 2007). People with type 2 diabetes were more likely to have a particular variant of the FTO gene, which was also shown to be linked to increased body weight. FTO comes in two varieties, and everyone inherits two copies of the gene. The variant making people fatter differed from the other version of the FTO gene by a single mutation in the DNA sequence. It was found that 16% of people have two copies of the high-risk variant, 50% have one high-risk and one low-risk, and 34% of people have two low-risk variants.

The study found that people with two copies of the particular 'fat gene' variant had a 70% higher risk of obesity than those with two copies of the other variant and weighed 3kg (6.5lb) more. In each case, the extra weight was entirely accounted for by more body fat, not greater muscle or extra height. The 50% of subjects who inherited one copy of each FTO variant had a 30% higher risk of obesity.

These findings must be treated with caution: FTO will not be the only gene that influences obesity, and inheriting a particular variant will not necessarily make anyone fat. Again, correlation does not prove causation. Except in very rare cases such as Prader-Willi syndrome, obesity is not therefore caused directly by genes but it may explain how people with apparently similar lifestyles differ in their propensity to put on weight.

An even more contentious theory is that obesity may be 'caught'. Exposure to adenovirus-36 (Ad-36), which is commonly associated with coughs and colds, can induce stem cells from fat tissue to become fat cells. In laboratory experiments, mice and chickens infected with the virus put on much more fat than uninfected animals. The same virus is more prevalent among overweight people, a strong indication that it may also cause obesity in humans.

With the exception of infectious diseases, no other chronic disease has increased so rapidly as obesity (see Chapter

3). Notwithstanding these emerging genetic and contagion explanations, the primary biological explanation is the imbalance between calories consumed and calories expended, with the excess of calories ingested being turned into fat. Lifestyle factors such as changes in diet and exercise patterns are the most likely candidates as causal factors for the rise in obesity levels. The availability of processed food from a variety of different countries may be one factor; reduced physical activity due to sedentary work and leisure patterns may be another. In America, reliance on energy-dense fast-food meals tripled, and calorie intake quadrupled, between 1977 and 1995 (Lin et al., 1999). Genetic explanations or contagion theories that explain perceptions of hunger or satiety or fat deposition may in the future offer the possibility of screening or treatment but in the meantime lifestyle and environmental change offer the only realistic ways of tackling obesity.

Summary

- For most people, health is associated first and foremost with a physical state of being. Having a knowledge of biological frameworks, pathways and mechanisms contributes to our understanding of this physical state of being

- The scientific discipline of biology helps us to uncover universal mechanisms that regulate the body (homeostasis)

- People's interpretation of bodily symptoms and states is highly varied and is related to many other non-physical factors, such as social factors and cultural beliefs. Biology provides a means of arriving at a common baseline understanding of what is occurring inside the human body by means of rigorous scientific methods

- Biology contributes in many ways to human health. Once processes have been understood, effective interventions may be proposed and refined. Biology is, however, distinct from medicine, its investigations and research being neither limited nor dictated by medicine

- Understanding biological concepts, frameworks and research methods enables us to discover the complexity and self-regulating nature of the human body. This in turn assists us in understanding what is happening in altered states of health, whether caused by assaults from the external world (for example infection or an extremely hostile environment) or internal errors in regulation (for example genetic conditions such as haemophilia). Understanding physical states of being is a crucial aspect of the wider task of understanding human health

Questions for further discussion

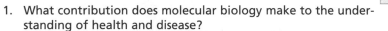

1. What contribution does molecular biology make to the understanding of health and disease?

2. Are genes the primary determinants of disease?

3. Is homeostasis the same as health?

Further reading and resources

Chalmers, A.F. (1983) *What is this Thing Called Science?* Buckingham: Open University Press.
A highly readable excursion into the nature of scientific research, gently exploding many of the myths about the nature of science.

Davey, B. (1994) The nature of scientific research: biomedical research methods, in K. McConway (ed.) *Studying Health and Disease*. Buckingham: Open University Press.
A useful summary of the main issues in general scientific and biological research relating to health in particular.

Wolpert, L. (2000) *The Unnatural Nature of Science*. London: Faber and Faber.
A witty and entertaining book on the origin of science and what science is; intended for the general reader.

The Wellcome Foundation website contains details of the human genome project: www.wellcome.ac.uk.

The Human Fertilisation and Embryo Authority is an excellent site to see the debates on stem cell research: www.hfea.gov.uk.

References

Becker, A.J., McCulloch, E.A. and Till, J.E. (1963) 'Cytological demonstration of the clonal nature of spleen colonies derived from transplanted mouse marrow cells'. *Nature* 197: 452–4.

Bernard, C. (1865) *An Introduction to the Study of Experimental Medicine*. First English translation by Henry Copley Greene, published by Macmillan (1927); reprinted in 1949. The Dover edition of 1957 is a reprint of the original translation with a new foreword by I. Bernard Cohen of Harvard University.

Brunner, E.J. (2000) Toward a new social biology, in L.F. Berkman and I. Kawachi (eds) *Social Epidemiology*. New York: Oxford University Press.

Cedar, S.H. (2006) 'Stem cell and related therapies: nurses and midwives representing all parties'. *Nursing Ethics* 13: 292–303.

Cedar, S.H., Cooke, J.A., Luo, Z. et al. (2006) 'From eggs to embryonic stem cells: biopolitics and therapeutic potentials'. *Reproductive Biomedicine* 13(5): 725–31.

Chalmers, A.F. (1983) *What is this Thing Called Science?* Buckingham: Open University Press.

Finley, M.I. (1963) *The Ancient Greeks*. Harmondsworth: Penguin.

Flier, J. (2004) 'Obesity wars: molecular progress confronts an expanding epidemic'. *Cell* **116**(2): 337–50.

Folsom, A.R., Kaye, S.A., Sellers, T.A. et al. (1993) 'Body fat distribution and 5-year risk of death in older women'. *Journal of the American Medical Association* **269**(4).

Frayling, T.M., Timpson, N.J., Weedon, M.N. and Zeggini, E. (2007) 'A common variant in the FTO gene is associated with body mass index and predisposes to childhood and adult obesity'. *Science* **316**(5826): 889–94.

Galton, F. (1883/1907/1973) *Inquiries into Human Faculty and its Development*. New York: AMS Press.

Kuhn, T. (1962) *The Structure of Scientific Revolutions*. Chicago: University of Chicago Press.

Lin, B.H., Guthrie, J. and Frazao, E. (1999) Nutrient contribution of food away from home, in E. Frazao (ed.) *America's Eating Habits: Changes and Consequences*. Agriculture Information Bulletin No. 750, US Department of Agriculture, Economic Research Service, Washington DC, pp. 213–39.

Morgan, T.M., Krumholz, H.M., Lifton,R.P. and Spertus, J.A. (2007) 'Nonvalidation of reported genetic risk factors for acute coronary syndrome in a large scale replication study'. *Journal of the American Medical Association* **297**(14): 1551–61.

Popper, K. (1959) *The Logic of Scientific Discovery*. London: Hutchinson.

Simpson, J.A., MacInnis, R.J., Peeters, A. et al. (2007) 'A comparison of adiposity measures as predictors of all-cause mortality: the Melbourne collaborative cohort study'. *Obesity* **15**: 994–1003.

Toates, F. (1998) *Stress: Conceptual and Biological Aspects*. Chichester: Wiley.

Weeks, J. (1989) *Sex, Politics and Society: the Regulation of Sexuality since 1800* (2nd edn). London: Longman.

Wolpert, L. (2000) *The Unnatural Nature of Science*. London, Faber and Faber.

Yusuf, S., Hawken, S., Ounpuu, S. et al. (2004) 'Effect of potentially modifiable risk factors associated with myocardial infarction in 52 countries (the INTERHEART study): case-control study'. *Lancet* **364**: 937–52.

Zhang, X., Shu, X.-O., Gong, Y. et al. (2007) 'Abdominal adiposity and mortality in Chinese women'. *Archives of Internal Medicine* **167**: 886–92.

LOUISE HILL CURTH

Chapter

History of health and illness

2

LEARNING OUTCOMES

This chapter will enable readers to:

- Understand what it is meant by history and how it can be applied to health

- Gain an overview of the discipline and development of the history of health and illness, including its theoretical and methodological approaches

- Reflect upon the insights that history can give to our understandings of health, illness and healthcare

state and feelings of the patient. The mid-eighteenth-century definition of disease was that of 'the state of a living body wherein it is prevented from the exercise of any of its functions' (Allen, 1765). A hundred years before, the word 'distemper' was used in place of disease, meaning 'any excess of heat or cold in the body of man' (Anon, 1657). This definition also focuses on the person, rather than what caused it and can only be properly understood in relationship to contemporary views on health and illness, which will be discussed later in this chapter.

As we have already seen in the Introduction, the term 'health' can be even more difficult to define because it can be both a subjective and/or an objective phenomenon. It is also a term that differs according to the people, the society, the culture and time in which they live. Many recent definitions have emphasized the element of adaptability and coping. Kovacs (1989, p. 261), for example, has suggested that health is a 'physical or mental state ... which is capable of adapting to the natural and social-environmental surroundings of the individual with the appropriate advantage or disadvantage ratio for the body and spirit'. In the mid-eighteenth century, the surprisingly similar definition was 'a proper disposition of the several parts to perform their respective functions, without any impediment or sensation of pain' (Anon, 1765). The unifying theme behind the diverse definitions seems to be that of being able to function in one's society to an appropriate degree (the meaning of which would be influenced by the place and time under study). Since social and cultural factors play a role in helping to form and reinforce different types of social behaviour, the ways in which this can be done will depend on the setting in which people live out their lives.

Views of what constitutes being healthy enough to carry out certain tasks can differ, for various reasons, across various social groups and over time. In some segments in modern British society, it is generally not considered to be morally or ethically wrong for someone to stay home from work if they feel unwell. However, before the advent of paid sick days in the early twentieth century, most workers would have had both economic and moral reasons for not staying home unless they were seriously ill. The concept of leaving work at a certain age (retirement) would also have been unfamiliar to people who considered themselves healthy enough to continue working as long as they were physically able. For the elderly, the threat of ending up in the poor house was partially removed by Lloyd George's introduction of old age pensions and the National Insurance Act of 1911.

In the past, religious beliefs played a major role in helping people to understand their state of health. It was widely thought that disease first appeared on earth as a direct consequence of 'original sin'. God was thought to be able to punish individuals, communities or even nations through causing epidemics as a message of displeasure. In order to stay healthy, therefore, people needed to try to live a good, sin-free life (Thomas, 1991). A popular literary device in the sixteenth and seventeenth centuries was to use the analogy of the body being a fortress under perpetual threat from the devil. This was likely to have been a familiar idea for readers accustomed to Christian imagery of the body protecting the soul from the devil. Furthermore, comparing the body to a fort constantly under attack was something that most people could empathize with in an age of recurring social upheavals, political conflicts and wars. Richard Saunders (1681) argued that:

> 'tis simple reason … to keep out an enemy, then to let him in, and afterwards to beat him out, so doubtless is men in the Government of their health would use Reason more, they would use the Physician less.

THINKING ABOUT

Does this analogy of your health under attack still make sense in early twenty-first-century Britain?

While it was clearly important to try to be a good, moral person, there were more practical guidelines about how to live a healthy lifestyle in earlier times. This rested on the idea of having a good health regimen, a concept that can be traced to the *Hippocratic Corpus*. This was a body of around 60 texts on health and illness written in the fourth century BC by followers of Hippocrates (often referred to as the 'father of medicine'). Although a vast range of topics were covered in these texts, the most important component in a good health regime was that of food and drink (Schiefsky, 2005).

The *Hippocratic Corpus* also introduced the idea that disease was caused by different types of imbalances of the four humours within the body. Although these humours were always in flux, the aim was to keep them as balanced as possible. As every living creature was thought to have a unique combination of humours, this was a complicated undertaking that required detailed medical knowledge and in-depth understanding of the individual in question.

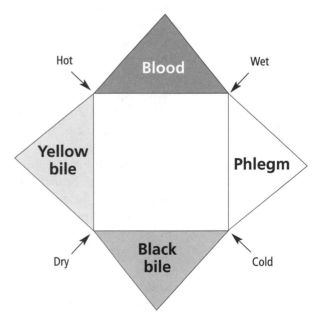

Figure 2.1 The four humours

Figure 2.1 illustrates the four humours of black bile, blood, yellow bile and phlegm and their related qualities. It was thought that all bodies had a predominance of one humour, depending on a variety of factors ranging from the time they were born to the place in which they first saw light. Each of the humours was linked to the four primary elements of fire, air, water and earth, which were further tied to the four material qualities of heat, dryness, coldness and wetness and the four seasons of the year. Autumn, for example, was thought to be cold and dry, as was the humour called black bile. This meant that if black bile was the predominant humour in a person's body, they would have a cold and dry constitution. Springtime was seen as hot and moist, as was air and the blood humour. Being cold and moist, winter was related to water and a phlegmatic body, while the hot and dry summer corresponded to yellow bile (Wear, 2000).

The relationship between health and the four humours was further refined by Galen of Pergamum (*c.* 131–200 AD). As a prominent physician and prolific writer, Galen is credited with rationalizing Hippocratic ideas on diagnosis and prognosis (French, 2003). Of most interest to this chapter, however, is the theory that he developed about the 'non-naturals'. The non-naturals were one of the three basic types of phenomena whose mixture would define whether an individual was healthy or diseased. These consisted of 'thynges naturall', 'thynges not naturall' and 'thynges ageynst nature'. The first included the four elements of earth, air, fire and water, which manifested themselves as the four humours. The second type was the 'non-naturals', which had the power to alter one's imbalance of humours, thereby destroying the desired state of health. According to Galenic thought, there were six non-naturals, which consisted of 'ayre', 'meate and drinke', 'slepe and watch', 'mevying and rest', 'emptynesse and replettion' and 'affectations of the minde'. The final category that could influence health consisted of 'contra-naturals', which literally meant against the naturals or 'thynges ageynst nature'. These consisted of pathological conditions made up of 'syckenesse, cause of syckenesse and accidents whiche foloweth syckenesse' (Niebyl, 1971; Gil-Sotres, 1998).

Although little could be done to alter either the naturals or the contra-naturals, it was believed that the non-naturals could be manipulated in order to protect the health of individuals. It was generally accepted that the most effective way to do this was by following a daily health regime based on living by 'Rule and wholesome Precepts', which would result in a stronger body and mind (Maynwaringe, 1669). Interestingly, the basic rules involved in this are almost identical to the 'modern' recommendations on living a healthy lifestyle. The following section, based on health regimen texts written in the sixteenth and seventeenth centuries, illustrates the importance of the non-naturals. Clearly, it was within the means of most people to follow at least some of these rules on getting fresh air, exercising, getting regular sleep, eating and drinking healthily, evacuating bodily waste and avoiding stress.

Defining health and disease: six non-naturals

Air

Although concern about the quality of the air we breathe often seems to be a modern issue, it actually dates back to Hippocratic writers who believed that plagues or epidemics were the result of breathing in noxious air (Longrigg, 1998). What we now refer to as 'air pollution' is said to emanate from a number of sources, including industry, agriculture, services, households, solid waste management, road, air and sea transport. With the exception of air transport, all these factors also featured in the creation of miasma. Toxic air could also be created through the work of butchers, tanners or farm workers, as well as from human or animal excrement. Battlefields full of rotting bodies were thought to exude dangerous fumes, as would swamps and muddy areas or stagnant water (Corbin, 1996).

During the Middle Ages and early modern period, it was widely believed that disease could be transmitted through the air. During the cholera outbreaks of the mid-nineteenth century, it was believed that there was a deadly concentration of miasmata, a noxious vapour, near the banks of the River Thames. The wide acceptance of miasma theory overshadowed the theory brought forth by John Snow in the 1840s that cholera was spread through water.

CONNECTIONS

Chapter 3 describes Snow's early epidemiological work in documenting the pattern of the disease.

While it would often be impossible to avoid areas with bad air in the course of daily life, it seems likely that most people would have tried to avoid polluted areas. Of course, the quality of air varied depending on location and outside conditions. In general, rural areas were thought to enjoy better air than congested, polluted towns. However, certain weather conditions, such as foggy or misty days, as well as thunder or lightning, were thought to cause ill health in town and country areas equally (Wear, 1992). Precipitation in the form of rain showers was not considered hazardous in itself, although the vapours they released were thought to be dangerous. It was said that 'they that come abroad soon after those Showers, are commonly taken with sickness'. The same held true for people who went outside 'where the Air is cold long after sun-rising, where the Air is long hot after sun set [and] where the Air is long, close, cloudy or thick' (Pond, 1687).

Motion and rest

There are obvious parallels between the perceived importance of exercise in early modern and twenty-first-century England. However, for many centuries, writers of popular medical texts included homilies such as 'Exercise is best,

account of the changes in the human body. There is a popular misconception that those who could afford it subsisted on large quantities of meat and little else. In fact, for many centuries, the word 'meat' was actually used in the generic sense of meaning all types of food. In the winter, 'strong meats' such as beef, accompanied by red wine, were considered to be part of a healthy diet. In the summertime, it was considered best to eat fish and salads, perhaps with a glass of light white wine. Fresh fruits, in season, were well liked and consumed in large quantities. Indeed, this was so much the case that many texts warned readers about the dangers of overindulging.

Wine, consumed in moderation, was thought to be an important ally in the fight against disease. According to Tobias Whitaker (1638), 'the bloud of the grape' was 'neerest to the nature of the Gods and their nature is incorrupt'. Wine was the most nutritious beverage available, being 'more pure and better concocted then any other juyce, either of milke, egges, corne, fruits, or the like'. People who regularly consumed the beverage could expect to be 'faire, fresh, plumpe, and fat', rather than water or beer drinkers, who 'look like Apes rather than men'.

In general, Whitaker and other writers considered red wine to have a more beneficial effect on health than white. Although there is ongoing debate about the differences between the two, many modern studies also suggest that this is true, due to the high amounts of polyphenols that red wine contains. Supporters of this theory argue that polyphenols give red wine higher levels of antioxidant and antimicrobial actions, as well as proving more beneficial to enzyme systems (Van de Wiel et al., 2001). Too much wine, of either type, was (and still is) believed to destroy a state of good health.

Evacuation and retention

It was widely accepted that good health was linked to the periodical removal of excessive humours. This was done by regularly purging the system as a preventive measure. The modern definition of purging refers to the emptying of the bowels, perhaps with the assistance of colonic irrigation. However, in the medieval and early modern period, this was only one of many different methods used to remove unwanted materials from the body.

There were a number of different ways in which to purge offensive matter from almost every natural or artificial bodily orifice. Generally, they began with phlebotomy, or blood-letting, which comes from the Greek words *phleps* or vein, and *tome* or incision. Vomiting, 'neesing' (sneezing) and gargarismes (gargles) were three popular methods for clearing the upper body. A more general, overall method was causing the body to sweat.

How science now understands the physiological pathways that regulate processes such as sweating is discussed in Chapter 1.

What might be called 'sexual evacuation' was also considered to be an important part of a good health regime. In moderation, and at the correct times of the year, sexual intercourse was an important part of good health. Galenic theory held that if the 'natural seed' were kept too long within the body, it would turn into poison. In fact, for married men, regulated and moderate sexual emissions played a major part in the preservation of health. Although most advice of this nature was aimed at men, some authors suggested that regular sexual intercourse was a necessity for women. On the other hand, too much sex would weaken the seed, and could result in stunted or deformed offspring (Stone, 1979; Crawford, 1994).

According to contemporary stereotypes, either abstinence or even moderation could be almost impossible for many married men. The reason and the blame for this lay with their physically demanding wives who were cursed with 'voracious sexuality', which could make them physically demanding whatever the season. Such behaviour could adversely affect their men, as too much sex was thought to weaken their seed and therefore their general health (Crawford, 1994; Fletcher, 1995). The physical reason for this had to do with Galenic theory, whereby men were thought to be hotter and drier than women. In some cases, women's urge to obtain sperm to counteract their colder and wetter complexions could spiral out of control (Weisner, 1998). Sexually transmitted diseases were another possible consequence of uncontrolled sex, then as now.

Passions and emotions

A final, yet important component of a healthy lifestyle involved keeping a rein over one's emotional state. Judging by the vast number of texts on the subject, there was a great deal of interest in learning how to avoid or suppress excessive feelings of pride, anger, envy, malice, sorrow and fear. Such themes are still evident today, both in the academic press and the multitude of popular 'self-help' books and articles printed in the mass media. Some studies suggest that such 'negative emotions' increase mortality rates following a myocardial infarction, or can even play a role in the onset of coronary disease (Kubzansky and Kawachi, 2000).

? Why is an understanding of past concepts of health and illness important?

Since all societies experience disease and illness, it follows that they also develop various practices to deal with them. Inherent in this framework would be people playing the role of a carer or 'healer', either on a formal or informal basis. It would also include the use of some type of organic and/or inorganic substances as medications. The study of medical history helps to provide insights into contemporary beliefs and practices, which, in turn, offer a greater understanding of how our current ideas have developed. In addition, the study of health and illness in the past can help to enhance current understandings of the theoretical, cultural and ethical bases of beliefs and practices.

Developments in medicine and healthcare

Since ideas about what constitutes health and illness are linked to the society and culture in which they take place, it is understandable that they will change over time. Developments in medicine too are a consequence of many developments – the pressures of the economy and need for trade, war and nationalism, developments in education and its institutions, religious beliefs and the relative importance of religious institutions, scientific and technological developments and developments in communication.

While biomedicine is the dominant model in the twenty-first century, it should not be used to judge or denigrate earlier belief systems. In fact, a great deal of our modern knowledge base can be traced back to much earlier times. As already mentioned, the theory of the four humours is attributed to the work of Hippocrates and Galen. Although the medieval period is no longer referred to as the 'Dark Ages', there is still a stereotype that there were few changes in medical knowledge between the sixth and fourteenth centuries. In fact, there is evidence that contemporary medical practice was influenced both by ancient Greek writings and the Byzantine Empire. This was also the period when medicine began to be taught at what would become great universities on the Continent and in England, such as Padua, Bologna, Paris, Montpelier and Oxford (Nutton, 1999). Although medicine continued to be based mainly on ancient Greek ideas into the early modern period, including the continuance of the practice of blood-letting based on the four humours, and religious ideas still held sway, the growth of 'new science' in the late seventeenth century began to have an effect on beliefs and practices and the influence of the Church declined.

The ideas of Thomas Sydenham (1624–89) led to a great advance in the treatment of patients. He recognized the importance of detailed observation, record-keeping and the influence of the environment on the health of the patient. During the eighteenth century, through a series of painstaking dissections, William Harvey was able to demonstrate that the body contains only a single supply of blood, and that the heart is a muscle pumping it round a circuit. Research into general anatomy and physiology led to new 'mechanistic' theories whereby the body was seen to be comparable to a machine. The development of the microscope enabled organisms to be studied and the study of microbes, or microbiology, and the increased knowledge of pathogenic microbes led to the development of new medicines to tackle infectious diseases. By the late eighteenth century, the use of infected matter from smallpox victims was being used as a preventive measure in parts of Europe, but the practice of inoculation is credited to Edward Jenner, a country doctor who injected patients with cowpox to protect them against smallpox. Surgery also made great advances in the nineteenth century. Industry could produce better surgical instruments and from the 1840s onwards, the discovery of the anaesthetics ether, chloroform and cocaine allowed surgeons to take more time over operations. During the Industrial Revolution, means of communication such as the telegraph and railways meant that scientists and doctors were able to read about each other's breakthroughs in medical journals like the *Lancet*.

Every society and culture attempts to pass on existing ideas about health and illness to succeeding generations. Depending on the people in question, this might include informal dissemination through kinship groups, or a more formal system of apprenticeship or organized education. For centuries, it was accepted that a 'healer' was anyone who helped to expedite recovery from illness. According to English common law, if the patient consented, anyone could prescribe medical treatment. (However, if the patient died, the practitioner could be tried for a felony.) Early modern ideas on health and illness resulted in a system whereby patients had many choices regarding what types of healers to consult or remedies to use. This was a largely unregulated setting, where surgeons (practitioners in the management of external lesions and treatment of broken bones), apothecaries (retailers of medicinal ingredients and producers of medicines) and physicians competed with traditional healers in a 'medical marketplace'. University-educated physicians were the smallest group of healers in this setting, although there were a large number of men who referred to themselves as 'physicians' who had probably learned their trade through an apprenticeship.

Many academics dislike the term 'medical marketplace', arguing that it implies that healthcare was limited to commercial services, ignoring the presence of various levels of healers who either bartered their skills or charitably offered them for free. In addition, the idea of a purely commercial marketplace also negates the overriding importance of 'domestic physick', which was probably the first port of call for most people, and, in many cases, the only medical assistance that they were likely to receive (Wear, 2000, pp. 17–34).

There were a relatively small group of university-educated practitioners in the early modern medical marketplace. Since their education consisted of what might now be referred to as 'medical philosophy', such men would have needed to learn 'practical' medicine through much the same channels that other healers did. In many cases, this would have occurred through taking part in some form of apprenticeship. However, from the late fifteenth century on, the most common medium for the transmission of medical knowledge was through printed literature.

Over the centuries, a great deal of lay medical knowledge would have been passed on through the oral culture, although there was a steadily rising stream of vernacular medical literature from which people could supplement their knowledge. Before the advent of mechanical printing in the late fifteenth century, manuscript sources in both Latin and English were available, although due to the small numbers produced and high costs, these were out of the reach of much of the population. The printing press allowed the mass production of such works, which increasingly included both translations of foreign-language texts and those initially written in the vernacular. During the course of the seventeenth century, there was a massive increase in this type of literature, including many different publications, ranging from small, cheap almanacs through to large, expensive medical tomes (Hill Curth, 2007).

Example 2.1

GRAY'S ANATOMY

One way of analysing a discipline is to study the major ideas that it produces over time. A prime example of this is *Gray's Anatomy*, written by Henry Gray, who was lecturer in anatomy at St George's Hospital Medical School in London, Although it was first published in 1858, it is still the bestselling anatomy book of all time and is now in its thirty-ninth edition. The first edition was lauded as being both a scientific and artistic masterpiece and had 750 pages and weighed 1.53kg. The current version is over twice that length in order to include our current knowledge and understanding of anatomy (Porter, 1999, p. 318).

There is some debate both about what is meant by the 'professionalization' of medicine and when it began. Some of the common features include the growth of formalized, centralized medical education and professional autonomy. John Henry (1991, p. 191) feels that this occurred during the Renaissance, pointing out that although medicine was established in the late Middle Ages as one of the higher university faculties alongside theology and law, it only became professionalized through early modern licensing. A more widely accepted view, however, is that professionalization is a phenomenon of the late eighteenth and nineteenth centuries (Brunton, 2004). This argument is backed by the debate about what this term actually means, and it is generally accepted that this is linked to the growth first of formalized, centralized, hospital medical schools, followed by the development of university-based programmes. According to many historians, medicine only began to be recognizable as a scientific discipline in the nineteenth century when the profession became 'professionalized' (Porter, 1999, pp. 173–4).

The 1858 Medical Act marked an important turning point in the professionalization of British medicine. There were three main aims to this Act: a uniformity of qualification; representative self-governance; and the exclusion of unqualified practitioners from the medical marketplace. Perhaps most importantly was the formation of the General Council of Medical Education and Registration or GMC, which was charged with putting together and maintaining a register of named practitioners whom the public could trust. The register facilitated the establishment of a group professional identity based on:

1. The emerging scientific paradigm that developed out of natural philosophy and which was taught at the universities

2. The doctor as 'gentleman', offering disinterested advice and eschewing the selling of drugs, advertising, canvassing for patients and using unqualified assistants for the doctor to enable a cheaper service to be provided

3. A solidarity and esprit de corps of those sharing a licence to practise.

CONNECTIONS
CONNECTIONS

Chapter 11 examines some recent developments including the unlicensed use of organs for transplantation or research that have called into question the basis of medical ethics.

Theoretical and methodological approaches

The development of the discipline

One hundred years ago, however, the field of medical history was dominated by men whose main interest was in the history of 'great doctors' and the (supposedly) unilinear path of scientific, medical progress. These were not academics, however, but 'physician(s), trained in the research method of history' (Sigerist, 1951). As a result, much of this early work displayed a tendency to transpose contemporary concepts and beliefs on to the past. Kenneth Dewhurst (1981) has argued that this was valid behaviour by those who have been 'nurtured on a more skeptical and scientific approach to medicine'. In fact, such a statement suggests, first, that patients and practitioners in the past were naive and perhaps even ignorant, and, second, that only 'scientific' medicine is good or right. Such ideas not only negate the validity or worth of earlier belief systems of health and illness, but the ways in which people chose to deal with them.

Fortunately, the tendency to negate earlier medical practices and practitioners is no longer the norm. Medical history is now a greatly expanded discipline with a far closer relationship with the social sciences, especially sociology and anthropology (Lindemann, 1999). This has resulted in a variety of new ways of looking at issues of health and illness, with many historians now focusing almost entirely on the close link between illness, society and healing (Brieger, 1981; Rosenberg, 1992; Wilson, 1993). These historians are joined by a vast range of academics from other disciplines, whose unifying feature is their interest in concepts of health and illness in the past, whether 10, 100 or 1,000 years ago.

History, as all the other disciplines described in this book, has its own approach to researching and explaining its core questions. Thucydides (*c.* 460 BC –*c.* 400 BC) is credited with having begun the scientific approach to history in his work *The History of the Peloponnesian War*. In his historical method, Thucydides emphasized chronology, a neutral point of view, and that the human world was the result of the actions of human beings not divine intervention. In the twentieth century, historians focused less on epic narratives, which often tended to glorify the nation or individuals, and more on realistic chronologies. As a result, there are a large number of different theoretical and methodological approaches that can be applied to the study of health in past times. We will focus on two: social history and Marxist history.

Social history

The later part of the twentieth century saw the burgeoning of a new type of 'social history' with highly segmented subdisciplines. Each of these has developed its own sources, methods, topics, problems and concerns. Taken literally, the term 'social history' refers to the history of societies, or social structures, processes and trends, a definition that illustrates the close links between sociology and history (Conze and Wright, 1967). The exact focus does, of course, depend on the place and time in which the research takes place. John Tosh (2002, pp. 125–6) feels that the focus has shifted between three main areas since the 1970s. It began with looking at how organizations such as charities and governmental bodies dealt with 'social problems', such as poverty or ignorance. This was followed by an examination of 'everyday life', both in the home and the workplace. The third stage focuses more on particular groups, such as members of the working classes or women. Although the main interest, at the moment, is on patients' points of views, there are many other medical historians who work in other areas, depending on their own academic background and interests.

Marxist history

It has been argued that Karl Marx was the 'single most influential theorist' of twentieth-century historians. His interpretation is generally referred to as 'the materialist conception of history' or 'historical materialism', which stressed the important relationship between economic production, social institutions and the everyday life of people (Green and Troup, 1999). Critics of the school have argued that Marxism attempted to 'reduce all of history to material causes ... overlooking the influence of ideas, emotions, personalities and emotions' (Appleby et al., 1994, p. 80).

Marxist studies on the history of health-related issues would be likely to focus on issues of political and economic power operating within a capitalist society. They would also look at the way in which the National Health Service 'mirrors the society's class structure through control over health institutions, stratification of health workers and limited occupational mobility' (Waitzkin, 1978).

One example of the use of Marxist theory can be found in a study of asylums and the evolution of mental health policy. As a Marxist historian, Andrew Scull disagreed with the commonly held view that the growth of mental asylums in the nineteenth century was linked to growing urbanization and industrialization. Instead, he argued that their phenomenal rise was related to 'the emergence of segregative control mechanisms and the growth of an ever more highly rationalized capitalist order' (Scull, 1977, p. 339).

The historical method

History is studied through the assessment and interpretation of **evidence** and thus entails using primary sources. In general, there are two main types of source materials used by historians. 'Primary' materials are those written or compiled by people living in the time period under study. These might include handwritten letters, journals or other accounts, printed pamphlets or books, newspapers or journals. If the subjects of interest were or are still alive, they might also include taped or transcribed interview notes. 'Secondary' sources, on the other hand, can date from any time after that period. These can include commentaries on earlier events, government reports or statistics, official documents, newspapers, journals or television or radio programmes.

Information about how to have a 'healthy lifestyle', for example, has been widely available through various types of popular literature for centuries. The earliest European manuals on a health regimen, or a 'salutis regimen', began to appear in the twelfth century (Rawcliffe, 1999). Unfortunately, although such manuscript texts on health continued to be produced by medieval scribes, they were too expensive for most people. However, the spread of the new technology of printing throughout Europe in the late fifteenth century meant that books were becoming increasingly accessible. Books on health regimes proved to be extremely popular and by the seventeenth century had become one of the most profitable components of the publishing trade (Smith, 2002). The genre remained popular through the following centuries and is, in fact, still thriving in the early twenty-first century. The following example illustrates almanacs, easily accessible texts on healthy living.

EXAMPLE 2.2

ALMANACS

Almanacs are one of the oldest known forms of literature, dating back to the manuscript texts on lunar and planetary motion from the third century BC (Parker, 1975). By the Middle Ages, the genre had grown into a highly popular annual means of using astrological calculations to predict events for the coming year. The first printed almanac was published by Johannes Gutenberg in 1448, eight years before his famous Bible. By the 1470s, large numbers of almanacs were being printed in various countries in Europe (Capp, 1979). The first domestically printed edition appeared in England in 1537, and quickly become what one historian has called a 'scientific bestseller' (Jones, 1999; Simons, 2001).

Printed in their hundreds of thousands every year, these cheap, annual publications targeted and were read by a wide cross-section of the public, making them the first true form of British mass media. Although their main purpose was to disseminate information about the movements of the stars and planets and their subsequent effects on all living things, most included a range of other interesting, useful and/or entertaining topics. Although their primary function was not to disseminate medical information, most provided a great deal of information on popular beliefs and practices (Hill Curth, 2007).

although rarely, with sulfites of copper (House of Commons, 1856).

The public outcry about food safety became so great that in 1869 Lord Eustace Cecil called upon Her Majesty's government to 'give their earliest attention to the widespread and most reprehensible practice of using false weights and measures and of adulterating food, drink and drugs'. In 1872, the first Food, Drink and Drugs Act was passed, to be followed by the Sale of Food and Drugs Act of 1875, which required local authorities to appoint public analysts as well as providing workable measures against adulteration (French and Phillips, 2000).

In addition to concerns about adulteration, there were concerns with the ways in which commercial bread was manufactured. The majority of London bakeries were situated underground, with 'conveniences' situated in one corner opposite the dough troughs in the other and with open drains running the length of the room. 'Sulphurous fumes' from the furnace mixed with flour dust and moisture from the bread would render the air almost impossible to breathe (*British Baker, Confectioner and Purveyor*, March 1894, p. 589).

Instead of skilled bakers, owners hired sweated labourers with poor personal hygiene who worked around the clock in overheated, filthy conditions. These men suffered a range of health problems from heat exhaustion to pneumonia, heart failure, chest and lung damage from the flour dust and uncomfortable rashes on their hands, known as 'baker's itch'. A study in 1848 found that out of 111 bakers examined by Dr Guy, none were in 'robust health' (Petersen, 1995).

Traditionally, bread has been made by hand out of a mixture of flour, water, salt and yeast. In addition to worries about the workers who were handling commercial dough, there were also worries about the effects that bread prepared with yeast could

have on health. This was due to a prevailing idea in mid-Victorian London that 'fermented bread has a tendency to ferment a second time in the stomach, and thus bring on acidity and other inconveniences' (Dodd, 1856). The contemporary discovery that carbon dioxide could be used instead of yeast gave rise to a new type of bread developed by Dr John Dauglish in the late 1850s. His products were referred to as 'aerated' bread, after the carbonated water he used as a raising agent instead of yeast. The product was also free of any adulterants and was produced almost entirely by machinery.

This new bread proved so popular that Dauglish was able to find investors to help build the Aerated Bread Company (ABC). One of the major reasons for the young firm's success was undoubtedly that it played on the public concern about food safety by developing a bread that would now be referred to as a 'health food'. The ABC advertised heavily in the daily newspapers, promising readers that its bread was 'untouched by hand in its entire manufacture'. Furthermore, it was not only 'most valuable' for 'sustaining the health of children' but it would even 'give great relief to persons suffering from acidity of the stomach, flatulence, heartburn and loss of appetite' (*Daily News*, 1886). Aerated bread was 'tried dietetically' at Guy's Hospital and by numerous London physicians who were willing to vouch for its health value (Lobb, 1860). Presumably, the growing popularity of aerated bread suggests that either consumers believed that its consumption aided their health or that it actually did so.

Although the ABC began simply as a manufacturer of bread, it soon developed into an outfit with multiple retailing outlets. As the size of its distribution network increased, so did its product line. ABC swiftly moved from simple white loaves into other types of baked goods. Within the first decade or so of its existence, it developed a new form of catering for light refreshments to provide additional outlets for its products. The company continued to grow through a mixture of good business practices, as well as adopting novel concepts and technologies. By the end of the century, an article in *The Master Baker* (1899) lauded the Aerated Bread Company as being 'the leading company, notwithstanding the ever-increasing competition of its younger, and perhaps more enterprising rivals'.

The Aerated Bread Company is an excellent example of an organization that developed in response to the increasing demand for variety and volume of cheap, unadulterated bread. As the original company prospectus stated:

> Wherever the aerated bread has been introduced it has obtained favour with the Public and support from the Medical Profession, by its perfect cleanliness and purity, and wholesome and nutritious qualities; and it must, when supplied in quantity, supersede the use of fermented bread. (Aerated Bread Company Prospectus, 1862)

Summary

- Views on what constitutes a state of health and/or illness are dependent on the society and culture, as well as the time period in which they take place

- Medical history is an interdisciplinary subject, heavily influenced by both social sciences and humanities

- While medical history was once concerned only with 'great doctors' and 'great discoveries', it now focuses mainly on the ways in which people understood and experienced states of health and illness

Questions for further discussion

1. Why do ideas about what constitutes 'health' differ over time?

2. What arguments would you use to justify including a historical perspective in health studies?

3. What accounts for the dominance of the biomedical model in the twenty-first century?

4. What influence can or should history have on the development of policy in relation to healthcare?

5. How does the study of medical history help us to understand modern ideas about health and illness?

Further reading

Bynum, W.F. and Porter, R. (eds) (1993) *Companion Encyclopedia of the History of Medicine*. London: Routledge.
This two-volume set contains a variety of essays on issues concerning health and illnesses in a range of societies and different time periods.

Conrad, L.I., Neve, M., Nutton, V. et al. (eds) (1996) *The Western Medical Tradition 800 BC to AD 1800*. Cambridge: Cambridge University Press.
The essays in this book provide an excellent overview of the types of holistic medical beliefs and practices that were dominant for well over 1,000 years before the advent of biomedical theory in the nineteenth century.

Loudon, I. (1997) *Western Medicine: An Illustrated History*. Oxford: Oxford University Press.
This book of essays is divided into three parts, covering different sides of medical history. The first part looks at the important role that art and visual representations can play in the study of medical history. This is followed by a chronological view of changing ideas of health and illness, with a final section on medical institutions and personnel over the centuries.

Porter, R. (1999) *The Greatest Benefit to Mankind: A Medical History of Humanity*. London: W.W. Norton.
Roy Porter, who died prematurely in 2002, was one of the foremost medical historians of the late twentieth century. In addition to this major tome, he produced a large number of texts on early modern history, all of which are highly recommended.

Webster, C. (ed.) (2001) *Caring for Health: History and Diversity*. Buckingham: Open University Press.
This is an excellent compilation of essays that provide an analytical overview of the historical development of Western models of health between the sixteenth and late twentieth centuries.

There are some journals and websites with a specific focus on history and health or medicine, for example *Journal of the History of Medicine and Allied Sciences, Medical History and Social History of Medicine*. Websites include:
- British Official Publications: www.nimr.mrc.ac.uk
- US National Library of Medicine: www.nlm.nih.gov/
- Wellcome Trust: www.wellcome.ac.uk

References

Allen, F. (1765) *A Complete English Dictionary*. London.

Allestree, R. (1680) *The Whole Duty of Man*. London.

Appleby, J., Hunt, L. and Jacob, J. (1994) *Telling the Truth about History*. London: W.W. Norton.

Arcangeli, A. (2000) 'Dance and health: the Renaissance physicians' view'. *Dance Research: Journal of the Society for Dance Research* 18: 3–30.

Arcangeli, A. (2003) *Recreation in the Renaissance: Attitudes toward Leisure and Pastimes in European Culture, c.1425–1675*. Basingstoke: Ashgate.

Ayas, N., White, D., Manson, J. et al. (2003) 'A prospective study of sleep duration and coronary heart disease in women'. *Archives of Internal Medicine* 163: 205–9.

Baker, A. (1858) An Address to Master and Journeymen Bakers Dedicated to the General Board of Health and the Medical Profession. London.

Black, J. and MacRaild, D.M. (2000) *Studying History*. Basingstoke: Palgrave – now Palgrave Macmillan.

Boyd, K.M. (2000) 'Disease, illness, sickness, health, healing and wholeness: exploring some elusive concepts'. *Journal of Medical Ethics* **26**: 9–17.

Brieger, G.H. (1981) 'Guest editorial: the history of medicine and the history of science'. *ISIS*, pp. 535–40.

Brunton, D. (2004) The emergence of a modern profession?, in D. Brunton (ed.) *Medicine Transformed: Health, Disease and Society in Europe 1800–1930*. Manchester: Open University Press, pp. 119–47.

Capp, B. (1979) *Astrology and the Popular Press: English Almanacs, 1500–1800*. London: Cornell University Press.

Conze, W. and Wright, C.A. (1967) 'Social history'. *Journal of Social History* **1**: 7–16.

Corbin, A. (1996) *The Foul and the Fragrant: Odour and the Social Imagination*. London: Papermac.

Crawford, P. (1994) Sexual knowledge in England 1500–1750, in R. Porter (ed.) *Sexual Knowledge, Sexual Science: The History of Attitudes to Sexuality*. Cambridge: Cambridge University Press.

Dannenfeldt, K.H. (1996) 'Sleep: theory and practice in the late Renaissance'. *Journal of the History of Medicine and Allied Sciences* **41**: 415–41.

Dewhurst, K. (1981) *Willis's Oxford Casebook*. Oxford: Oxford University Press.

Dodd, G. (1856) *The Food of London*. London.

DoH (Department of Health) (2005) Press release: 'Department of Health launches major oral history project', www.dh.gov.uk/en/Publicationsandstatistics/Pressreleases/DH_4104426, accessed 28 May 2007.

Fletcher, A. (1995) *Gender, Sex and Subordination in England 1500–1800*. London: Yale University Press.

French, R. (2003) *Medicine before Science: The Business of Medicine from the Middle Ages to the Enlightenment*. Cambridge: Cambridge University Press.

French, M. and Phillips, J. (2000) *Cheated Not Poisoned? Food Regulation in the United Kingdom 1875–1938*. Manchester: Manchester University Press.

Fulder, S. (1996) *The Handbook of Alternative and Complementary Medicine*. London: Vermillion.

Gale, C. and Martyn, C. (1998) 'Larks and owls and health, wealth and wisdom'. *British Medical Journal* **317**: 1675–7.

Gil-Sotres, P. (1998) The regimens of health, in M.D. Grmek (ed.) *Western Medical Thought from Antiquity to the Middle Ages*, trans. A. Shugaar. London: Harvard University Press.

Green, A. and Troupe, K (1999) *The Houses of History: A Critical Reader in Twentieth-century History and Theory*. Manchester: Manchester University Press.

Hardy, A. (1988) 'Diagnosis, death, and diet: the case of London, 1750–1909'. *Journal of Interdisciplinary History* 18(3): 387–401.

Harsgor, M. (1978) 'Total history: the Annales School'. *Journal of Contemporary History* 13(1): 1–13.

Henry, J. (1991) Doctors and healers: popular culture and the medical profession, in S. Pumfrey, P.L. Rossi and M. Slawinski (eds) *Science, Culture and Popular Beliefs in Renaissance Europe*. Manchester: Manchester University Press, pp. 191–221.

Heslop, P., Smith, G.D., Metcalfe, C. et al. (2002) 'Sleep duration and mortality: the effect of short or long sleep duration on cardiovascular and all-cause mortality in working men and women'. *Sleep Medicine* 3: 305–14.

Hill Curth, L. (2002) 'The commercialisation of medicine in the popular press: English almanacs 1640–1700'. *The Seventeenth Century* 17: 48–69.

Hill Curth, L. (2007) *English Almanacs, Astrology and Popular Medicine 1550–1700*. Manchester: Manchester University Press.

House of Commons Select Committee (1856) *Report from the Select Committee on Adulteration of Food*. London: HMSO.

Jones, P.M. (1999) Medicine and science, in L. Hellinga and J.B. Trapp (eds) *Cambridge History of the Book in Britain, 1450–1557*, vol. I. Cambridge: Cambridge University Press, pp. 433–9.

Kovacs, J. (1989) 'Concepts of health and disease'. *Journal of Medicine and Philosophy* 14(3): 261–7.

Kripke, D.F., Garfinkel, L., Wingard, D.L. et al. (2002) 'Mortality associated with sleep duration and insomnia'. *Archives of General Psychiatry* 59: 131–6.

Kubzansky, L. and Kawachi, I. (2000) 'Going to the heart of the matter: do negative emotions cause coronary heart disease?' *Journal of Psychosomatic Research* 48(4–5): 323–37.

Laurence, A. (1996) *Women in England 1500–1760*. London: Phoenix.

Lindmann, M. (1999) *Medicine and Sociology in Early Modern Europe*. Cambridge: Cambridge University Press.

Lobb, H.W. (1860) *Hygiene of Bread*. London.

Longrigg, J. (1998) *Greek Medicine from the Heroic to the Hellenistic Age: A Source Book*. New York: Routledge.

Malcolmson, R. (1973) Popular recreations before the eighteenth-century, in R. Malcolmson (ed.) *Popular Recreations in English Society 1700–1850*. Cambridge: Cambridge University Press.

Marx, K. (1976) *Capital: A Critique of Political Economy*. London: Penguin.

Maynwaringe, E. (1669) *Vita sana and longa: the Preservation of Health and Prolongation of Life*. London.

Neve, R. (1671) *Merlinus Verax, or, An Almanac*. London.

Niebyl, P.H. (1971) 'The non-naturals'. *Bulletin of the History of Medicine* 45: 486–92.

Nutton, B. (1999) The rise of medicine, in R. Porter (ed.) *Cambridge Illustrated History of Medicine.* Cambridge: Cambridge University Press, pp. 52–81.

Parker, D. (1975) *Familiar to All: William Lilly and Astrology in the Seventeenth Century.* London: Cape.

Peacham, H. (1622) *The Complete Gentleman: The Truth of our Times, and The Art of Living in London.* London.

Pelling, M. (1998) Attitudes to diet in early modern England, in M. Pelling, *The Common Lot: Sickness, Medical Occupations and the Urban Poor in Early Modern England.* London: Longman.

Petersen, C. (1995) *Bread and the British Economy c. 1770–1870,* edited by A. Jenkins. Aldershot: Ashgate.

Pond, E. (1687) *An Almanac.* London.

Porter, R. (1999) Medical science, in R. Porter (ed.) *The Cambridge Illustrated History of Medicine.* Cambridge: Cambridge University Press.

Porter, R. (2003) *Blood and Guts: A Short History of Medicine* (2nd edn). London: Penguin.

Rawcliffe, C. (1999) *Medicine and Society in Later Medieval England.* Stroud: Sutton.

Rosenberg, C. (1992) *Explaining Epidemics and Other Studies in the History of Medicine.* Cambridge: Cambridge University Press.

Saunders, R. (1681) *Apollo Anglicanus.* London.

Schiefsky, M. (2005) *Hippocrates on Ancient Medicine.* Leiden: Brill.

Scull, A. (1977) 'Madness and segregative control: the rise of the insane asylum'. *Social Problems* **24**(3): 337–51.

Sigerist, H.E. (1951) *A History of Medicine: Primitive and Archaic Medicine,* vol. I. Oxford: Oxford University Press.

Simons, R.C. (2001) ABCs, almanacs, ballads, chapbooks, popular piety and textbooks, in J. Barnard and D.F. McKenzie (eds) *The Cambridge History of the Book in Britain,* vol. 4. Cambridge: Cambridge, University Press.

Smith, W.D. (2002) *Consumption and the Making of Respectability, 1600–1800.* London: Routledge.

Stone, L. (1979) *The Family, Sex and Marriage in England 1500–1800.* Cambridge: Cambridge University Press.

Thomas, K. (1991) *Religion and the Decline of Magic.* London: Penguin.

Tosh, J. (2002) *The Pursuit of History* (3rd edn). London: Longman.

Trigge, T. (1681) *Calendarium Astrologicum.* London.

Turner, B. (1997) Medicine, diet and moral regulation: Foucault's impact on medical sociology, in D. Porter (ed.) *Social Medicine and Medical Sociology in the Twentieth Century.* Amsterdam: Rodophi, pp. 175–94.

Underdown, D. (1995) Regional cultures? Local variations in popular culture in the early modern period, in T. Harris (ed.) *Popular Culture in England, c.1500–1850.* Basingstoke: Macmillan – now Palgrave Macmillan.

Van de Wiel, A., Van Golde, P.H.M. and Hart, H.C.H. (2001) 'Blessings of the grape'. *European Journal of Internal Medicine* **12**: 484–9.

Venner, T. (1660) *Viva recta ad vitam longam*. London.

Waitzkin, H. (1978) 'A Marxist view of medical care'. *Annals of Internal Medicine* **2**: 264–78.

Wear, A. (1992) Making sense of health and the environment in early modern England, in A. Wear (ed.) *Medicine in Society*. Cambridge: Cambridge University Press.

Wear, A. (2000) *Knowledge and Practice in English Medicine 1550–1680*. Cambridge: Cambridge University Press.

Weisner, M. (1998) *Women and Gender in Early Modern England*. Cambridge: Cambridge University Press.

Whitaker, T. (1638) *The Tree of Humane Life, or, The Bloud of the Grape*. London.

Wilson, A. (1993) A critical portrait of social history, in A. Wilson (ed.) *Rethinking Social History: English Society 1570–1920*. Manchester: Manchester University Press, pp. 1–25.

Epidemiology and health

This chapter will enable readers to:

LEARNING OUTCOMES

- Define different epidemiological approaches and be aware of their importance to healthcare

- Understand where epidemiology stands in relation to other disciplines in healthcare

- Describe the different research designs used by epidemiology

- Gain an appreciation of the concepts of health and sickness as they are used in epidemiology

Overview

Epidemiology is the study of how diseases are distributed among different groups of people and the factors that affect this distribution. Accurately recording who in a defined population contracts a disease (the disease rate) also makes it possible to explore factors that might affect disease acquisition. Disease patterns are traditionally studied in relation to time, place and person. For example: Does the disease occur during particular seasons? In certain geographical locations? Age groups? Do those who become sick differ in their lifestyle habits from those who remain healthy? In this way, epidemiology tries to predict conditions (risk factors) that might lead to disease, and thus identify strategies that might be used to prevent its occurrence. Moreover, once someone has contracted a disease, epidemiology can help to identify prognostic factors, which indicate how quickly or severely the disease may progress. The natural history of diseases (how they develop and progress over time) is thus central to epidemiology. Since it is concerned with rates, epidemiology focuses on populations of people rather than single individuals. The first part of the chapter explores the approach of epidemiology to health-care problems and how health and disease are conceptualized in epidemiology. The second part of the chapter describes how epidemiological data are collected and analysed. It concludes with a case study discussing how epidemiology informs public health issues such as obesity by analysing its distribution and seeking to explain its causes.

Introduction

Epidemiology (from the Greek *epi* – upon, *demos* – people, *logos* – science) is the science of how often and why diseases occur in different groups of people. It is concerned with the who, what, where, when and how of disease causation (Valanis, 1999). This focus on health and disease in human populations, as opposed to individuals, is central to epidemiological theory and the research methodologies that it uses. Epidemiologists are concerned with the experience of groups, the differences between groups and whether chance might have affected these differences or whether they provide clues to the **aetiology** or cause of disease.

Four questions drive the discipline:

● Who becomes sick or is most likely to be affected by a disease or condition?

● Why do particular people become sick?

● When are people most likely to be affected?

● How effective are the available treatments and preventive strategies?

In many ways epidemiologists are like detectives trying to understand if a disease occurs at particular times, in particular groups and what might be the reasons for this. The focus of epidemiology has traditionally been a concern with disease. The study of the distribution of disease (mortality and morbidity) – descriptive epidemiology – has been central to public health strategy. It identifies and quantifies ill health problems in communities, whether nations or smaller groups within nations, and assesses the scope for prevention. The assessment of population health is not, however, straightforward. A wide range of data is available to illustrate different aspects of a population's health – the illnesses and diseases experienced, how many people are born and die, and the lifestyles and health behaviours of the population. This chapter argues that, as health is not easily defined, a broader view of epidemiology is needed that uses methodologies incorporating lay perceptions and perspectives. In identifying health problems, social epidemiology focuses not just on biomedical causes but also on socioeconomic factors.

The contribution of epidemiology to health studies

For hundreds of years, certainly long before the founding of the discipline, people have been trying to make sense of why disease occurs at certain times, in certain places and in certain people. Some early commentators suggested that supernatural events caused sickness, whereas others, such as Hippocrates, related disease to lifestyle and environmental conditions. Although the cause of disease was often historically unknown, links between certain conditions (perhaps something to do with the climate or geography) and the occurrence of disease were made.

Example 3.1

JOHN SNOW AND THE BROAD STREET PUMP

During the early nineteenth century, severe cholera epidemics threatened London, and John Snow, a doctor, became interested in the cause and transmission of the condition. In 1849, he published *On the Mode of Communication of Cholera*, which suggested that cholera was a contagious disease caused by a poison in the vomit and stools of cholera patients. He believed that the main means of transmission was water contaminated with this poison. This differed from the commonly held theory that diseases were transmitted by inhaling vapours or miasmas.

In 1854, 500 people died in the Soho area of London. By plotting the geographical location of each case, shown in Figure 3.1,

Snow deduced that the deaths occurred in people living close to a water pump in Broad Street, yet a workhouse with 535 inmates close to the pump had had only four fatalities. On investigation, Snow found that the workhouse had its own water pump and had not used water from the Broad Street pump. Snow made sure that the handle of the pump was removed, and from then on the number of new cases declined. Although the epidemic was probably self-limiting, this showed the importance of mapping mortality.

Snow later provided further convincing evidence to support his theory and clarified the mode of transmission of cholera. Carefully documenting the incidence among subscribers to the city's two water companies, he showed that the disease occurred much more frequently in the customers of one of them, which took its water from the lower Thames where it had become contaminated with London sewage.

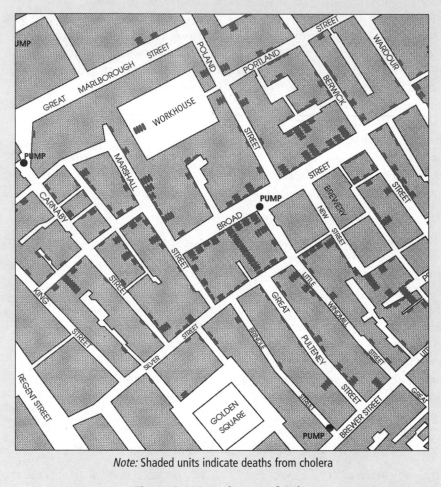

Note: Shaded units indicate deaths from cholera

Figure 3.1 Snow's map of Soho

Much early epidemiological work centred on identifying the causes of infectious diseases and, in the mid-nineteenth century, involved the initiation of a public health movement based on the work of sanitary inspectors and engineers. Although the public health movement recognized the link between environmental conditions and health, the motives of reformers such as Edwin Chadwick were not so much to improve the conditions of the poor but to maintain economic and moral stability. With the acceptance of the germ theory of disease (rather than the theory of miasma, 'bad air', which was previously dominant), the therapeutic era of public health began. This focused more on treatment than on prevention. The foundation of the

National Health Service (NHS) and the professionalization of medicine further contributed to the emphasis on therapeutic medicine.

Chapter 2 examines early understandings of health and disease and developments in scientific understanding.

In the 1970s, however, this perspective was challenged by McKeown's (1976) observations that immunization and therapy had shown little effect on mortality compared with socioeconomic factors. The modern view of disease causation relies on multifactorial explanations. It is now recognized that there may be a particular agent of disease (for example a microorganism or a dietary substance such as fat), but a complex of social factors may lead people to behave in particular ways, and these behaviours (for example smoking or a lack of exercise) contribute to disease. The physical environment may also have a bearing on health. Thus a new public health movement has emerged that recognizes health to be a function of physical, psychological and social environments (Ashton and Seymour, 1991).

Evidence of the inverse relationship between health and socioeconomic status is discussed in Chapter 4.

Such sentiments were enshrined in 1980 in the Black Report (Townsend et al., 1988), which reported the differential health experiences associated with different social classes. The report was largely suppressed by the ruling Conservative government, but the links between social class and health have re-emerged under the Labour administration elected in 1997 (Acheson, 1998; DoH, 1997, 1999, 2003, 2004, 2006).

Although epidemiology and public health have always played a part in the health service, their role has waxed and waned according to prevailing health problems, the ways in which society perceives those problems and the subsequent government policy devised to counteract them. In addition to recognizing the importance of socioeconomic factors in the genesis of disease, epidemiologists have had to respond to changing problems as the incidence of infectious disease has (at least in the Western world) declined. The simplistic one agent/one disease model had to be abandoned as epidemiology struggled both with more complex problems, such as heart disease and cancer, which have no obvious single cause, and with mental as well as physical illness.

Epidemiology has gained increasing importance as a result of:

- the need to collect data to plan services and to ascertain quality of services

- the emergence of the evidence-based healthcare movement and the desire for evidence-based health policy

- the acknowledgement that ill health is linked to socioeconomic factors and the continuing focus on tackling health inequalities.

The emergence of new infectious disease threats, such as HIV/AIDS, MRSA (methicillin-resistant Staphylococcus aureus – an antiobiotic-resistant infection commonly found in hospitals), SARS (severe acute respiratory syndrome) and A/H5N1 ('bird flu') have kept the surveillance role of epidemiology in the news headlines. The *World Health Report 2007, A Safer Future: Global Public Health Security in the Twenty-first Century*, calls for global cooperation in surveillance to control outbreaks (WHO, 2007). The emergence of major threats to life expectancy in both high- and low-income countries from the lifestyles we adopt adds a new focus to the epidemiological work on more complex health problems such as cancer and heart disease.

Common to many healthcare systems in high-income countries has been an increasing emphasis on the provision of a service to consumers and a demand for quality care that was cost-effective. As part of strategic planning, health authorities have instituted mechanisms to determine the need for health services in their local community and the extent to which that need was being met. Epidemiology and demography (the study of population size, density, growth and distribution) provide the tools to collect the 'hard' data that are used to plan services and ascertain quality. All health authorities now collect large data sets of demographic, fertility, mortality and morbidity trends, which can be used to identify geographic variations and local patterns. (See, for example, the use of such data to tackle public health issues at the Association of Public Health Observatories at www.apho.org.uk and the Office for National Statistics at www.statistics.gov.uk.)

The emergence of the evidence-based healthcare movement

Over the past 20 years, a strong movement towards the use of more evidence in healthcare has been promoted by both the government and the professions (DoH, 1993, 1996). It is argued that if healthcare professionals based more of their decisions on evidence, the quality of care could be both standardized and improved, in some instances also saving costs. There is thus a drive towards increasing clinical effectiveness. For many, such evidence takes the form of research, such as surveys and clinical trials, which produces quantitative data. Many of these designs have a foundation in epidemiology.

The rise of **evidence-based healthcare practice** was strongly influenced by a group of clinicians who advocated the principles of clinical epidemiology (Sackett et al., 2004; Fletcher and Fletcher, 2005). In their interactions with clients, most healthcare professionals go through a process of gathering information about, for example, physical and psychological symptoms, the results of investigations, social circumstances, cultural histories and so on. In medicine, such information is required to answer certain questions – Is this person sick? Do I need to do further tests? What is the optimal treatment for this condition? The answers to these questions form the basis of the subsequent action taken by the doctor. Clinical epidemiology aims to provide a scientific basis for this process of decision-making.

NICE, the National Institute for Health and Clinical Excellence (www.nice.org.uk), is another user of evidence, including epidemiological evidence, to inform decisions about whether the NHS should provide certain treatments. In reality, economic constraints also limit what is provided by the NHS.

THINKING ABOUT

One of the consequences of the evidence-based movement is the increased availability of information for the public. How able do you feel to evaluate treatment choices when you are unwell?

CONNECTIONS

Chapter 10 explores the economic basis for healthcare decisions and Chapter 11 discusses the ethical dilemmas posed by such decision-making.

Example 3.2

SCREENING FOR PROSTATE CANCER

The question of whether men should be routinely offered a screening test for prostate cancer provides an example of where the science of epidemiology can be applied at the level of individual patient encounters.

There are clearly few advantages to instituting a screening procedure for a condition for which no treatment exists, or in which early treatment is no better than late treatment. From a socioeconomic viewpoint, it also is reasonable only to screen for conditions that have a relatively high incidence and that cause a considerable burden of suffering, although any one individual may naturally take a different view on this. The acceptability of screening tests and the potential of reaching those at most risk is also important. It is, for example, well known that those who take up **screening** for cervical cancer are in fact those least at risk of this disease. Finally, it is important to establish the trustworthiness of any screening test.

Substantial increases in incidence have been reported in many countries over the last 20 years. This apparent rise may be due to increased detection and/or increasing

numbers of at risk men due to the ageing population. There is also, however, controversy over the accuracy of the screening procedure, which consists of a blood test, a rectal examination and an ultrasound scan (see www.info. cancerresearchuk.org for some of the main arguments).

In deciding whether a test is trustworthy and suitable for use, doctors must consider the following question: how often does the test produce a false-positive result (when a person would be wrongly classified as having the disease) or a false-negative result (when a person would be wrongly classified as being disease free)? Diagnostic tests are discussed later in the chapter.

There is also an ethical problem of identifying individuals as 'diseased' when their condition in fact causes few problems. Screening for prostate cancer may identify individuals with early disease that may remain unsymptomatic and untroubling. Such individuals may even die 'with' the disease rather than 'of' the disease (Mettlin et al., 1991).

The UK National Screening Committee (www.nsc.nhs.uk) regularly reviews whether evidence supports the introduction of new screening, including, for example, for ovarian cancer and and osteoporosis.

? When the Birmingham City Council Scrutiny Committee produced its 2004 report *Children's Nutrition: Obesity*, they found no hard data on the levels of childhood obesity in Birmingham. The report said:

> The committee ... believes that it is vital that local data on childhood obesity prevalence is collected and analysed, both to monitor the size of the problem and also to estimate the impact of actions to reduce obesity on population health. (cited at www.screening.nhs.uk/childhealth)

How might such data be collected?

The link between ill health and socioeconomic conditions

The early history of epidemiology illustrates how it recognized the association between socioeconomic status and ill health, but with the rise of a powerful medical establishment, the public health function and preventive medicine were upstaged by an emphasis on therapeutics. However, the new public health movement renewed an interest in social epidemiology that focuses on the relationship between socioeconomic factors and health. More recently, three reports (Acheson, 1998; DoH, 1999, 2003) have highlighted the significance of social inequalities and poverty in the genesis of disease and thus emphasized the central role of epidemiology. The new social epidemiology goes beyond establishing that associations exist between static socioeconomic factors and ill health, to examining why they exist and how to begin to tackle these inequalities.

Traditionally, epidemiology has valued most highly information interpreted within the scientific medical model. Lay and medical interpretations of risk differ and this may help to explain why lay people do not slavishly follow widely promoted public health messages such as smoking cessation messages. The recognition by public health professionals of lay epidemiology may be important in understanding and overcoming barriers to public health and implementing health programmes especially preventive programmes such as smoking cessation programmes (Hunt and Emslie, 2001; Lawlor et al., 2003). People's understandings of and explanations for their own health and illness and how information fits with their beliefs and experiences clearly have a role in the promotion of health.

Lay interpretation of risk is sometimes termed 'lay epidemiology' (Hunt and Emslie, 2001). It is a term used to describe the processes through which health risks are understood and interpreted by lay people (Allmark and Tod,

2006). Other authors have extended the scope of lay epidemiology to include lay information-gathering, so lay epidemiology is the process whereby lay people gather evidence and use experts in their midst to understand the epidemiology of diseases. It is a process often associated with political activism.

LAY INTERPRETATIONS OF RISK

Medical or epidemiological and lay constructions of the factors contributing to a person having a family history of heart disease acknowledge the importance of the number, age at death, and biological relationship of the person to affected relatives. However, there are also important differences in: notions of what constitutes a 'premature' death; the fluidity and ambivalence that many people (particularly men from manual backgrounds) feel about whether or not they have a family history; and the distinction commonly drawn by people between having a family history and whether or not this puts them at increased personal risk.

Source: Adapted from Hunt et al. 2001

The pursuit of epidemiological knowledge by lay people is triggered by their dissatisfaction with the explanations provided by the conventional scientific community. It is often fuelled by environmental concerns or the failure of governmental responses or public inquiries to satisfy ordinary people. Examples of lay epidemiology in action are the Camelford water contamination incident (Example 3.4) and the recognition of Gulf War syndrome after a long struggle between Gulf War veterans and the scientific and military communities.

LAY EPIDEMIOLOGY AND THE CAMELFORD WATER SUPPLY

This example illustrates the way in which the scientific evidence of ill health may differ from people's lived experience.

In the UK, the contamination of the water supply in Camelford, Cornwall in July 1988 triggered the emergence of the locally organized Camelford Scientific Advisory Panel, which undertook its own investigation independent of the governmental inquiry led by Dame Barbara Clayton. This action was precipitated by the divergence of opinion between the conclusions of the scientific inquiry (that persistent effects on health from aluminium contamination were unlikely) and the views of the local population.

At the heart of the dispute lay the claim to validity of the different types of evidence that each party held. The lay epidemiologists of Camelford carefully collected data gleaned from people's experience, whereas Clayton's committee collected objective scientific evidence from toxicological studies and clinical measurements. Each party considered their evidence to be equally valid; unfortunately, however, only one party (that which was legitimized through the government and the adherence to the principles of scientific epidemiology) was in a position significantly to influence the outcome of the event.

However, health for these people was clearly not simply constructed through a narrative of biological dysfunction. The official Clayton Report stated:

In our view it is not possible to attribute the very real current health complaints to the toxic effects of the incident, except in as much as they are the consequence of the sustained anxiety naturally felt by many people. (Cornwall and Isles of Scilly DHA, 1989)

Thus these health problems were not only denied a 'biological' cause, but also relegated to a community diagnosis of 'sustained anxiety'. As Williams and Popay (2006) note, this explanation of the community's beliefs 'was a way of indicating its unreliability and, therefore, its distance from the standards of scientific discourse'. Yet a recent scientific research study has found in favour of the community's views, concluding that the people exposed suffered considerable damage to their cerebral functioning that was not related to anxiety (Altmann et al., 1999).

Concepts of health and disease in medical epidemiology

Before we can fully understand the contribution that epidemiology makes to healthcare, it is necessary to explore how concepts such as health, disease, normality and abnormality have traditionally been conceptualized. For many of those working in healthcare, epidemiology is a discipline that remains firmly associated with medicine and the methods of natural science. The following definition reflects this link with biology and physiology, stating that epidemiology is

> the study of a disease or a physiological condition in human populations and of the factors which influence that distribution ... Thus epidemiology can be regarded as a sequence of reasoning concerned with biological inferences derived from observations of disease occurrence and related phenomena in human population groups. (Lilienfeld and Stolley, 1994, p. 4)

Epidemiology has, however, begun to expand to encompass other perspectives that are based on world views and theories drawn from other disciplines within the social sciences.

In medicine and epidemiology, health has been defined as the absence of disease. This is, however, quite a simplistic definition, and the World Health Organization (WHO, 1946) has specified that health is 'a state of complete physical, mental and social well-being and not merely the absence of disease and infirmity'. Even this definition has attracted criticism as commentators search for a broader, more positive concept of health (Seedhouse, 2002). The major problem with this definition is that disease or physiological status does not fully embrace the image of health held by most people. Many other factors – social, psychological, spiritual and environmental – are involved in perceptions of health. Hence, the term **quality of life** is often used to describe a person's health state.

Illness can be defined as a state of poor health, subjectively perceived, regardless of whether a person has a disease. A person may simply feel unwell. In medicine, disease means a diagnosable condition of abnormality. It can be used broadly to mean any condition that causes discomfort or dysfunction (**morbidity**) and/or death. A person with undetected high blood pressure who feels in good health would be diseased, but not ill.

CONNECTIONS

Chapter 1 outlines the biomedical definition of health as an organism's ability to efficiently respond to challenges (stressors) and effectively restore and sustain a state of balance, known as 'homeostasis'.

In its studies of populations, epidemiology becomes concerned with categorizing people into groups according to whether they are normal (that is, disease free) or abnormal (that is, diseased). Reference is usually made to particular physical and biochemical parameters, for example blood count, body weight, concentration of liver enzymes, absence of cellular changes and so on, in order to define normality. Each of these characteristics will have a normal range, below or above which disease may be indicated.

THINKING
ABOUT

Can you think of any tests or investigations you have undergone that used definitions of normality?

One example is the test for anaemia. If your haemoglobin level were found to be below 12 mg/100 ml, you would be recalled for further measurements and might be recommended an iron supplement. The recognition of normality and abnormality within epidemiology is often based on precise measurements of the type made in the biological and physical sciences. It is important that such measurements are both *valid* (that is, they measure what you think they are measuring) and *reliable* (repeated measurements coming up with the same result). Validity and reliability are much easier to measure when dealing with numerical data, which can be easily compared with a gold standard.

It is a short step, then, to see how, in this sort of system, phenomena that are readily measured and observed, for example serum cholesterol concentration, are attributed greater 'reality' than other phenomena such as nausea or wellbeing, which are more difficult to measure and for which normal ranges are less likely to have been defined (although scales have been developed to achieve this; see Bowling, 2004).

? Why might it be difficult to identify and distinguish a 'normal' state?

Even when epidemiology and medicine confine themselves to using such objective, hard measures, difficulties may arise, for although in some cases there is a clear distinction between the values that are normal or abnormal in a population, more often than not the values for the diseased population overlap with those of the normal population, giving a 'grey' area. Difficulties then arise in trying to determine where the cut-off point between the two categories lies and thus the point above or below which disease may be defined. There may also be controversy between doctors over what the normal range should be. A good example here is that of blood pressure, for which, over the years, the 'normal range' has changed. Furthermore, the normal range may vary across different populations and different age ranges (see Fletcher and Fletcher, 2005).

By recognizing the differences and similarities between cases, epidemiologists are able to classify diseases. They have traditionally based such classifications of disease on the medical model. As we saw above, the medical diagnosis has become centred on science through the use of tests and technological procedures. The work of early scientists such as Pasteur and Koch suggested that each disease had a single, specific and objective cause, which, given the right treatment, could be selectively destroyed (as with the use of antibiotics to destroy infecting microorganisms). In the medical model, the classification of disease is based on demonstrable physical changes in the body's structure or function. If these deviate from the norm, the patient 'has' a disease.

Each disease possesses certain recognizable characteristics that distinguish it from other diseases. Moreover, such diseases are considered to be universal in form and content, that is, they 'appear' in the same way in different people in different locations and at different times. Routine mortality statistics are based on this classification of the recorded cause of death. The WHO produces the *International Statistical Classification of Diseases and Health Related Problems* (ICD), which is used in most countries to classify and code mortality and morbidity.

Social epidemiology

Despite the apparently objective measures of disease, its assessment in a person is a social valuation, often with social consequences. Parsons (1951) put forward the theory that the sick role is a form of 'deviance' that is legitimized in the social world. People designated as sick are exempted from normal activities and responsibility for their condition, but there is an expectation that the sick will acknowledge that the sick role is undesirable and seek help. The anthropologist Frankenberg (1980) suggests that the social environment or milieu is central to understanding what health and sickness are. He defines disease as a malfunction of structure or function; illness as a person's perception and experience of socially devalued states; and sickness as the social recognition of disease and illness.

What these sociological and anthropological perspectives have in common is their insistence that ill health is not just a malfunctioning of the physical body, but is instead closely affected by societal and cultural factors. In this respect, the views and ideas that lay people have on how, when and why they become sick become important (Stacey, 1988; Stainton Rogers, 1991; Mulhall, 1996).

CONNECTIONS

Chapter 4 discusses the social construction of illness in detail and Chapter 6 explores how health and illness are perceived differently in different cultures.

Since epidemiology is concerned with measuring the rate of health and ill health in populations and determining the reasons for it, it is clearly important that it takes full account of the different ways in which such concepts have been constructed.

? If there are different perspectives on what constitutes health and sickness, how will this affect ideas of abnormality and disease?

The sociocultural view of abnormality suggests that although disease may be seen as a biological deviation, what is normal and abnormal is a social and moral judgement. Lewis (1993) contends that the diagnosis of abnormality is not confined to the medical domain but is a departure from some 'standard' of normality. He suggests that such standards are set by both individuals and the society in which they exist. 'Normal' then becomes relative to circumstances and individuals – it is not a universal phenomenon that can be applied across all cultures and all occasions.

Example 3.5

THE SOCIAL CONSTRUCTION OF ILLNESS

Schizophrenia provides an example of a socially constructed definition of mental illness. Statistics collected for a study in the Republic of Ireland showed that, on one day in 1971, 2% of males in western Ireland were in a mental hospital. However, through an exploration of community definitions, it can be shown how abnormality and normality are 'constructed' by the community. Quiet and eccentric individuals are tolerated, but those who violate the strong sanctions against expressions of sexuality, aggression and disrespectful subordination to parental or religious authority are perceived to be nonconformists and thus 'prime candidates for the mental hospital'. Thus, a large number of young bachelors had been labelled as mentally ill and institutionalized.

The medical view is that nature produces diseases in constant and distinct ways. Diseases are not entities or things but a particular set of attributes characteristically shown by people who fall ill in this way. Diseases as such do not exist in nature but are produced by the conceptual schemes imposed on the natural world. Thus, some states of the body are valued and others are not, being deemed abnormal. Biological changes are undoubtedly a material fact, but the sociocultural viewpoint is that it is the significance of these changes that matters.

Sources: Scheper-Hughes, 1978; Dingwall, 1992; Lewis, 1993

This section has illustrated how epidemiology has traditionally used medicine as the basis for its way of knowing about sickness and health – for building up its understanding of these concepts. The idea that diseases are entities defined through the methods and technologies of biology is, however, challenged by the sociocultural view. If epidemiology focuses only on the malfunctioning of the corporeal body, it is in danger of ignoring other aspects that are important in the generation of ill health. Moreover, it needs to take account of these other viewpoints in order to understand the considerable impact that the socioeconomic and physical environments have on people's health. Social epidemiology has been defined as the branch of epidemiology that studies the social distribution and social determinants of health and makes explicit their association with health and illness (Berkman and Kawachi, 2000).

Theoretical and methodological perspectives

Epidemiology predominantly uses the conceptual framework of medicine to direct its activities, although other perspectives drawn from the social science disciplines may also be illuminating. When it comes to looking at the practical ways in which epidemiology might contribute to healthcare, both these perspectives need to be considered. However, since epidemiologists have traditionally based their methods on medicine, rather more examples exist of activities within this sphere of influence.

Using medicine as its conceptual backdrop, epidemiology has been used in diverse ways (Valanis, 1999):

1. determining the natural history of diseases

2. identifying risks

3. classifying diseases

4. diagnosing and treating diseases

5. surveillance of health status

6. planning health services

7. evaluating health services.

The natural history of disease

In attempting to determine who, when and why certain people become sick, epidemiologists are interested in the entire natural progression of a disease, whereas many healthcare professionals, particularly those working in hospitals, are more focused on specific stages of the disease process, for example when the condition has been deemed serious enough by the patient to seek their advice. The natural history of a disease is generally described as the course it takes without medical intervention, whereas the clinical course is defined as that which evolves under medical treatment.

The natural history of a disease is useful in prognosis, which involves the prediction of events to come. In other words, it tells sufferers and their carers what they might expect in the future in terms of recovery, remission symptoms and their ability to 'carry on as normal', either now or at some time in the future.

Descriptions of the course of diseases reported in the literature may be susceptible to sampling bias. This is because such accounts are usually derived from specialist centres whose patients may not be representative of the whole spectrum of patients cared for in primary and secondary settings. Fletcher and Fletcher (2005) provide the example of multiple sclerosis to illustrate this. From the viewpoint of hospitals, multiple sclerosis must appear to be a lethal disease. A prognostic survey conducted in the community (Percy et al., 1971), however, demonstrated that 50% of diagnosed patients were alive 50 years after the onset – the same number as would have been expected to survive even if they did not have multiple sclerosis. Studies of the natural history of a disease must therefore take into account the full spectrum of people who might be afflicted.

THINKING ABOUT

Think about an illness that you and someone you know have both had. Did your illness follow the same course? Did you have the same treatment?

Biological and physiological knowledge enables epidemiologists to understand more clearly how diseases are caused and thus hopefully how they might be prevented. Information concerning the early natural history of conditions is essential to the planning of timely interventions and the identification and treatment of high-**risk groups**.

Identifying risk

Risk refers to the likelihood that someone free of a condition but exposed to certain **risk factors** will subsequently acquire that condition. In today's society, we seem to be unable to escape from the idea of risk – the risk of toxic waste, climate change, infectious agents, bad driving, contaminated food, war, famine, our genetic inheritance.

For infectious diseases, it is quite simple to identify the relationship between the exposure to risk and an adverse outcome. However, in most chronic diseases, such as cancer and heart disease, the relationship between risk and disease is less clear. In these cases, it is difficult for clinicians to develop estimates of risk based on their own limited experience. An individual doctor will perhaps see neither the resulting outcome following an exposure nor enough patients to determine which of many possible risk factors are the most important. It is here that epidemiology, through its study of populations rather than individuals, can provide vital knowledge. Through the use of case control and cohort studies (see below), risk and prognostic factors can be determined, which allows screening programmes and health promotion strategies aimed at changing risk behaviours to be established.

Classifying disease

Epidemiological data are used for the classification system (the ICD) that is central to modern Western medicine. The ICD was primarily disease oriented and a means of assigning the cause of death, but it now includes a wider range of health problems. The current version of ICD is ICD-10, which came into use in 1994 and is available online at www.who.int/classifications/icd/en/. It encompasses infectious and parasitic diseases, diseases and their location in the body – malignant neoplasms (cancers), for example, being linked to sites such as the breast or pancreas – as well as a category on the factors influencing health status and contact with the health services.

? In what situations might the use of the ICD be limited?

Using the ICD can be problematic because:

- death certificates give no information about contributory behaviours such as smoking

- mental health problems are not identified because malfunctioning of the physical body is not present

- a wide range of factors, including environmental (for example housing), socioeconomic (for example poverty) or lifestyle (for example drinking), could contribute to the cause of death but these are not recorded on the ICD.

Diagnosing and treating disease

Diagnosing what is wrong with people is a central activity in medicine, often involving the application of diagnostic tests. The interpretation of these tests is actually quite difficult. Figure 3.2 illustrates some properties that clinicians may use to determine the usefulness of diagnostic tests. Test results may present four possible scenarios. Two are correct – a positive test in the presence of disease and a negative test in the absence of disease. Where tests mislead is when they present results that are false-positive (that is, a person is wrongly identified as having a disease) or false-negative (that is, a person is wrongly identified as being free of the disease). It would not be too serious if a false-positive test indicated that a patient had a urinary tract infection and should be treated with antibiotics. However, if a patient with breast cancer were given a false-negative result, the disease might progress beyond the stage amenable to treatment. In this latter case, we would want a test with high sensitivity that is unlikely to miss cases of disease. We would also, however, need a specific test, since it would be traumatic if people without breast cancer were told they had this disease and wasteful to treat people unnecessarily. Highly specific tests are unlikely to classify people without the disease as having it. New diagnostic tests should be compared with a gold standard (the best possible assessment of whether the condition is present or not, for example an expensive 'scan') to determine their appropriateness for use in different situations.

How accurate and reliable are diagnostic and screening tests? The 2 x 2 matrix below illustrates the relationship between the results of a diagnostic test and the actual presence of disease.

Disease

		Present	Absent	
Results of diagnostic test	**Positive**	True positive a	False-positive b	$a + b$
	Negative	False-negative c	True negative d	$c + d$
		$a + c$	$b + d$	$a + b + c + d$

Properties of the diagnostic test:

Sensitivity is the proportion of those with the disease who test positive

Sensitivity = $a/(a + c)$

Specificity is the proportion of those who do not have the disease who test negative

Specificity = $d/(b + d)$

Figure 3.2 Screening tests

Surveillance and the planning and evaluation of health services

Surveillance and planning are interrelated. In epidemiology, surveillance involves the collection, analysis and interpretation of data about who is most at risk of contracting a disease, and where and when diseases are most frequently observed. Data on the incidence and prevalence of disease in a population are collected routinely, for example cancer registers, hospital episode statistics and general practice research databases.

Monitoring conditions in this way can alert health professionals to trends or unusual clusters of events. In many developed countries, infectious diseases must be notified to the appropriate authorities in order that outbreaks may be identified and confined. The surveillance of other conditions such as birth defects may identify possible causal agents. A knowledge of the distribution of disease in communities according to geographical location, age, ethnic origin, socioeconomic group and so on is obviously vital to the planning of healthcare services; epidemiology can provide the tools for such analyses.

The collection and analysis of data does not, however, occur in a social vacuum, and producing knowledge in a numerical form does not guarantee its objectivity. Statistics are collected and presented in different ways for all sorts of different reasons and to fit all kinds of different agendas. Whenever you are presented with health information data, some simple questions should be asked:

- Which population do the data represent?

- Is there any missing information?

- How have categories such as 'child' and 'elderly' been constructed (that is, how are they defined and by whom)?

- Who collected the data and why?

- Do the data attempt to provide evidence to substantiate a particular viewpoint (for example the government's)?

THINKING ABOUT

Can you think of an example in which data have been manipulated to present a particular picture, or where data may not be accurately recorded?

Example 3.4 concerning the contamination of the water supply at Camelford is an example of data manipulation. In this case, the ethnographic data collected by a support group and a scientific advisory group of lay academics were afforded less credence than the scientific data collected through the official inquiry. Similarly, despite Snow's epidemiological studies on the transmission of cholera, the British authorities continued as late as 1885 to insist that cholera was 'non-communicable, non-specific and endemic in Egypt'; the government did not wish to accept that cholera originated in India because this would have disrupted Britain's substantial commercial and trading interests with that country.

Methodologies used by epidemiology

Every discipline goes about its research in a particular way according to the paradigm within which its practitioners work. A **paradigm** is perhaps best understood as a world view based on a set of values and assumptions that are shared by a particular group. Epidemiology has strong historical links with medicine, practitioners in both these disciplines tending to work within the natural science paradigm. The scientific paradigm is also often called the positivistic paradigm.

The main tenets of this paradigm are as follows:

- Scientists believe that the social world and the physical world are physically real and objective and can therefore be known

- There are universal laws that predict and explain phenomena

- The data collected are usually quantitative.

CONNECTIONS

Chapter 1 demonstrates how the disciplines of biology, physiology and the study of the natural world are located in a scientific paradigm.

The assumptions that underpin the positivistic paradigm have certain consequences for research that is conducted through this perspective. Thus natural scientists:

- seek cause and effect relationships

- attempt to generalize these relationships to populations other than the one under study

- ensure that researcher **bias** is carefully controlled

- reduce social situations down into smaller parts (perhaps two variables) for study.

Epidemiologists often use research designs that simply observe events as they happen in a population rather than as they might happen in a controlled experiment. As a result, they are concerned with factors (other than the one under investigation) that might affect the outcome of the study or bias its results. Bias is the result of any process that causes observations to differ systematically from their true values. Think of your bathroom scales: because they are not regularly calibrated, they might consistently tell you that you weigh five pounds less than when you were weighed at the gym. This is a case of *measurement bias*.

Another source of bias may occur when subjects are recruited for a study. Many epidemiological studies compare the experiences or outcomes of two groups, one of which has been exposed to a risk factor and the other which has not. Since we are interested only in the effect of that risk factor, it is important that the two groups being compared do not differ in other significant ways that might affect the outcome.

Selection bias occurs when the way in which subjects are selected distorts the outcome of the study. A study might, for example, be interested in finding out whether meditation reduces stress levels. A programme of meditation seminars is offered to the directors of a large City bank. The stress levels of those who undertake the programme is then compared with stress levels in those directors who chose not to attend. Selection bias is present if these two groups differ in other respects that may affect the degree to which they suffer stress. For example, those who volunteer for such programmes may be particularly 'health conscious' and be undertaking other strategies such as regular exercise, which might affect their stress level. In other words, the two groups are not comparable with respect to factors that might affect the outcome of the study.

Confounding bias occurs when two factors are associated and the effect of one is confused with the effect of the other. An example is provided in a study of urinary tract infections in patients with catheters (Crow et al., 1986). When analysing the results of this study, it was found that females who were catheterized by doctors suffered fewer urinary tract infections than those catheterized by nurses. This might have led us to believe that nurses were less skilled at catheterization. However, the data also showed that doctors usually inserted catheters in the operating theatre and that women undergoing an operation were likely to receive antibiotics. These factors – the person doing the catheterization, the place of catheterization and the receipt of antibiotics – were therefore confounding, and it was difficult to know which factor was really responsible.

Another factor that may affect the results of epidemiological studies is chance. Chance is random error. Unlike bias, which results in an observation being consistently above or below a value, chance is just as likely to deflect a measurement below as above its true reading. The probability of chance or random error accounting for the results of a study are estimated using statistics (the **p-values** or probability values that you may have seen in research papers relate to this).

These two sources of error – bias and chance – are always carefully considered in the design and analysis of epidemiological studies.

Experimental studies

One of the principal aims of epidemiology is to identify cause and effect relationships, for example does asbestos cause small cell lung cancer?

A certain factor is sometimes the direct cause of a disease, and early epidemiologists who focused on infections certainly had considerable success in pinpointing their cause and thus controlling outbreaks. However, the focus of epidemiology is now firmly on chronic diseases. Most of these have multiple causes, and in their turn these causes may have multiple effects. Heart disease, for example, has been seen in **association** with smoking, stress, obesity and high blood pressure, but smoking also causes chronic obstructive airways disease, bladder cancer and lung cancer. This intricate relationship between several factors, some known and some unknown, has been termed the 'web of causation'.

Bradford Hill (1897–1991), a British medical statistician, established certain criteria as a way of determining the causal link between a specific factor (for example cigarette smoking) and a disease (such as emphysema or lung cancer). Bradford Hill's criteria form the basis of modern epidemiological research and are outlined in Table 3.1 and explained in detail with examples in Chapter 28 of Bradford Hill and Hill (1991).

Table 3.1　Cause and effect relationships

Using the following criteria, it is possible to weigh up the evidence from a number of studies to try to decide whether a strong case exists for a particular factor being the cause of a disease even when it has not been possible to undertake experimental studies. Consider the example of sun exposure as a cause of skin cancer.

1. *Strength:* the stronger the association, the more likely it is to be causal, that is, the higher the relative risk of skin cancer is for those with high sun exposure compared with those with low exposure, the more likely the association is to be causal.

2. *Plausibility:* does it seem likely, according to what is known about the pathology and natural history of skin cancer, that sun exposure could be a causal factor?

3. *Temporality:* common sense would suggest that a cause needs to precede its hypothesized effect, that is, does exposure to the sun precede skin cancer?

4. *Dose–response:* if an increasing level of exposure leads to an increased incidence of disease, the case for cause and effect is strengthened, that is, are those who are most exposed to the sun (sunbathers or outdoor workers) more likely to get skin cancer?

5. *Reversibility:* if the removal of a risk factor reduces the incidence of disease, it may be its cause, that is, if sun exposure is reduced (through skin protection creams, covering up and not going out, as in Australia), does the incidence of skin cancer drop?

6. *Consistency:* if several studies all come up with the same answer, this provides strong evidence that the relationship is causal.

The best way of establishing cause and effect relationships is through experimental research in which the investigator has a considerable degree of control over what is happening. In simple terms, in experimental studies, two groups of participants are assembled, one group receiving an intervention of some kind, perhaps a new drug treatment, the other group receiving nothing and acting as a control. In such studies, researchers have control over who is and who is not exposed to the intervention. Human populations cannot, however, always be easily studied in this way because of logistical or ethical problems. It would not, for example, be ethical to expose groups of people to potential risk factors for a disease. Nor is it feasible, over a period of time, to expose one group to a risk factor while ensuring that another group, similar in all other respects, is not exposed to a risk factor. Much epidemiological research is conducted with naturally occurring populations, when it is not always possible to undertake experiments. It is important to assess the evidence from these other types of studies carefully.

CONNECTIONS
CONNECTIONS ....

Clinical trials used to test drugs are described in Chapter 1.

Two types of experimental study are used in epidemiology – clinical trials and preventive trials. In a clinical trial, the effect of a specific 'treatment' on people who already have a particular condition is studied. In this sense, 'treatments' may include not only drugs, but also equipment (for example different wound dressings) and 'procedures' (such as different ways of organizing the accident and emergency clinic). Preventive trials investigate the effect of a potential preventive measure in people who do not have the condition in question. A preventive trial might, for example, examine the effect of two different ways of conveying health promotion messages about smoking to teenagers. A schematic diagram of a typical trial is shown in Figure 3.3.

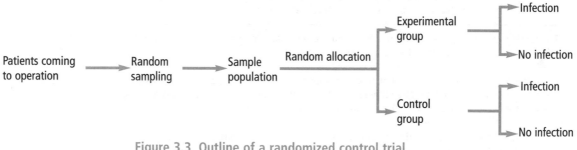

Figure 3.3 Outline of a randomized control trial
Source: Mulhall, 1996

Trials are considered by many to produce 'strong' (that is, valid and reliable) evidence about cause and effect relationships. This is because the investigator retains control over who does and does not receive the intervention (sometimes called the 'independent variable'). Table 3.2 provides a checklist of some features you should look out for when assessing the validity of randomized controlled trials.

? Consider a study to investigate whether patients washing with an antibacterial soap before an operation suffer fewer postoperative wound infections:

- Why is it important to have two groups of participants?

- Why is it important that the two groups are similar in characteristics (such as age, sex and disease severity)?

- What factors could influence the outcome of this study and make it hard to tell whether washing does reduce the incidence of postoperative infections?

Since in trials we are interested in trying to pinpoint the relationship between just two variables – the intervention and the outcome – it is important to try to minimize the effect of any other factors. For example, if the patients in the control group in Figure 3.3 were younger than those in the experimental group, they might naturally suffer fewer postoperative wound infections. This would then interfere with the design of the trial and bias its results. To prevent this happening, trialists attempt to assemble two groups of participants whose characteristics (such as age, sex and disease severity) closely resemble each other. This is achieved by randomly allocating people into either the experimental or the control group, hence the name randomized controlled trial (RCT).

Table 3.2 Checklist for assessing the validity of randomized controlled trials

- Is the randomization of the participants into each group blinded? If clinicians have a choice of which subjects enter which group in the trial, it is highly likely that the two groups that emerge will not be comparable

- Is the assignment of participants to the treatment groups really random? Checking whether the two groups are roughly comparable in terms of various characteristics such as age, sex and so on helps to determine whether the two groups are similar

- Are those assessing outcomes blind to the treatment allocation? If clinicians and/or subjects are aware of which group they are in, this may bias the outcome results

- Are the groups treated identically other than for the named intervention? In all trials, it is important to try to prevent other factors interfering with the outcome of the trial

One of the most contentious issues surrounding the use of experiments is informed consent – in other words, do people know what they are letting themselves in for when they agree to enter a trial? Although all good trials pay particular attention to this, the gap between the knowledge and language of healthcare professionals and lay people often militates against the latter really gaining a good understanding. This is well illustrated in a study by Snowdon et al. (1997) that examined informed consent by exploring the parental reaction to a random allocation of their sick babies to treatment or control groups in a UK collaborative trial of extra corporeal membrane oxygenation. The researchers illustrated how the nature of the trial or the trial treatment, particularly the concept of randomization, was poorly under-stood by parents. In only 12 out of 21 interviews were they sure that at least one parent was aware of the random nature of the allocation of their baby to standard or trial treatment.

Observational studies

Observational studies involve studying population groups and events as they occur naturally. Thus, epidemiologists might take a group of people who have been exposed through the course of life events to a risk factor, say an occupational exposure to carcinogens, and compare them with another group who have not suffered such exposure to determine whether the exposed group have a higher incidence of cancer. Mortality experience of different groups in the populations is often compared using mortality rates, some common examples of which are given in Table 3.3.

Table 3.3 Common rates used in epidemiology

Crude rates	These refer to the entire population, for example the **mortality rate** for Greater Manchester, but tell us nothing of the characteristics of the underlying population
Specific rates	These measure the number of events occurring in a subgroup of the population, for example the mortality rate of female children in social class I in two different districts of Manchester
Standardized rates	These take account of the structure of a population. This is important when comparing rates because we know that certain characteristics of a population will affect the disease incidence, for example a population with a high proportion of elderly people will have a correspondingly high mortality rate. By determining how many deaths might be expected in a population and then comparing this with how many deaths actually occur, we can gain an idea of whether the experience of the population has been the same as the standard experience. The standardized mortality ratio is the ratio of: $$\frac{\text{number of observed deaths}}{\text{number of expected deaths}} \times 100\%$$ This figure is easy to understand since ratios over 100% indicate an unfavourable 'mortality experience', whereas those below 100% indicate a favourable experience. Coggan et al. (2003) provide a worked example of standardization

Epidemiologists undertake three main types of observational research:

- cohort studies
- case control studies

● prevalence studies.

In each of these designs, attempts must be made to recognize, and deal with, the potential differences that might arise between comparison groups.

Cohort studies

Cohort studies are sometimes called 'longitudinal' or 'prospective' studies, indicating that they continue over a period of time and that the participants are usually followed into the future. A **cohort** is a defined group of people who have a characteristic in common (for example have the same disease, live in the same town or work for the same organization), who are then followed over time to find out what happens to them. Examples might be the survival rate for Hodgkin's disease, or the development of cardiovascular disease among Whitehall civil servants: the cohort study would be used to study prognosis in the case of Hodgkin's disease and to study risk factors for the development of cardiovascular disease in the study of civil servants. Cohort studies are often used to study risk.

Cohort studies provide the next best available evidence when it is not possible to undertake experiments. This is because the design of such studies aims to minimize the effect of the three types of bias (selection, measurement and confounding; see above). There are, however, disadvantages to cohort studies:

● the length of time that may be necessary to conduct the study

● the subsequent costs that will accrue

● the necessity for large-scale studies when the outcome of interest occurs infrequently, for example the Framingham heart study (Dawber, 1980) followed 5,000 adults over many years.

As a result of these disadvantages, another type of research design for assessing risk – the case control study – has been developed.

Case control studies

In case control studies, a group of people with the particular condition of interest, for example breast cancer, are assembled (the cases) and compared with an otherwise similar group without the condition (the controls). Thus, in contrast to a cohort study, the cases already have the outcome of interest, a search being made for factors in the past that may explain the outcome. Case control studies are therefore always retrospective. Figure 3.4 outlines a typical case control study.

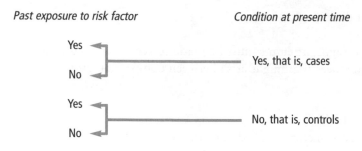

Figure 3.4 Outline of the design of a case control study
Source: Mulhall, 1996

The advantages of such a design relate to the fact that the investigator identifies cases at the current time. This is simpler and economically cheaper than the situation in the cohort design where one has to observe a large group of unaffected individuals and wait for cases to occur. In other words, the natural frequency of the disease (which may be very low) does not constrain the identification of cases.

Case control studies are more prone to bias than cohort studies. Since the 'case' and 'control' groups are chosen by the investigator, selection bias may occur. It is important that cases and controls have had an equal chance of being exposed to the factor of interest. Furthermore, there is a strong chance of measurement bias, which may occur when cases recall exposure differently from non-cases. Not surprisingly, sick people have generally reflected more than healthy controls on past events (either medical, for example drug history, or non-medical, for example working conditions) that may have affected their condition.

Prevalence studies

The final observational design is the cross-sectional or **prevalence** study. In a prevalence study, a defined population is surveyed and its disease status determined at one point in time. This gives us a snapshot at a certain moment of who has and has not got the condition of interest within a particular population (the point prevalence). This is different from incidence. Prevalence studies are particularly useful in planning healthcare services and informing policy issues.

Incidence is the proportion of a group free of a condition who develop it over a given period of time (a day, a year or a decade, for example). It measures the rate at which new cases arise in a population, as opposed to prevalence, which measures the proportion of a population that have the condition at any one point in time.

CASE STUDY Trends in obesity

This case study illustrates how trends in obesity can be identified from routine data sources; how we can strengthen our argument about increasing trends in obesity by looking for replication of national patterns both at local and international levels. From a health perspective, rising trends in obesity only become an important issue if they are accompanied by increases in ill health, so the case study will show how this can be investigated. Finally, to illustrate how some of the study designs discussed earlier in the chapter can be put into action to tackle health problems, the case study will consider possible intervention studies and how they might change the trend.

How do we measure obesity?

If we are to examine trends in obesity over time, we need to consider how obesity is defined and measured and to be sure that measure is used in the same way over time and in different countries. The World Health Organization (WHO, 2000, p. 6) defines obesity as 'a condition of abnormal or excessive fat accumulation in adipose tissue, to the extent that health is impaired'. However, as discussed in Chapter 1, there is little consensus on how to measure fatness. Obesity is most commonly measured by body mass index (BMI), which is defined as weight (kg) divided by height squared (m^2). People with a BMI above 25 kg/m^2 are classified as overweight, while those people whose BMI exceeds 30 kg/m^2 are classified as obese. These categorizations are universally agreed and accord with the recommendations of WHO. BMI is a measure that has been consistently applied over time, so is useful for examining trends over time as we know we are looking at the same measure at each time point.

As BMI relies only on accurate measurement of height and weight, it is relatively simple to use and has been reliably collected for many years and in many countries. However, a difficulty with using BMI to measure fatness is that those people who exercise build up muscle mass and because muscle weighs more than fat, a super fit athlete may have a high BMI. In children, there are additional difficulties with interpreting BMI as a measure of fatness complicated by growth and there is no universally accepted BMI-based categorization of obesity. In the UK, BMI measurement in children is related to the UK 1990 BMI growth charts to give age- and gender-specific information and a child above the 91st centile is classified as overweight and a child over the 98th centile as obese. Thus, although BMI is the most widely used measure of obesity and has been consistently applied over time, it can be a misleading measure of fatness, particularly in children, so there may be a bias. Other measures of fatness can be used such as skin fold thickness or waist to hip ratio but these are more difficult to measure reliably and are less routinely measured than weight and height, so are usually only available in research studies.

Is obesity increasing?

To answer this question, we need to consider how we can access information about BMI for the population over several years. In the UK, height and weight are measures that general practices make for each patient, usually when they register at the practice and then weight will be periodically measured. In theory, if all practices did this and we could gather the information from all GP practices, we could calculate BMI for a large proportion of the population. In reality, the data are not collected at a regular time and there is currently no way of pooling the data across practices, so this routine source will not be helpful for answering our question.

Fortunately in the UK, there are a number of large national surveys conducted each year, many of which gather some health measures and although this information is only on a sample of the population, we will be able to use this to examine national trends. The Health Survey for England, accessible from www.dh.gov.uk/en/ Publicationsandstatistics/PublishedSurvey/ HealthSurveyForEngland/index.htm, is conducted with a large stratified random sample of the population of England and BMI is part of the information collected. From the Health Survey for England, we know that in 1993, 13.4% of adult males and 17.8% of adult females in England were obese (BMI > 30) and that 44.4% of adult males and 32.2% of adult females were overweight (BMI 25–30). In the same survey in 2005, 23.5% of adult males and 24.8% of adult females in England were obese and 43.4% of adult males and 32.9% of adult

females were overweight. The trend in obesity for adult males and females is shown in Figure 3.5.

To consider the prevalence of obesity in local areas and compare this to the national picture, information is available through the local community health profile, accessible from www.communityhealthprofiles.info. All the information in the community health profiles for 2007 is based on the Health Survey for England for the period 2000–2002. The average proportion of obese adults is 21.8% and the range for local authorities in England is 14.6–31.0%, so there is evidence of significant local variation, even within regions. For example, the community health profile for Lambeth in London for 2007 shows the proportion of obese adults is 17.1%. In neighbouring Southwark, the prevalence of adult obesity is 18.5%, both significantly below the average for England. However, in Barking and Dagenham (another London borough), the prevalence of adult obesity is 23.4%, significantly above the average for England. Local community health profiles first became available in 2006 and as this series becomes established, it will become much easier to monitor local trends over time. In 2004 in England an obesity **target** for children was introduced to halt the year-on-year rise in obesity in children under 11 by 2010.

Is there evidence of increasing trends in obesity in other countries?

National and state-based obesity prevalence data for America is available on the website of the Centre for Disease Control and Prevention (www.cdc.gov) based on data from the National Health and

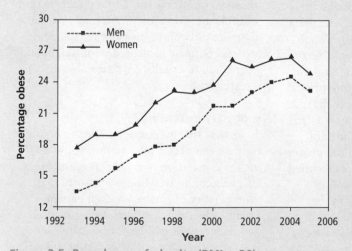

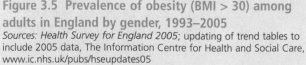

Figure 3.5 Prevalence of obesity (BMI > 30) among adults in England by gender, 1993–2005
Sources: Health Survey for England 2005; updating of trend tables to include 2005 data, The Information Centre for Health and Social Care, www.ic.nhs.uk/pubs/hseupdates05

Nutrition Examination Survey. In 1998, the median prevalence of obesity (BMI > 30) across the 51 states was 18.3%; by 2006, the median prevalence of obesity was 25.1%. Ezzati et al. (2006) provide an analysis of trends in US national and state-level obesity and show patterns of increasing obesity that are similar to those shown in Figure 3.5 for England. Morabia and Costanza (2005) report a similarly increasing trend in obesity in Switzerland. Many studies of individual countries have noted increases in childhood obesity in recent years. There are also reports of increasing obesity trends in older people, for example the Australian Institute of Health and Welfare (2004) shows that the rate of obesity among older Australians has trebled over the last 20 years. Even in low-income countries, malnutrition and obesity can coexist in the same communities due in part to high-fat and carbohydrate diets but also to the ways in which fatness is viewed favourably as a sign of socioeconomic status (Kruger et al., 2005).

The WHO online Global InfoBase (www.infobase.who.int) allows comparison of obesity rates between different countries. While obesity rates are high in the UK compared to France, they are significantly lower than many other parts of the world. The highest prevalence rates for obesity are in Nauru in the South Pacific where 80.5% of women and 80.2% of men are obese (BMI > 30).

What has caused the increase in obesity?

While we cannot answer this sort of question definitively from cross-sectional survey data, if we examine information from surveys such as the Health Survey for England, we can look for trends over time in levels of physical activity and changing diet. This clearly indicates a pattern of decreasing levels of physical activity over the same period that Figure 3.5 indicates increasing

levels of obesity. It is tempting to conclude that decreasing levels of physical activity cause the increase in obesity, but all that it is strictly possible to say from this cross-sectional data is that there is an association. To be able to say decreasing physical activity causes the rise in obesity, we would need to follow people through time and first see a decrease in their physical activity and then observe that this is followed by an increase in obesity in a cohort study. In addition, to be sure a drop in physical activity was the cause, we would need to carefully monitor their diet. If diet also changed, then we will potentially have confounding variables and it will be difficult to identify whether the main cause is changing diet or changing physical activity unless we conduct an experiment.

What are the health effects of increasing obesity?

There is now considerable evidence that obesity is associated with a range of health problems (NAO, 2001). Table 3.4 shows the extent to which obesity increases the risk of developing a number of diseases relative to the non-obese population.

More recent evidence suggests some of these risks are even higher, for example the Medical Research Council Human Nutrition Research website (www.mrc-hnr.cam.ac.uk/research/obesity/diabetes.html) suggests that at a BMI of 35 kg/m2, a woman is more than 80 times and a man more than 40 times more likely to develop type 2 diabetes than at a BMI of 22 kg/m2.

If we examine diabetes and cardiovascular disease rates over time, we find that the increasing rates of diabetes and cardiovascular disease mirror the rises over time in the prevalence of obesity. If we look at the international pattern for rates of diabetes, we find that the countries with the highest rates of obesity also have the highest rates of diabetes. Nauru has the highest prevalence of obesity in the world and also has the highest prevalence of diabetes in the world – almost a third of the entire population live with diabetes. Again this cross-sectional information can only indicate association and we require more complex studies to confirm that obesity is a major cause of diabetes.

Table 3.4 Estimating increased risk for the obese of developing associated diseases, taken from international studies

Disease	Relative risk: women	Relative risk: men
Type 2 diabetes	12.7	5.2
Hypertension	4.2	2.6
Myocardial infarction	3.2	1.5
Cancer of the colon	2.7	3.0
Angina	1.8	1.8
Gall bladder diseases	1.8	1.8
Ovarian cancer	1.7	–
Osteoarthritis	1.4	1.9
Stroke	1.3	1.3

Source: ©NAO, 2001, para. 2.17, Figure 5

Who is at risk?

The *Health Survey for England 2004* found that those considered to be particularly at risk of obesity in the UK include black African, black Caribbean and Pakistani women and black Caribbean men (HSE, 2004). Also children from families where one or both parents are overweight or obese (Parsons et al., 1999) and those giving up smoking are at increased risk. High birth

weight may also be associated with an increased risk of obesity later in life (Parsons et al., 1999). The risk of obesity is associated with social class and household income. The *Health Survey for England 2003* estimated that 18% of women in the National Statistics Socioeconomic Classification (NS-SEC) managerial and professional group were obese, compared with 19.6% in NS-SEC intermediate group and 29% in NS-SEC routine and manual group. However, the pattern of association was less clear for overweight women, and for obese and overweight men. In terms of household income, in 2003, the prevalence of obesity in women decreases as income increases, but the pattern is less clear for men (HSE, 2003).

What evidence is there of successful interventions?

Having established that there is a real increase in obesity and a related health problem, the next step is what to do about it. Interventions may focus on preventing obesity such as nutrition education with children, or focus on reducing the problem in those who are already obese in order to decrease their health risk. Evidence is needed to decide which interventions are most effective. Randomized controlled trials are the best method for demonstrating effect. For example, Sahota et al. (2001) carried out a randomized controlled trial of a primary school-based intervention to reduce risk factors for obesity and Moore et al. (2003) carried out a cluster randomized trial of an intervention to improve the management of obesity in primary care. NICE has recently published the first national guidance on the prevention, identification, assessment and management of overweight and obesity in adults and children in England and Wales (www.nice.org.uk). In common with many systematic reviews of the evidence relating to effective interventions, it concludes that many studies of interventions to prevent and manage obesity were of short duration, with little or no follow-up, were conducted outside the UK and were poorly reported.

Summary

- Epidemiology has traditionally relied on a medical model as its basis for theory and practice

- Its key questions are who becomes sick and why particular people become sick. From this, it is possible to identify the risk factors for diseases and the healthcare needs of the population

- It also questions how effective curative and preventive healthcare services are. From this, more effective strategies for health may be identified

- Epidemiology employs the scientific method of enquiry to answer these questions and uses a variety of large data sets

- Epidemiology is increasingly embracing different perspectives from the social sciences to arrive at a more complete picture of health needs

Questions for further discussion

1. How and should epidemiological data be used as the basis for government policy? Are epidemiological data objective?

2. How would you describe the impact of a disease or health problem on health and health services, either in the UK or internationally. How and by whom should healthcare priorities be determined?

Further reading

Coggan, D., Barker, D.J.P. and Rose, G. (2003) *Epidemiology for the Uninitiated* (5th edn). London: BMJ Publishing.
Provides succinct explanations for the novice of the major concepts and research designs used in epidemiology. A quick reference guide.

Moon, G., Gould, M., Brown, T. et al. (2000) *Epidemiology: An Introduction*. Buckingham: Open University Press.
A clear, readable introduction to the principles and methods of epidemiology.

Mulhall, A. (1996) *Epidemiology, Nursing and Healthcare*. Basingstoke: Macmillan – now Palgrave Macmillan.
This book explores the knowledge base, ideology and practice of epidemiology. It provides an

account of traditional medical epidemiology but contrasts this with other approaches to the discipline that are more informed by the social sciences.

Numerous websites will provide summaries and analyses of health trends including www.statistics.gov.uk and the health observatories at www.pho.org.uk. The NHS Information Centre at www.ic.nhs.uk provides access to information from the Health Surveys for England and statistics relating to health and lifestyle from a variety of other sources. Current evidence on effective interventions and guidelines for the management of health conditions can be found at the NICE website www.nice.org.uk and the NHS Centre for Reviews and Dissemination website at www.york.ac.uk/inst/crd/.

References

Acheson, D. (1998) *Report of the Independent Inquiry into Inequalities in Health*. London: Stationery Office.

Allmark, P. and Tod, A. (2006) 'How should public health professionals engage with lay epidemiology?' *Journal of Medical Ethics* 32(8): 460–3.

Altmann, P., Cunningham, J., Dhanesa, U. et al. (1999) 'Disturbance of cerebral function in people exposed to drinking water contaminated with aluminium sulphate: retrospective study of the Camelford water incident'. *British Medical Journal* 319(7213): 807–11.

Ashton, J. and Seymour, H. (1991) *The New Public Health* (3rd edn). Milton Keynes: Open University Press.

Australian Institute of Health and Welfare (2004) *Obesity Trends in Older Australians*, Bulletin 12. Canberra: Australian Institute of Health and Welfare.

Berkman, L.F. and Kawachi, I. (2000) A historical framework for social epidemiology, in L.F. Berkman and I. Kawachi (eds) *Social Epidemiology*. New York: Oxford University Press, pp 3–12.

Bowling, A. (2004) *Measuring Health: A Review of Quality of Life Measurement Scales* (3rd edn). Buckingham: Open University Press.

Bradford Hill, A. and Hill, I.D. (1991) *Bradford Hill's Principles of Medical Statistics* (12th edn). London: Edward Arnold.

Coggan, D., Barker, D.J.P. and Rose, G. (2003) *Epidemiology for the Uninitiated* (5th edn). London: BMJ Publishing.

Cornwall and Isles of Scilly DHA (1989) *Water Pollution at Lowermoor North Cornwall: Report of the Lowermoor Incident Health Advisory Group* (chair: Professor Dame Barbara Clayton). Truro: CISDHA.

Crow, R.A., Chapman, R.G., Roe, B. and Wilson, J. (1986) *A Study of Patients with an Indwelling Urethral Catheter and Related Nursing Practice*. Report to the Department of Health. London: DoH.

Dawber, D.R. (1980) *The Framingham Study: The Epidemiology of Atherosclerotic Disease*. Cambridge, MA: Harvard University Press.

Dingwall, R. (1992) Don't mind him, he's from Barcelona. Qualitative methods in health studies, in J. Daly, I. MacDonald and E. Willis (eds) *Researching in*

Healthcare: Designs, Dilemmas and Disciplines. London: Routledge, pp. 161–75.

DoH (Department of Health) (1993) *A Vision of the Future: The Nursing, Midwifery and Health Visiting Contribution to Health and Healthcare.* London: DoH.

DoH (Department of Health) (1996) *Promoting Clinical Effectiveness: A Framework for Action in and through the NHS.* Leeds: NHSE.

DoH (Department of Health) (1997) *The New NHS: Modern, Dependable.* London: HMSO.

DoH (Department of Health) (1999) *Saving Lives: Our Healthier Nation.* London: Stationery Office.

DoH (Department of Health) (2003) *Tackling Health Inequalities: A Programme for Action.* London: Department of Health Publications.

DoH (Department of Health) (2004) *Choosing Health: Making Healthy Choices Easier.* London: Department of Health Publications.

DoH (Department of Health) (2006) *Tackling Health Inequalities: Status Report on the Programme for Action* – 2006 Update of Headline Indications. www.dh.gov.uk/en/Publicationsandstatistics/Publications/ PublicationsPolicyAndGuidance/DH_062903.

Ezzati, M., Martin, H., Skjold, S. et al. (2006) 'Trends in national and state-level obesity in the USA after correction for self-report bias: analysis of health surveys'. *Journal of the Royal Society of Medicine* **99**(5): 250–7.

Fletcher, R.H. and Fletcher, S.W. (2005) *Clinical Epidemiology. The Essentials* (4th edn). Philadelphia: Lippincott Williams & Wilkins.

Frankenberg, R. (1980) 'Medical anthropology and development: a theoretical perspective'. *Social Science and Medicine* **14B**(4): 197–207.

HSE (2003) *Health Survey for England 2003.* Available at www.dh.gov.uk/ assetRoot/04/09/89/11/04098911.pdf

HSE (2004) *Health Survey for England 2004: Health of Ethnic Minorities – Full Report.* Available at www.ic.nhs.uk/statistics-and-data-collections/health-and-lifestyles/health-survey-for-england/health-survey-for-england-2004:-health-of-ethnic-minorities—full-report.

Hunt, K. and Emslie, C. (2001) 'Commentary: the prevention paradox in lay epidemiology – Rose revisited'. *International Journal of Epidemiology* **30**(3): 442–6.

Hunt, K. Emslie, C. and Watt, G. (2001) 'Lay constructions of a family history of heart disease: potential for misunderstandings in the clinical encounter?' *Lancet* **357**: 1168–71.

Kruger, H.S., Puoane, T., Senekal, M. and Van der Merwe M. (2005) 'Obesity in South Africa: challenges for government and health professionals'. *Public Health Nutrition* **8**(5): 491–500.

Lawlor, D.A., Frankel, S., Shaw, M. et al. (2003) 'Smoking and ill health: does lay epidemiology explain the failure of smoking cessation programs among deprived populations?' *American Journal of Public Health* **93**(2): 266–70.

Lewis, G. (1993) Some studies of social causes of and cultural response to disease, in C.G.N. Mascie-Taylor (ed.) *The Anthropology of Disease*. Oxford: Oxford University Press, pp. 73–124.

Lilienfeld, D.E. and Stolley, P.D. (1994) *Foundations of Epidemiology* (3rd edn). New York: Oxford University Press.

McKeown, T. (1976) *The Role of Medicine: Dream, Mirage or Nemesis*. London: Nuffield Provincial Hospitals Trust.

Mettlin, C., Lee, F., Drago, J. and Murphy, G. (1991) 'Findings on the detection of early prostate cancer in 2425 men'. *Cancer* **67**(12): 2949–58.

Moore, H., Summerbell, C., Greenwood, D. et al. (2003) 'Improving management of obesity in primary care: cluster randomised trial'. *British Medical Journal* **327**(7423): 1085–8.

Morabia, A. and Costanza, M.C. (2005) 'The obesity epidemic as harbinger of a metabolic disorder epidemic: trends in overweight, hypercholesterolemia, and diabetes treatment in Geneva, Switzerland 1993–2003'. *American Journal of Public Health* **95**(4): 632–5.

Mulhall, A. (1996) *Epidemiology, Nursing and Healthcare: A New Perspective*. Basingstoke: Macmillan – now Palgrave Macmillan.

NAO (National Audit Office) (2001) *Tackling Obesity in England*. London: Stationery Office.

Parsons, T. (1951) *The Social System*. London: Routledge & Kegan Paul.

Parsons, T., Power, C., Logan, S. and Summerbell, C. (1999) 'Childhood predictors of adult obesity: a systematic review'. *International Journal of Obesity* **23**: S1–107.

Percy, A.K., Norbrega, F.T., Okazaki, H. et al. (1971) 'Multiple sclerosis in Rochester, Minn. A 60 year appraisal'. *Archives of Neurology* **25**(2): 105–11.

Sackett, D.L., Haynes, R.B., Guyatt, G. and Tugwell, P. (2004) *Clinical Epidemiology. A Basic Science for Clinical Medicine* (3rd edn). Philadelphia: Lippincott Williams & Wilkins.

Sahota, P., Rudolf, M., Dixey, R. et al. (2001) 'Randomised controlled trial of primary school based intervention to reduce risk factors for obesity'. *British Medical Journal* **323**(7320): 1027–9.

Scheper-Hughes, N. (1978) 'Saints, scholars and schizophrenics: madness and badness in Western Ireland'. *Medical Anthropology* (part 3): 59–93.

Seedhouse, D. (2002) *Health: The Foundations of Achievement* (2nd edn). Chichester: John Wiley & Sons.

Snowdon, C., Garcia, J. and Elbourne, D. (1997) 'Making sense of randomisation: responses of parents of critically ill babies to random allocation of treatment in a clinical trial'. *Social Science and Medicine* **45**(9): 1337–55.

Stacey, M. (1988) *The Sociology of Health and Healing*. London: Unwin Hyman.

Stainton Rogers, W. (1991) *Explaining Health and Illness*. London: Harvester Wheatsheaf.

Townsend, P., Davidson, N. and Whitehead, M. (1988) *Inequalities in Health: The Black Report and the Health Divide.* London: Penguin.

Valanis, B. (1999) *Epidemiology and Healthcare* (3rd edn). Stamford: Appleton Lange.

WHO (World Health Organization) (1946) *Preamble of the Constitution of the World Health Organization.* Geneva: WHO.

WHO (World Health Organization) (2000) *Obesity: preventing and managing the global epidemic.* Report of WHO consultation. WHO Technical Report Series **894**(3): 1–253, Geneva: WHO.

WHO (World Health Organization) (2007) *World Health Report 2007, A Safer Future: Global Public Health Security in the Twenty-first Century.* Geneva: WHO.

Williams, G. and Popay, J. (2006) Lay knowledge and the privilege of experience, in D. Kelleher, J. Gabe and G. Williams (eds) *Challenging Medicine* (2nd edn). London: Taylor & Francis, pp. 122–45.

NORMA DAYKIN and MAT JONES

Sociology and health

This chapter will enable readers to:

- Identify the key characteristics of sociology as a discipline

- Understand key sociological concepts and debate their relevance to health and healthcare

- Understand research evidence exploring the social patterning of health and disease

- Debate various theoretical explanations for the social patterning of health and disease

- Understand theories and concepts relating to the social impact of healthcare and the social roles of the healthcare professions

LEARNING OUTCOMES

Overview

When we become ill, it sometimes seems that bad luck has singled us out for special attention, yet an extensive body of evidence suggests that health and disease are patterned in complex ways that defy notions of luck or chance, indicating a more systematic process of disease causation. In the first part of this chapter, the social patterning of health and illness is explored. Evidence linking social divisions, such as class, gender and ethnicity, with experiences of health and healthcare is examined. Finding adequate explanations for the persistence of social inequalities, as well as strategies to eliminate or reduce them, is an important goal of health policy and one to which sociology can make a distinctive contribution. The second part explores the methodological approaches of sociology to understanding the ways in which people interpret and manage ill health in their lives. The attempts of health professionals to manage and cure ill health have come under sociological scrutiny. In particular, sociologists have looked beyond the altruism often assumed of health professionals to examine the individual, group and social impact of professional practice. The final case study illustrates the breadth of sociology. The social causation perspective is applied to issues regarding social and dietary inequalities, while the social constructionist perspectives is used to explore issues regarding risk and social anxieties concerning diet.

Introduction

In contrast to disciplines such as biology and psychology, which focus on health at the individual level, sociology examines the social dimensions of health, illness and healthcare. Sociology is a broad discipline including diverse approaches and perspectives. Some of the key questions addressed by sociologists researching health and illness include:

- What accounts for socioeconomic inequalities in health and illness?
- How do social structures, institutions and processes affect the health of individuals?
- What are the characteristics of healthcare work?
- What is the nature of professional–client relationships?
- How do ordinary people make sense of health and illness?
- What impact do healthcare services have on individuals and society?

The ideas and practices surrounding Western scientific medicine have been a central concern within sociology. These ideas are often taken for granted as the basis upon which much healthcare provision is organized.

However, they only emerged alongside the economic and cultural changes brought about by the spread of industrial capitalism during the eighteenth and nineteenth centuries (Stacey, 1988). This period was characterized by urbanization and a changing class structure. The growth of the middle classes provided new markets for healthcare, which supported the newly established profession of medicine.

These events were underlined by a widespread support for the ideas as well as the practices of medicine. However, support for scientific medicine reached a peak in the postwar period and subsequently medicine's dominance in healthcare has been challenged. Scientific medicine is seen as limited, in that it draws on the belief that mind and body are separate entities. This notion of Cartesian dualism, named after the philosopher Descartes, is seen as problematic for at least two reasons:

● It leads to a rather mechanistic approach in which illness and disease are treated as mechanical malfunctions

● It leads to a reductionist approach (that is, it reduces diseases to a single, usually physical, cause).

This form of scientific medicine is challenged by complex, chronic conditions that affect an increasing number of people. For example, there is no real agreement on the existence of physical causes for conditions such as repetitive strain injury and myalgic encephalomyelitis (ME). Scientific medicine has, however, always coexisted with a number of rival or alternative approaches. In recent years, the support for such alternatives seems to have grown, with an increasing number of people seeking help from complementary therapists as well as, or instead of, medical professionals.

The contribution of sociology to health studies

Sociologists have sought to understand these diverse perspectives on health. They have examined the conditions of healthcare provision and the social relationships between healthcare providers and recipients. Healthcare institutions and their social context have been an important focus of study for sociologists. Social factors such as **gender**, for example, seem to exert a powerful influence upon the make-up of the various health professions, particularly nursing and medicine.

Sociology provides a number of well-established approaches to questions such as those about the social patterning of health and disease and the social impact of healthcare interventions. While sociology overlaps with other disciplines such as epidemiology, psychology and social policy, sociology is also a distinct discipline with its own theoretical and methodological frameworks. For example, while sociologists draw on epidemiological data to analyse patterns of health and illness, they are concerned to understand the social processes affecting illness and healthcare rather than with the mapping of aggregate population risk. Similarly, while sociologists increasingly share with psychologists a concern with subjective experiences of ill health, they emphasize social and cultural rather than individual aspects of these.

Sociological writings are infused with key concepts such as social class, social context, social structure and social process. There is no single shared understanding among sociologists about the definitions of these concepts, although notions of power are central to many sociological accounts of health and illness. Recently, in response to wider socioeconomic and cultural changes, new debates and perspectives have emerged. Changing experiences of work, the impact of globalization on economic and cultural life, and changing ideas about gender roles and emerging patterns of family life have all influenced sociological writings. The debate is reflected in increasing concerns with, for example, identity, consumption, the body and the emotions. Sociologists have also debated whether these changes reflect an intensified late modern society or herald a new postmodern condition. At the same time, central themes such as social divisions of **class**, gender and **ethnicity**, remain central to sociology of health and illness.

Socioeconomic inequalities in health

A key area that sociology has investigated in relation to health is that of **social inequalities** and their impact on health. During the last century, life expectancy in relatively affluent countries such as the UK, the US and Europe has risen steadily, yet there remains a strong inverse relationship between mortality and morbidity rates and socioeconomic status (Townsend and Davidson, 1982; Adler et al., 1994; Roberts and Power, 1996; Drever and Bunting, 1997; Mackenbach et al., 1997; Acheson, 1998; Kunst et al., 1998; van Rossum et al., 2000; Lantz et al., 2001).

CONNECTIONS

See Chapter 3 for more details about data collection and the interpretation of epidemiological data.

In the UK, the report of the Working Group on Inequalities in Health (Townsend and Davidson, 1982), known as the Black Report, examined standardized mortality ratios for different social classes in order to assess the scale of inequality and monitor changes over time. The working group used occupational class as a measure of inequality, adopting the Registrar General's classification of social class I (professional occupations) to social class V (unskilled manual occupations). The well-known findings of the Black Report include a marked and persistent difference in mortality rate between the occupational classes, for both sexes and at all ages. A steep class gradient, showing that the risk of death increases with lower social class, was observed for most causes of death. The pattern for respiratory diseases was particularly strong. Babies born to parents in social class V were found to be at double the risk of death in the first month of life compared with the babies of professional-class parents.

The authors concluded that the introduction of the NHS, which aimed to provide free healthcare to all regardless of income or social status, had not eliminated health inequalities. Furthermore, patterns of relative inequality seemed to have changed little over time despite an overall improvement in life expectancy. In relation to infant mortality, social class differences had actually increased during key periods. Mortality alone was acknowledged as a crude indicator of population health. Evidence from sources such as the General Household Survey was presented to show that patterns of morbidity followed a similar class gradient to that of mortality, with people in lower socioeconomic groups reporting higher levels of ill health than those in higher socioeconomic groups. Finally, inequalities were also found to exist in the utilization of health services, working-class people making less use of services and receiving less good care than their middle-class counterparts.

The Black Report received a rather frosty reception from the then Conservative government, which seemed reluctant to embrace the notion of health inequality. More recently, the changing public health agenda has encouraged a renewed focus on socioeconomic influences on health. This has been underlined by a concern with widening income inequalities and the growing problems of poverty and homelessness. In 1998, the Labour government commissioned an Independent Inquiry into Inequalities of Health (the Acheson Report). The report found that the patterns of health inequality identified in the Black Report continued into the 1990s. Other factors, such as ethnicity and housing status, were also found to be associated with increased risk of mortality and morbidity. Socioeconomic status is also linked to health-related behaviours such as cigarette smoking and dietary habits. The percentage of smokers among men in the unskilled manual classes was more than two and a half times that seen in professional classes.

Table 4.1 shows trends in life expectancy in England and Wales for the years 1997–2001 from the Office of National Statistics' Longitudinal Survey. During this period, a boy born into the professional and managerial classes (social classes I and II) could expect to live for approximately six years longer than a boy born to parents in the semi-skilled or unskilled manual classes (social classes IV and V). There was a smaller gradient for women, with life expectancy at birth for a girl born to parents in the professional and managerial groups 4.6 years longer than for a girl born to parents in the partly skilled or unskilled occupations (ONS, 2007). (Note: the social class classification system has since changed, and now includes new categories for the self-employed and long-term unemployed. The current classification system can be accessed by visiting the website www.statistics.gov.uk.)

Table 4.1 Life expectancy at birth by gender and social class 1997–2001

Social class	Males	Females
I higher professional	79.4	82.2
II managerial and technical	77.8	81.7
IIIN skilled non-manual	76.8	81.3
IIIM skilled manual	74.6	79.3
IV partly skilled	73.3	78.6
V unskilled	71.0	77.6
All	75.4	80.1

Source: ONS, 2007

The additional years gained from increased life expectancy are not always lived in good health. Data from the 2001 census (Office for National Statistics, General Register Office for Scotland, Northern Ireland Statistics and Research Agency) indicate the following:

● one in six people in the UK (10.3 million) living in a private household reported having a limiting long-term illness (LLTI)

● among those aged 60–74, 41% of men and 38% of women report an LLTI

● the lowest rate of illness is found among those working in higher managerial and professional occupations (7%), compared with 15% for those working in routine occupations

● people who had never worked or were long-term unemployed had the highest rate of LLTI (37%) of any socioeconomic group.

Explaining health inequalities

Sociologists are not interested simply in mapping patterns of health inequality, they also seek to provide explanations for these patterns. These explanations have important implications for the planning and delivery of health and social services.

? What accounts for the socioeconomic patterns of health and disease?

A range of different explanations was debated within the Black Report and in subsequent publications. The debate has centred on four different types of explanation for inequalities in health:

- artefact
- social selection
- cultural
- material/structural.

The artefact explanation

Following the publication of the Black Report, there was a debate on the nature, definition and measurement of social class. For some, the apparent widening of health inequalities was a product of the methods of measurement used (Illsley, 1986). This approach questions the validity of comparing death rates between social class groupings whose size and composition are changing over time. Economic developments and changes in employment have led to the diminishing size of social class V, which contains traditional unskilled groups such as manual workers.

In order to overcome the difficulties suggested by the artefact explanation, several studies have adopted alternative methodologies and drawn on different data sets to examine the evidence (Bartley et al., 1998; Shaw et al., 2000). Researchers have increasingly made use of longitudinal data to explore the relationship between deprivation and health over the life course (Bartley, 2004). The evidence suggests that there is a persistent inverse relationship between health and socioeconomic status regardless of how socioeconomic status is measured.

THINKING ABOUT

Do you think people's health affects their employment and if so, in what ways?

The social selection explanation

The social selection explanation suggests that the poorer health status of those in the lower social classes reflects a tendency towards downward mobility of people with ill health rather than an outcome of class inequality. The healthiest members of each socioeconomic group may be absorbed into higher groups, leaving those with the greatest number of health problems behind.

Longitudinal research, which follows people over a long period in order to identify which emerges first, ill health or downward social mobility, is needed to test this theory. Such research suggests a complex relationship between health and social mobility (Bartley et al., 1998; Bartley, 2004). Poor health can often serve to disadvantage people in employment and other areas. However, the selection explanation cannot account for the whole pattern of health inequality, and selection processes themselves may apply differently to different groups. People in more advantageous social positions, with more resources and support, seem to be better able to overcome the effects of early health problems than do those in disadvantaged circumstances.

Cultural explanations

Cultural explanations suggest that the social distribution of ill health is linked to differences in health behaviours such as smoking and alcohol consumption and to different groups' attitudes to their health. These behaviours are complex and situated in particular circumstances. For example, cigarette smoking may be a response to specific needs arising from poverty and deprivation, as Hilary Graham's work with mothers caring for young children has shown (Graham, 1987, 1998). The authors of the Black Report did not accept cultural factors as an adequate explanation for health inequalities.

Materialist/structural explanations

The authors of the Black Report favoured explanations of health inequalities that focused on the **material** causes of ill health, such as living and working conditions. This generated research on the impact of factors such as nutrition, housing, transport, environmental and occupational hazards on health. This research took as its starting point that these impacts are a product of the way society is organized, the result of material deprivation and structural inequality. Deprivation is both absolute (the inability to obtain a defined level of resources necessary to sustain health) and relative (the inability to obtain socially valued resources and to participate in society), and both are important influences on health.

The debate since the 1990s

The debate about the relative merits of these explanations, particularly between cultural and materialist explanations, became somewhat polarized during the 1990s. For many, lifestyle explanations favoured by some politicians were seen as overemphasizing personal responsibility for health. This polarization was in part a response to the entrenched nature of politics in the years of the Thatcher government (Williams, 2003). The years following the election of the Labour government in 1997 saw a shift in public policy, heralding a greater willingness to recognize the impact of poverty and deprivation as well as lifestyle choices on health inequalities (DoH, 1992, 1999).

Nevertheless, there is an ongoing debate about how to theorize health inequalities and address these in practice. This stems in part from different understandings of social inequality. While the notion of social class is central to the study of socioeconomic inequalities in health, there are diverse perspectives among sociologists about what class is and how it can be measured (Drever and Whitehead, 1997; Williams, 2003). Marxist sociologists such as Navarro (2004) view class as a relational concept based on exploitation. However, in many empirical studies that shape policy, social class is loosely defined, used as a summary indicator of a range of dimensions of inequality such as income, housing status and educational level.

The post-Thatcher years also saw a greater willingness among researchers to recognize the complex relationships between material and cultural factors affecting health. For example, Wilkinson (1996) has offered a psychosocial explanation of health inequalities that identifies connections between stress, health and relative inequality. The data presented by Wilkinson mapped levels of life expectancy against the gross national product (GNP) of advanced capitalist societies, indicating that the rate of health improvement attained by a particular country is not determined simply by its level of development. Rather, health outcomes are influenced by the extent of income and status differentials in a particular country. More egalitarian societies characterized by a narrow income differential enjoy a greater improvement in overall life expectancy than more unequal societies at a comparable stage of economic development. This may be because unequal societies are characterized by chronic social stress, while societies with a narrow income differential are characterized by greater levels of social cohesion and community support.

Other authors have also explored the influence of status, social cohesion and self-esteem on health outcomes (Marmot, 2004). These studies have opened the way for a neo-Durkheimian exploration of the role of social cohesion and the impact of social structures on patterns of health (Williams, 2003). One example of this is the increasing use of the concept of **social capital** in relation to health. The notion of social capital has its origins in Durkheim's (1952) findings that a lack of social integration was associated with an increased risk of suicide. Recent proponents of social capital include Coleman, Bourdieu and Putnam. Bourdieu defines social capital in terms of the actual or potential resources that are linked to membership of a group (Everingham, 2001). Putnam (1995, p. 66) defines social capital positively as 'features of social organization such as networks, norms and trust, that facilitate coordination and cooperation for mutual benefit'. Coleman's definition of social capital is anything that facilitates individual or collective action (in Portes, 1998). Authors therefore use different definitions, ranging from subjective perceptions of engagement to tangible economic resources. While most authors see social capital as a positive force, it is not inevitably so, and several authors call for caution in addressing the issue (Baum, 1999; Lynch et al., 2000). The Mafia and the 'old boys' network' are two examples of strongly cohesive groups with high social capital that are not necessarily beneficial for health and may actively operate to reduce the health status of others outside the network.

Kawachi et al. (1997) contend that it is social capital (in this case defined as levels of trust and networking) rather than income that is responsible for improved health status, or vice versa. Any positive effects of social capital on health are hard to demonstrate, given the dominance of the individual and the randomized controlled trial in medical trials and evidence bases. However, there is a growing body of research and evidence which strongly indicates that social capital is linked to improved health, and that strategies to support social capital may be more cost-effective than the traditional manipulation of individual **lifestyles** and behaviours.

> **?** What do you think accounts for the fact that women live longer yet report more ill health than men?

Gender and health

Until recently, the debate on gender and health has centred on the apparent paradox that although women tend to live longer than men, they seem to experience higher levels of ill health. Recent trends suggest that these patterns are not fixed and that the relationships between sex, gender and health are increasingly complex. Early research on gender and health also focused on women's health. The debate in the 1970s and 80s was largely driven by activism by women to improve their health and healthcare (Doyal, 2001). This approach was a response to long-standing imbalances that had led to male health concerns dominating research and policy interventions. There is evidence that gender bias continues to affect contemporary research and health policy. For example, conditions such as coronary heart disease and stroke are often assumed to be 'male' diseases despite their significance for women in industrialized and developing countries (Doyal, 1995). More recently, men have begun to focus on the implications of masculinity and gender for their health.

In most countries, women's life expectancy exceeds that of men, although levels of socioeconomic development and the degree of discrimination against women also impact on this finding (Arber and Thomas, 2001). Statistics for 2005 show that in some countries, for example Afghanistan, where life expectancy at birth is 42 years, there is no difference between males and females; whereas in the Russian Federation, female life expectancy exceeds that of males by 13 years (WHO, 2007).

In developed countries such as the UK and the US, women's life expectancy exceeds that of men by about five years, and this pattern is now apparent in some developing countries. There is some evidence that the gap between men and women in these societies is narrowing, perhaps as a consequence of changing patterns of employment as well as the increasing adoption by women of 'risk' behaviours such as smoking and alcohol consumption. In industrial countries like the UK, male deaths from circulatory diseases (including heart disease and stroke) have tended to exceed those of women, particularly between the 1950s and 1980s (Lawlor et al., 2001). However, circulatory diseases along with cancer are the commonest cause of death for both sexes (ONS, 2007). Cancer death rates among females rose to a peak in the late 1980s, declining during the 1990s, while among males, rates increased substantially to the late 1970s and then declined more rapidly from the 1990s (ONS, 2007).

Researchers have also examined differences in ill health between men and women, finding complex interactions between sex, age and socioeconomic status (Bartley et al., 2004). In the 2001 census, men were more likely than women to report good health, however, self-reported rates of good health decrease steadily with age, with 40% of those identifying themselves as not in good health being aged 65 and over. The overall difference between the sexes was small once the age distribution of the population was taken into account. Similarly, up to age 59, there were few differences in rates of LLTI between males and females. However, in the 60–74 age group, men had a higher prevalence of LLTI than women; the situation was reversed for those aged 75 and over, with more women than men reporting an LLTI (ONS, 2007). These data suggest that as a consequence of their greater life expectancy, women in developed countries are more likely than men to experience a range of conditions that lead to chronic impairment and disability. While ageing does not inevitably lead to ill health and a loss of independence, older women are more likely than older men to suffer from disabling conditions and to need help in performing basic activities such as bathing and shopping (Arber, 1998).

Other areas where gender differences have been examined are mental health (Payne, 1998), the use of health services (Doyal, 1998) and patterns of health-related behaviour. In relation to mental health, the prevalence of the most common mental health conditions, neurotic disorders, is higher among women than for men. On the other hand, suicide rates are higher among men (ONS, 2007). In relation to the use of health services, data from the General Household Survey on GP consultation rates show that consultations tend to be higher among women, with 16% of females having visited a GP in the 14 days prior to the interview compared with 11% of males. However, these differences disappear in the oldest age groups. Finally, patterns of health-related behaviour have also been examined in relation to gender. Data from the General Household Survey suggest that there may be some convergence in male and female patterns: between 1988 and 2005, the prevalence of smoking reduced from 30% to 25% among men and from 26% to 23% among women (ONS, 2007).

? What do you think accounts for gender differences in health status and reported ill health?

Explaining gender inequalities in health

As in the case of socioeconomic inequalities in health, a number of explanations for gender differences in health have been put forward. These include biological explanations, materialist and structural explanations, and cultural and social constructionist accounts.

Biological explanations

Biological explanations focus on the different reproductive roles of men and women, which impact on health. Sociologists traditionally tended to reject biologically based notions of gender identity. More recently, however, they have begun to engage more critically with notions of the body, which has led to a more inclusive focus and an engagement with biological discourse. This shift is also reflected in feminist research, which has explored the interaction between biology and society and the influence of biological factors on male and female health (Doyal, 1995, 2001).

Materialist/structural explanations

Materialist and structural explanations look at health outcomes for men and women, and how these may be determined by social factors. Researchers have drawn attention to differences in the social roles of men and women as well as differences in their access to resources such as income, employment, housing and leisure. Such research has uncovered persistent inequalities that can influence health. For example, segregation in the labour market means that women continue to be concentrated in low-paid employment and in roles such as caring and service work (Doyal, 1995; Arber and Khlat, 2002). They also continue to bear the bulk of responsibility for unpaid caring and domestic work (Lloyd, 1999; Moss, 2002). This means not only that women have less access than men to health-promoting resources, but that women and men may face different hazards and risks in both paid and unpaid work settings.

Cultural explanations and social constructionist accounts

Cultural explanations focus on the way in which health outcomes are influenced by roles, relationships, norms and expectations at macro- and micro-levels (Moss, 2002). **Social constructionist** accounts of gender go further than this, implying that gender is not a fixed category, questioning the notion that traits associated with masculinity and femininity are *essential* characteristics inherited at birth. Instead, gender roles are seen as being continuously negotiated (Cameron and Bernades, 1998). Hence, creating and performing an appropriate gender identity is a continuous task, and masculinity and femininity may both be associated to a varying degree with individual men and women (Annandale and Hunt, 1990).

THINKING ABOUT

Can you think of an example where how you feel about your gender has impacted on your health or health-related behaviour?

Research has explored the impact on health of expectations, attitudes and behaviours concerning approved forms of gender identity. A key area is that of sexual health: expectations about gender clearly help to shape interaction and the negotiation of sexual activity. The social construction of gender therefore provides the context for, and sometimes constrains, strategies to reduce a number of risks, such as unwanted pregnancies and sexually transmitted diseases. For example, one study found that the explicit pursuit of sexual pleasure is often approved of for males, whereas girls can be stigmatized for displaying sexual knowledge even if this knowledge can protect them from risk (Thomson and Holland, 1994).

Earlier research explored the effects of stereotyping of female patients in healthcare services (Doyal, 1998; Payne, 1998). More recently, it is suggested that certain notions of masculinity may have a negative effect on men's health. This research distinguishes between different forms of masculinity. It is traditional or hegemonic masculinity, with its emphasis on risk-taking, self-reliance and dominance, which is viewed as potentially dangerous, for example it can discourage men from seeking help for health problems (Cameron and Bernades, 1998). These issues have been explored in studies of the relationship between masculine identities, risk-taking and health promotion (Courtenay, 2000; DeVisser and Smith, 2006; Gough and Conner, 2006; Robertson, 2006). Finally, research has identified emerging trends in women's health that have arisen as a consequence of the adoption by women of traditional 'masculine' practices such as cigarette smoking (Graham, 1998) and alcohol consumption (Bloomfield et al., 2006; Wilsnack et al., 2006).

The different explanations of gender inequalities in health are not necessarily mutually exclusive, rather they focus on different aspects of gender such as the impact of reproductive roles, psychosocial factors, occupational factors, cultural trends and social structuring (Arber and Thomas, 2001). Health outcomes are increasingly recognized as part of a complex relationship between macro- and micro-level social factors spanning geopolitical environment, cultural norms and the distribution of risks and resources within households (Moss, 2002).

The combined impact of these factors is illustrated by changing patterns of risk in HIV/AIDS. The impact of gender on HIV/AIDS risk is discussed by Türmen (2003). In the early stages of the pandemic, infection was predominantly among men but by the early years of the twenty-first century, women represented 48% of new infections and, in developing countries, 67% of newly infected individuals aged between 15 and 24. This shift is attributed to a number of factors including women's greater biological susceptibility to infection than that of men, as well as social and cultural factors that increase the risk of HIV infection among women. These include high levels of sexual violence against women, lack of education and knowledge about risk, poverty and dependence on male partners, and lack of negotiating power in rela...

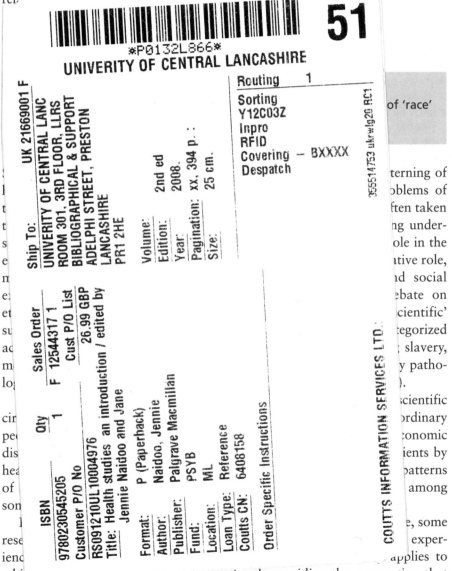

...terning of ...oblems of ...ften taken ...ng under-...ole in the ...ative role, ...d social ...ebate on ...cientific' ...tegorized ...slavery, ...y patho-...).

...scientific ...ordinary ...conomic ...ients by ...patterns ...among

...e, some ...exper-...applies to white p... ...well as black people, thereby avoiding the assumption that only the ethnicity of black people needs to be examined. In practice however, the term 'ethnicity' is often used as a euphemism for 'race', and most studies of ethnicity and health focus only on ethnic minorities.

Example 4.1

'RACE', ETHNICITY AND HEALTH

- The evidence linking ethnicity with health is complex and apparently contradictory, the picture being further limited by a number of methodological problems. UK studies have, however, shown excess mortality for men born in Bangladesh, Ireland, Scotland and West/South Africa (Davey Smith, 2003).
- An excess coronary heart disease mortality has been found in people born in the Indian subcontinent, and a relatively high mortality from stroke has been found among people of Afro-Caribbean origin. Research has examined ethnic differences in risk factors, especially in relation to alcohol use in the white population and weight in the black population (Dundas et al., 2001).

- The mortality rates of common types of cancer, such as breast and lung cancer, appear to be relatively low among people from the Caribbean and the Indian subcontinent (Harding and Rosato, 1999).
- A higher rate of infant mortality is found for most migrant groups, a particularly high level being seen among the babies of Pakistan-born mothers (Davey Smith, 2003).
- The members of minority ethnic groups perceive their health in poorer terms than do the general population. Middle-aged Irish and Pakistani men, and older Indian and Pakistani women, show significantly higher rates of common mental disorders than their white English counterparts (Weich et al., 2004).

The Black Report's framework, developed by Davey Smith (2003), has been used as a starting point to explain these data. As with social class, artefact explanations focus on the problems caused by the use of particular measurement tools (Manly, 2006). Challenges in ethnicity and health research stem from the problematic use of country of birth as a measure of ethnicity, half of the UK's ethnic minorities having been born in the UK. Other problems include treating ethnicity and class separately, and failing to recognize the heterogeneous nature of ethnic majority populations.

Biological explanations focus on factors such as genetic variations and the role of inherited conditions such as blood disorders in relation to conditions such as thalassaemia. These explanations have been criticized for overestimating the impact of genetic factors on the causation of disease and for reinforcing biolological conceptualizations of 'race' (Frank, 2001). Cultural explanations tend to focus on particular lifestyles, behaviours, religious practices and beliefs associated with different ethnic groups. On the one hand, the increasing diversity of societies like the UK and the US has stimulated demands for 'culturally and linguistically competent healthcare' (Shaw-Taylor, 2002). On the other hand, the focus on cultural differences as a cause of health outcomes has been challenged: the cultural characteristics of minority ethnic groups are often portrayed in negative terms, and the positive influences of culture on health are sometimes overlooked.

Material and structural explanations emphasize the direct effects of socioeconomic factors, such as poor housing and unemployment, on members of minority ethnic groups (Nazroo, 1997). Members of minority ethnic groups are disproportionately represented in lower socioeconomic groups. While material disadvantage impacts negatively on the health of minority ethnic groups, it is unlikely that social class alone can explain the excess mortality observed in minority ethnic groups (Nazroo, 2001).

Racism has been used to explain patterns of ethnicity and health. Racism can affect the health of minority ethnic groups in a number of ways. Discrimination in employment causes psychosocial distress as well as limiting access to income and resources needed for health. A recent study by Bhui et al. (2005) found a strong association between perceived discrimination in the workplace and common mental disorders such as depression. Finally, ethnicity is associated with different patterns of access and use of health services. Racism can also affect the responsiveness of health authorities to the particular needs of minority ethnic groups. Public services have been seen as responding more punitively to ethnic minorities than to other groups. Rates of admission to mental health wards are three or more times higher than average in black African, black Caribbean, and white and black Caribbean mixed groups, and people from these groups are more likely than others to be compulsorily detained (Healthcare Commission, 2006).

Theoretical and methodological approaches

Sociology – the study of human social life – involves a conscious distancing of the sociologist from the object of study, whether that involves personal emotions (for example bereavement or ill health), social institutions (for example the family, or healthcare services) or group life (for example health professionals' peer group norms and pressures). Sociological study often involves investigating what appears at first sight to be natural, universal or common sense, only to discover that such behaviours or practices are fundamentally affected by specific social factors and influences. Sociology offers a wide range of theoretical and methodological approaches for the study of health. This brief introduction presents an overview of selected issues in the sociology of health that illustrates key theoretical and methodological approaches.

These approaches begin with different starting points when considering issues such as the impact of health services. While health services seem self-evidently beneficial, some have questioned this, even arguing that the harm done by modern medicine outweighs the benefits. We can explore this debate by distinguishing between consensus and conflict approaches. Both acknowledge that health professionals, particularly doctors, enjoy a significant amount of power. They can sanction a number of benefits such as employees' sick leave, claimants' eligibility for welfare payments and patients' entitlement to services. They also endorse controlling and restraining actions such as the incarceration of individuals defined as mentally ill.

Consensus approaches accept the necessity of these functions for the smooth running of modern societies. Furthermore, they suggest that members of regulated professions are, because of their extensive training and commitment to ethical conduct, well placed to carry them out. In contrast, conflict perspectives question professional power, highlighting issues of professional domination and social control, and the oppressive impact of some practices.

Recent developments, such as the advancement of nursing and other professions, increased managerialism in the NHS and the growth of complementary therapies, suggest that power, particularly medical power, is not exercised without challenge and resistance. Theorizing these trends, recent accounts suggest that traditional approaches may be limited by a rather narrow and mechanistic understanding of power. Rather than being delegated by society or imposed on individuals and groups, power is increasingly viewed as fluid and diffuse, capable of being mobilized in many ways and from a range of sources.

The sociology of lay–professional relationships: functionalist approaches

The **functionalist** sociology of Talcott Parsons (1951, 1975) provides a well-known and influential example of a consensus model. Parsons was concerned to demonstrate the ways in which practices such as medicine contribute to the maintenance of the social order. Illness not only disturbs individual functioning, but is also socially dysfunctional, undermining the values, activities and roles that support productivity and social stability. In order to prevent such a disruption, mechanisms are needed that render illness an undesirable and temporary social state. Parsons identified such a mechanism in the form of the **sick role**, into which people ideally enter when they become ill. The sick role confers both rights and obligations. The rights are:

● an exemption from responsibilities such as work and social obligations, which needs to be legitimized by a physician in order to be valid

● that the sick individual avoids any blame or responsibility for their condition.

The two obligations are:

● the sick person must want to get better

● the sick person must seek competent help, usually from a trained physician.

? How adequate is the sick role in accounting for:
1. Someone with food poisoning?
2. Someone with depression?

3. Someone with asthma?
4. Someone who is HIV positive?

Sociologists have debated the relevance of the concept of the sick role in relation to contemporary patterns of health and illness. One of the issues that arises is that access to the sick role may not be enjoyed equally by all. The sick role concept may apply relatively closely to acute illnesses such as influenza, but even in these cases there are some social obligations (such as caring for others) from which exemption may be difficult to gain. In the case of chronic conditions, the rights associated with the sick role concept apply less clearly, and social obligations may be difficult to escape in the longer term. Furthermore, some conditions (for example HIV/AIDS) carry a stigma. This means that assumptions of responsibility and blame may influence how the person is seen and treated by others.

The obligations associated with the sick role concept are also more complex than at first appears. These obligations render the doctor much more powerful than the patient in professional–client interactions. Functionalists such as Parsons accept the asymmetrical nature of the doctor–patient relationship on the grounds that doctors, as modern professionals, are required to be altruistic and ethical practitioners as well as knowledgeable. These attributes are seen as ensuring that a doctor's personal feelings towards a patient do not influence the consultation or treatment offered. The physician is expected to put the welfare of the patient above any personal interest.

CONNECTIONS

Chapter 11 discusses the ethical principles underlying professional practice and the lay person's obligations.

The power imbalance between doctors and patients becomes more problematic if professionals are seen as a group seeking to influence the organization of services and rewards. Further, patients can often become experts in their condition and may feel frustrated if they are not listened to by doctors. A more critical perspective would suggest that professionals' interests may conflict with those of service users, and would question the degree of trust that society grants to doctors (evidenced by their high degree of autonomy and the lack of external surveillance of many procedures).

Hence, Parsons' concept of the sick role has been criticized as being naive in relation to issues of power, although the debate continues. The **empowerment** model (Crossley, 1998), for example, has developed as an alternative way of conceptualizing professional–client relationships. This model suggests that doctors' technical competence may be more limited than traditional beliefs concerning the efficacy of scientific medicine suggest. This can be seen in relation to conditions such as repetitive strain injury or ME for which there appears to be little medical consensus on the cause of the problem or appropriate treatment, or HIV, in which there is little possibility of a cure. The obligation to seek technically competent help from a physician makes little sense if technical competence is beyond the physician's scope. Instead, the empowerment model seems to enhance the status and authority of the experiential knowledge of the sufferer in the face of doctors' limited capacity to respond to complex chronic conditions.

Crossley warns, however, that the empowerment perspective underestimates the benefits of medicine. Whereas scientific medicine has not been able to provide a cure for many conditions, the medical management of chronic illness is constantly developing. Furthermore, the empowerment model is seen as offering a weak basis for practice because it lacks any notion of duty or social obligation to accompany the 'rights' associated with chronic illness.

The sick role concept, although criticized, has provided useful insights into the experience of illness and the role of medicine and has paved the way for a broader debate on the nature of medical authority and the relationship between medicine and social control.

Medicalization and social control

During the 1960s and 70s, a number of critical perspectives on medical power emerged. These often drew on the **medicalization** thesis, in which medicine is seen as expanding its social jurisdiction and replacing earlier mechanisms of social control such as religion. While Parson's functionalist model emphasized the benign and productive aspects of medical power, critical perspectives have identified some undesirable social costs of medical expansion.

The medicalization of society has been seen as taking place at a number of levels (Zola, 1972):

● Medicine has expanded its concerns to encompass areas of life not previously regarded as illness

● Medicalization has resulted in the concentration of control over technical procedures among doctors

● Doctors' authority has expanded to encompass areas of moral decision-making.

Medicalization involves the pursuit of medical, individual and technical solutions to an expanding range of problems. Where these problems are social in origin, medicalization can be seen as obscuring their social causes, inhibiting the development of alternative solutions.

Example 4.2

MEDICINE AS A THREAT TO HEALTH

In one well-known critique, Illich described medicalization as a major threat to health. Modern medicine was portrayed as generating iatrogenic disease, that is, illness that would not have come about without medical intervention. It was also suggested that society would be better off without professions such as medicine, which encourage dependency rather than self-reliance.

During the 1990s, feminist researchers highlighted the negative impact of conventional healthcare on women, suggesting that the benefits of modern medicine to women are oversold and its harmful effects understated. As patients, women are constrained in their ability to make rational choices, partly because doctors are themselves unaware of many of the risks attached to accepted forms of medical treatment. Furthermore, when doctors are aware of the risks, they may assume that female patients will not be able to cope with the information, and therefore keep their knowledge to themselves.

The notion of medicine as a threat to health remains influential. Contemporary journalism often seeks to expose the 'dangers of modern medicine', while the increasing popularity of complementary therapies and self-help sources such as the internet reveals apparent widespread disillusionment with conventional medical approaches.

Sources: Illich, 1977; Foster, 1995; McTaggart, 1996

While it is important not to overstate the benefits of medical practice, these theories may understate medicine's benefits; empirical evidence is needed in order to evaluate the impact of different health interventions. Without such evidence, these theories could potentially undermine efforts to improve health and reduce inequalities in health. Given that, for many people in the world, access to basic healthcare remains limited, it seems important to emphasize widening access to beneficial practices and resources as well as to re-examine questionable aspects of medical practice.

These theories do, however, highlight the impact of medical decision-making and point towards the need for a greater involvement of patients and lay people in such activity. In the face of such challenging claims about medicine, it seems that consumers need to make more and more complex and difficult choices concerning their healthcare. This theme is explored in the following sections, which examine a number of different approaches to understanding the relationships between medicine, health professions and society.

CONNECTIONS

Chapter 8 reviews policies designed to increase service user involvement in health and social care provision.

Marxist and political economy perspectives

Marxist and political economy perspectives also highlight the negative impact of medical power. However, rather than seeing professionals as the main problem, Marxist theory suggests that professional power is a product of a deeper set of power relations. Political economy perspectives draw on

Marxist theory to suggest that the structuring of society around the needs of capitalism as an economic system is the starting point of any analysis of health and healthcare. This theory suggests that capitalist societies are organized around the generation of profit, which is created by the exploitation of labour power.

Political economy writers such as Navarro (1979) drew broadly on this theory and applied it to health in a number of ways:

- The processes of industrial capitalism cause ill health directly, for example through occupational disease, industrial accidents and the manufacturing and marketing of harmful consumer products

- This burden of disease is disproportionately felt by those in lower socioeconomic groups

- Society does not do enough to prevent these problems or promote health because society's resources are channelled towards the maintenance of production over and above the social goal of securing and improving public health.

> **?** Consider the political economy of tobacco. How do you account for its continued manufacture and advertising?

Governments' reluctance to ban the manufacture and advertising of this dangerous product could be explained in terms of the dominance of the interests of tobacco producers over those of other groups and the economic benefits derived by governments from tobacco tax.

The political economy perspective also offers a critique of the role of medical and health services. According to Navarro, doctors are often seen as serving the interests of the dominant class, partly because of their own class position and partly because of their social role. Hence the role of medicine is seen as helping to minimize disruption to the economic functioning of society, even if this means supporting exploitative and oppressive economic and social relationships.

> **?** How relevant is the view that capitalism is a major threat to population health?

The global nature of capitalism perhaps makes it impossible to identify examples of societies and cultures unaffected by it. However, critics have argued that other (non-economic) social processes are equally influential. These include the cultural discourse of ideas and concepts. Furthermore, critics have argued that Marxism places too much emphasis on class divisions as the driving force of social change, ignoring the independent impact of other social relations, including gender and ethnicity.

CONNECTIONS
CONNECTIONS

Chapter 6 discusses the cultural construction of concepts of health and illness.

In response to these criticisms, political economy perspectives have taken a broader view than those of traditional Marxism, widening their scope to examine other aspects of power relationships such as gender and ethnicity. Political economy perspectives have exercised a strong influence over the sociology of health and illness, although this influence declined during the 1980s and 90s as new economic and social trends, such as changes in employment, leisure and lifestyle, emerged to challenge core assumptions concerning identity and class. Political economy perspectives may still evolve to meet these challenges. In the meantime, however, their legacy can still be seen, for example in relation to the inequalities in health debate, where material and structural explanations continue to hold sway.

Health professions and interprofessional relationships

Since the 1970s, a great deal of attention has been given to the role of health professions, with early discussions focusing on whether it is possible to identify core traits such as knowledge, training, practices of regulation and autonomy that set a 'profession' apart from other occupational groups (Freidson, 1970). Much of this research focused on the profession of medicine. More recently, the scope of the discussion has widened to include the roles and relationships between other groups including nurses (Davies, 1995; Porter, 1999).

Some of this writing has been influenced by *neo-Weberian* approaches, which focus on the characteristics of different professional groups in relation to social class and other hierarchies, as well as examining the strategies adopted by occupational groups to gain influence and control (Johnson, 1993). These professionalization projects involve professional groups in negotiating their relationship with the state as well as with other professional groups in situations where healthcare resources are increasingly limited (Witz, 1992; Johnson, 1993, 1995). Professionalization strategies have been identified such as that of 'dual closure' (Witz, 1992). This has two elements: usurpation to renegotiate role boundaries with more powerful groups; and demarcation to organize their relationships with less powerful groups. *Foucauldian* perspectives have also been brought to bear on this debate, identifying ways in which discourses of health, illness and care are used to shape professional roles and interprofessional relationships (Foucault, 1976; Armstrong, 1995; Lupton, 1995; Wicks, 1998).

Example 4.3

PROFESSIONALIZATION IN THE NHS

These issues were explored in a study by Daykin and Clarke (2000) of interprofessional relationships between nurses and healthcare assistants in the NHS. A training programme sought to enhance the roles of healthcare assistants, providing them with the skills to undertake tasks previously undertaken by nurses such as bedside observations. At the same time, the staffing ratios were to be changed to reduce the number of qualified nurses on the wards. The project was in part a response by managers to ongoing difficulties of recruitment and retention of qualified nursing staff and an attempt to reduce the rising costs of employing agency nurses to cover the work of this group.

The nursing and care staff had mixed views about the project, with some welcoming the changes and others seeing them as a dilution and fragmentation of care. For these nurses, the training of healthcare assistants was a 'task-oriented' approach that undermined the more holistic 'nursing process' discourse (Porter, 1992) that was key to their professional identity and job satisfaction. Others recognized the importance of the division of labour in healthcare and saw the changes as an opportunity for themselves and healthcare assistants to enhance their roles. The research identified among nurses a dual closure strategy of usurpation in relation to doctors and demarcation in relation to healthcare assistants. Some participants saw managers as being able to bridge these differences and divisions in order to overcome resistance to the changes in the care they proposed and to avoid the challenge of providing adequate resources to support alternative solutions to the problems of care delivery.

Sources: Porter, 1992; Witz, 1992; Daykin and Clark, 2000

Interactionist perspectives and the experience of illness

The perspectives discussed so far concentrate on the impact of illness, health and healthcare on society as whole. Sociologists have also examined the nature and meanings of the illness experience at the individual level, analysing this experience in the context of the interaction between people and exploring its implication for notions of identity and self. This tradition draws on the work of George Herbert Mead (1934), who saw human beings as distinctive, in that they are able to reflect on their own thoughts and actions. This approach, sometimes referred to as 'symbolic **interactionism**', emphasizes the ways in which people gain a shared understanding of the meanings attached to objects and phenomena. Meanings are not seen as pre-existing or intrinsic, but emerge from an interpretative process between people in which language is an important element. A nurse's uniform, for example, suggests femininity, caring, altruism and sacrifice – meanings reaffirmed by countless media portrayals.

Sociologists have applied these insights to the study of changes in identity, which occur when people become chronically ill or impaired. Goffman's work on stigma (1963) provides a well-known example of such an approach. According to Goffman, a person's sense of identity is formed in interaction with others and is reflected back to the individual through verbal and non-verbal communication. When someone possesses a distinguishing attribute that is perceived negatively by others, his or her identity is to some extent 'spoiled' or stigmatized. People attribute a range of negative characteristics, unrelated to the original attribute, to the individual. Wheelchair users, for example, are often assumed to be physically and intellectually dependent. Stigma may be attributed to people on the basis of physical attributes or personal and social characteristics, such as being gay or lesbian.

Goffman suggested that stigmatized individuals may react in a number of ways. They may attempt to 'pass', maintaining a performance of self in which the stigmatized attribute is disguised or hidden. They may also respond in ways that seem to confirm society's stereotyped views. Alternatively, they may create meanings that turn their experience into a positive one, for example reflecting on the lessons that their experiences have taught them. They may feel that they have grown in wisdom or sensitivity or somehow become a 'better person' because of their circumstances.

Goffman's theory was developed during the early 1960s and reflects the social values and norms of that time. In contemporary society, it seems that a wider range of options is available to stigmatized groups. These include activism and campaigning to transform social attitudes and end discrimination. Examples of this can be seen in the disability rights movement and in the responses of the gay community, which have challenged negative social attitudes and found collective sources of solidarity.

Interactionist perspectives may be limited, in that they focus attention on the victim rather than examining the reasons for discrimination against particular groups. Nevertheless, they do draw attention to the stress that can accompany stigmatizing experiences, including illness and disability. They also highlight the need for coping strategies in response to the challenges to identity that these experiences may represent. As a consequence, interactionist perspectives have had a strong influence on research in medical sociology, much of which is focused on interactions between professionals and patients, and the experiences of people with particular conditions.

Questions of identity and illness are increasingly important in sociological research. Increasing life expectancy and technological advances mean that an increasing number of people are surviving for a longer period, and are more likely to be living with a chronic condition. This in turn means that an increasing number of people may find that they cannot sustain the values of independence and achievement that they assumed would carry them through adult life. The onset of chronic illness may represent a profound threat to personal identity. Bury (1982, 2001) illustrates this through the notion of illness as a *biographical disruption*, disrupting the patterns of daily life and social relationships, and generating a range of tasks. These tasks may relate to practical needs such as symptom management, but also to maintaining a sense of identity and preserving one's cultural competence in the eyes of others.

The intimate relationship between illness and identity has led to a rethink of the body from a sociological standpoint. Evidently, our bodies form the physical locus within which we experience and interpret health and illness.

Sociology has traditionally been highly 'disembodied', seeing the body as a matter of intellectual concern for biology and biomedicine. At the same time, sociologists have also questioned whether there are any essential physical experiences that are not mediated by culture and social context. In this way, the body had almost become invisible within sociological discourse. Authors such as Frank (1991) have argued for a renewed focus on the body, drawing upon the concept of embodiment, or the lived experience of our bodies in the world. A concern with embodiment provides a bridge between structure and agency, between macro-social processes and micro-personal experience. For example, tiredness is clearly a physical sensation of the body. From an embodied perspective, tiredness can be seen to encompass both a temporary exit from a productive, socially structured role and a loss of willpower. While an episode of tiredness will hold specific personal biographical meaning, it is also the bodily expression of patterned and value-laden ideas current in society.

Chapter 1 focuses on the physical concepts of health and disease.

Recent interest in the body is unsurprising in the context of modern consumer society. What we eat, what we wear and whether we are fit are all cultural markers, locating our identities. Frost (2003) suggests that the emphasis on individualistic models of health, for example the focus on personal responsibility for a healthy diet and fitness, has made the body the object of self-discipline. While this disciplining of the body may seem to imply a continuous round of self-denial in order to restrain any appetite for excess, it also opens the way for more tangible forms of consumption. The plethora of health and fitness magazines, slimming aids, sportswear and membership of gym clubs are but a few of the goods and services available to assist the quest for a managed body. Giddens (1991) argues that the pace of social change is such that people lack traditional reference points for identity within a fragmented and shifting social order. Instead, the self, or body, becomes a project, the seat of identity and a source of stability, albeit in an ever-changing and unfinished form.

Social constructionist perspectives and beyond

So far we have explored perspectives that examine the impact of social processes on the meanings of phenomena such as health and illness. These perspectives suggest that health and illness cannot be understood as fixed and unchanging entities. Instead, the meanings attributed to health and illness may differ at different historical periods and between different cultures. Within Western medicine, for example, homosexuality is no longer perceived as a disease. At the same time, new diseases and syndromes, such as 'attention deficit disorder' and 'premenstrual syndrome', describe behaviour that would in previous decades have been understood in very different terms.

Sociologists have also explored the formation of ideas about health and illness, examining the role of different groups, such as professionals and scientists, in the production of discourses of health. These debates have implications for the study of lay perspectives, which may differ significantly from scientific and professional views. There has been a general shift away from approaches assuming that medical science is 'right' and other views 'wrong'. Instead, there is a growing recognition that professional and lay views are both socially constructed, meaning that they cannot easily be categorized as 'right' or 'wrong' because they both arise from the experiences and circumstances of different groups within society.

The writings of Foucault (1976, 1979a) have been studied by sociologists seeking to explore further this process of the social construction of medical knowledge. The notion of the 'gaze' has been used to explain the processes that enabled a medical understanding of the body to emerge during the eighteenth century. This perspective draws attention to the surveillance and control that are exercised through medical practices. Today, the bodies of healthy as well as sick people are seen as being increasingly under surveillance. Medical practice is no longer concerned with just the treatment of disease but has been extended into new areas such as prevention and health promotion. These practices, while apparently beneficial, may have negative consequences. While apparently exercising care, health professionals may also be exercising power and control.

Sociologists of late modernity have focused on the way in which social control and surveillance have spread throughout society. Beck (1992) first coined the term 'risk society' to describe the expansion of risk within modernized societies. Modernization is linked to particular risks as temporal and spatial limits no longer apply. Global climate change is a good example of the increased risks associated with modernization.

One response to the perception of increased risk is to try to control and avoid exposure to risk (Jones, 2004). The most effective strategy is to persuade people to practise risk avoidance voluntarily rather than try to enforce it. Foucault (1979b) used the notion of the gaze and surveillance to describe the modern trend for self-regulation and control. This has its origins in the panopticon, Jeremy Bentham's late eighteenth-century prison design incorporating a central watchtower. The argument was that prisoners would not know if they were being watched, so would develop self-discipline. Today, modern society is increasingly under surveillance, with computerization opening up new avenues for monitoring and regulation. The increased use of CCTV is often cited as symptomatic of modern life. Increasingly, people have been persuaded that surveillance is a good thing, to the extent that they voluntarily take on the task and self-surveillance and self-monitoring in all aspects of life are rapidly escalating. Examples of this include routine monitoring of blood pressure at home, self-monitoring regarding alcohol intake, and parental use of mobile telephones to monitor the activities of children and young people. There is also general compliance with the increased levels of surveillance, evident in everything from the use of pin codes on bank cards to the routine recording and playing back of phone calls to businesses.

What examples of surveillance in professional life can you think of? Do you think this degree of surveillance is positive or negative? Why?

This degree of monitoring and self-regulation is often linked to the 'risk-averse' nature of society. It has been argued that this process is unhelpful and leads to negative outcomes. For example, risk aversion has been linked to professional defensiveness, as the fear of litigation in cases of negligence or unprofessional practice spurs greater professional closure. The result of this process is arguably greater social distance between practitioners and patients. It also leads to more resources being directed towards providing evidence of actions taken and consent procedures (the audit paper trail), at the expense of direct action undertaken to care for clients and patients.

CASE STUDY Food and health

There seems little doubt that diets and eating practices in the West are undergoing major transformations. Caraher and Coveney (2004, p. 592) suggest that 'we in the developed world can expect to eat a different and better diet than did our predecessors 100 years ago'. Dietary improvements have meant that we live longer, are taller, and rarely suffer diseases of deprivation.

Furthermore, consumers live in an environment that appears to offer unprecedented food security. The major retail stores offer thousands of food lines, reliably sourced on the global market and with little seasonal variation. For those lacking the time or inclination, there is an expanding market for eating out and eating in with ready-prepared foods. Average households have greater disposable incomes, and food expenditure in real terms accounts for a smaller slice of personal spending than it did two decades ago (Hitchman et al., 2002). Given these conditions, this section examines

how two perplexing issues have attracted sociological enquiry: why diet-related health inequalities continue to exist in the West; and what accounts for the high level of social anxieties surrounding food and eating practices.

These two areas can be used to illustrate different traditions of sociological thought:

1. The *social causation* perspective is drawn upon to understand food insecurity and social inequalities in diets. This approach is similar to the materialist/structural approach developed by the authors of the Black Report (Townsend and Davidson, 1982) and is adopted by researchers working within a Marxist or political economy perspective.
2. The *social constructionist* perspective is adopted to explore perceptions of risk, trust and anxiety in relation to food. This approach is concerned to explore the conditions under which ideas and meanings are generated. Social

constructionism therefore builds upon the interactionist tradition in sociology, and questions commonplace assumptions about the relationship between language and objective knowledge.

Social causation of food insecurity and dietary inequalities

Research from a variety of Western nations indicates that there are clear socioeconomic differences in diets and diet-related ill health. Lower income groups tend to eat less fruit, vegetables and food rich in dietary fibre, have a lower intake of foods containing antioxidants, some minerals and vitamins, and have a higher salt intake. As part of a general social trend, lower income groups increasingly consume processed and energy-dense foods (high-sugar, high-fat foods). These dietary patterns are strongly linked to higher rates of obesity, increased risk of coronary heart disease and circulatory problems, some diet-related cancers and dental decay (Acheson, 1998; Shaw et al., 2000; Cummins and Macintyre, 2006; Kamphuis et al., 2006). Social causation perspectives have sought to explain these patterns with reference to a variety of societal processes. These draw together the changing character of global and local economic systems and the material conditions of people on low incomes in industrialized countries.

Lang and colleagues (Lang and Heasman, 2004; Lang, 2005) hold that global transformations of the food industry account, in part, for contemporary inequalities in diets. Lang (2005) argues that there has been a revolution within the food system in all aspects, from production, processing, distribution and retail through to consumption. Within this system, leading retailers assume a pivotal position. For example, in 15 EU states, 3.2 million farmers feed 250 million consumers, but this supply and demand is funnelled through only 600 supermarket chains with 110 key buying desks (Lang, 2005).

Retailers, along with a small number of leading brand processing corporations, now exercise unprecedented leverage over consumer tastes. Investment in marketing and promotion by these organizations considerably outstrips the health promotion budgets of national governments (Lang, 2005). The two leading commercial ad-spend budgets of the world each amount to £837 million a year, which is vastly more than the entire health education budgets of governments (Lang, 2005).

According to Lang, weak government controls have allowed a largely unfettered promotion of highly processed and energy-dense foods. These changes have had greater impact on the diets of lower income groups. In part this is simply because high-fat, high-sugar and high-salt foods have been marketed at a lower cost than 'healthier alternatives'. But the effects are amplified for poorer groups because of links with other social processes. Since the 1970s, the retail geography of industrialized countries has changed dramatically. The decline of high-street and neighbourhood food retailers has been mirrored by an expansion of large, often out-of-town, supermarkets. These changes have left many low-income communities with a dearth of retail outlets (Caraher and Coveney, 2004). Given that low-income households are less likely to own a car, these groups may encounter additional difficulties accessing supermarkets with poor public transport links.

The decline of local retail outlets has given rise to the claim that many low-income neighbourhoods in industrialized countries have become 'food deserts'. Cummins and Macintyre's (2006) review of food availability and pricing studies found that in the US and Canada, 'healthier' foods were less available and more costly in low-income neighbourhoods. In the US, income inequalities also appear to coincide with racial divisions. One study found that supermarkets were on average 1.15 miles further away for residents in black compared to white neighbourhoods (Cummins and Macintyre, 2002, p. 100). However, these associations are less clear in other industrialized countries such as the UK, Australia and the Netherlands. For example, a Glasgow study found that 57 foods representing 'a modest but adequate diet' were slightly more available in areas of deprivation and that prices varied little by area. However, it was also notable that high-fat and high-sugar foods were cheaper in poorer areas of the city (Cummins and Macintyre, 2002).

While many low-income areas have seen a decline in retail grocery outlets, fast-food outlets appear to have become more prevalent and more accessible in comparison to affluent areas (Cummins and Macintyre, 2006). Fast food is becoming an increasingly important part of people's diets in industrialized countries (Millstone and Lang, 2003). This has dietary implications because these foods tend to be high in animal fats and are up to 65% more energy dense than the average diet. In England and Scotland, McDonald's restaurants are more likely to be located in more areas of social deprivation (Cummins et al., 2005). There is some evidence to suggest that these associations may explain the higher rates of obesity in these neighbourhoods.

Other studies emphasize how food accessibility is more than just a question of proximity to shops. Hitchman et al.'s London-based study found that people on low incomes in the same streets had very different levels of access and patterns of shopping. Older people's diets were particularly sensitive to local shop closures. Given the personal nature of local shops, their closure also represented the loss of a social resource, which in turn reduced their

everyday support networks. Street crime, vandalism and personal threats deterred older people from using public transport and shopping further afield. Dietary inequalities therefore connect to wider social issues. Hitchman et al. (2002, p. 9) argue that 'the geography of food poverty cannot simply be drawn on a map'.

Poor diets and food insecurity also have a relationship to gender dynamics within low-income households. While women have increasingly become active in the labour market, gender roles around domestic work have been slower to change. British Social Attitudes Surveys show that in 70% of households, women make the evening meal and continue to do the majority of routine shopping (Lupton, 2000).

The interviewees who took part in Hitchman et al.'s study (2002) often suggested that men were unskilled at shopping efficiently within a budget. Regular and often unsociable working hours for many working women on low incomes meant it was difficult to prepare and coordinate regular family meals. Participants also reported how these pressures combined with the demands of family members to meet individual taste preferences. Hitchman et al. (2002, p. 9) found that cooks (usually women) did not lack awareness of 'healthy diets' nor did they lack skills in food preparation, but rather that 'achieving a nutritious diet on a low income requires extraordinary levels of persistence, flexibility and awareness'. The social causation perspective has therefore sought to identify the sum of social influences that determine poor diets in industrialized countries.

Social constructionist perspectives on food, risk and insecurity

The second group of theoretical approaches has been concerned with the social meaning of diets and eating practices. Here we consider how this approach has been used to explore perceptions of diet-related choice and food anxieties.

Giddens (1991) has noted how, for many people in the West, diets involve a bewildering array of choices of what and where to buy, how to cook and how to consume. Increasingly, these choices are not informed by tradition but are perceived to be 'expressions of identity': eating has become one very visible aspect of personal decision-making. While these choices appear to present unparalleled possibilities for self-expression, Giddens and, in a similar vein, Beck (1992) argue that they also entail new forms of insecurity. For example, eating disorders among young people could be seen to have their origins in the profound opportunities and strains of contemporary life. According to Frost (2003), eating practices, especially for young women, have become intimately associated with creating an ideal body image and moral strength of character. Yet the very freedom to self-create the body – and by inference one's identity – carries a burden that propels some young people into dietary disorders and self-starvation.

Where established beliefs and practices are less salient, it also becomes less clear where we invest trust. For both Beck and Giddens, individuals under conditions of late modernity have become increasingly conscious of food hazards produced by the technologies of the era. Food scares associated with, for example, BSE, genetically modified (GM) foods and salmonella mean that everyday foods are associated with health threats. Given that many of these risks are not readily perceptible, our food decisions are reliant on expert – and often medical – advice. Lupton (2005, p. 449) suggests that food advice has become 'deeply medicalized in its association with health, illness and disease'. However, this advice is often difficult to interpret or inconsistent in nature. For example, it may be difficult to make dietary choices based

upon complex information about 'good' and 'bad' fats, or the glycaemic index (GI) of carbohydrates.

Our management of food hazards thus involves the individual in complex assessments and the balancing of diverse sets of 'risks' and benefits. We have to eat, but it can feel like a risky business. Clear decisions cannot readily be reached simply through the application of more knowledge or greater scientific awareness. Under these circumstances, social constructionists have sought to explore how people interpret food risks as part of everyday experience. Green et al.'s study (2003) found that overt expressions of insecurity were exceptions rather than the norm. Everyday decision-making around food safety was presented as a routine endeavour – aided by a number of 'short cuts' or 'rules of thumb'. Similarly, Shaw's study (2004) of microbiological safety and BSE found that participants were able to locate their decisions in different contexts and, in so doing, brought competing logic to bear on risk decisions.

Discourse that surrounds food uncertainties can also be seen to serve ideological functions. Green et al. (2003) suggest that the language of safety was recurrently used by white study participants to explain reasons for avoiding 'ethnic (that is, Indian and Chinese) restaurants'. The researchers suggest that this 'risk speak' provided an apparently neutral framework for expressing disparaging and often racialized judgements of other social groups.

Food risk discourses are therefore often based in what Bourdieu (1984) described as 'processes of distinction'. That is, they act as vehicles for marking out and making judgements of group identity. Thus Green et al. (2003, p. 50) found that older age groups expressed active unconcern about risks:

For older consumers, demonstrating their resistance to risk ... contributed to their rhetorical construction of 'modernity' as overly concerned and anxious about risk, and themselves as 'survivors' who were to some extent invulnerable to risk.

Although a lot of social constructionist work has concentrated on individual perceptions of food risks, more recent studies have explored interpersonal negotiations and, notably, family dynamics of dietary behaviours. Drawing on parental perceptions and understandings of 'normal weight' and 'overweight' young teenagers living in poorer socioeconomic circumstances, Backett-Milburn and colleagues (2006) explored the negotiations between parents and their children and notably argue that parents lacked a discourse to talk about weight and overweight among their teenage children. Dietary issues were 'a fairly low priority in the hierarchy of health-relevant and other risks facing their teenagers' (Backett-Milburn et al., 2006, p. 624).

Backett-Milburn et al.'s study (2006) illustrates how social constructionist approaches can complement social causation theory. For many people on low incomes, weight-related issues have to be understood in the context of other risks that are perceived to be of greater importance.

Conclusion

This case study has provided a discussion of the ways in which sociological perspectives might apply to the study of food and diets. Although there are considerable differences, social causation and social constructionist approaches share some concerns common to most sociological enquiry. Both have an interest in the socially patterned nature of food consumption and the socially embedded character of individual choice. While it is commonplace to believe that dietary beliefs and practices are essentially personal matters, sociological accounts have sought to locate them in a wider social context.

Summary

- Sociology – the study of human social life – has addressed many issues concerning people's experiences of health and illness, and the organization of healthcare services

- A key theme in this area is the social patterning of health, ill health and premature death. Groups with less access to money and other material resources experience poorer health and a higher premature death rate. Societies with more egalitarian structures enjoy better health than more unequal societies

- There are several different sociological perspectives, ranging from those such as functionalism, which emphasizes the value of social consensus and continuity, to those such as Marxism and political economy, which emphasize the sources of social conflict and change

- Sociologists have explored the links between medical power and other social stratification variables such as gender and ethnicity

- Sociology involves both the critical examination of data (such as mortality rates) and the testing of theoretical frameworks and propositions

Questions for further discussion

1. Analyse the emergence of HIV/AIDS as a health issue using both social causation and social constructionist approaches.

2. Think back to recent encounters with the medical establishment. Critically analyse these encounters using sociological concepts.

3. To what extent are health-related behaviours socially determined? Illustrate your answer with reference to a specific behaviour, for example alcohol consumption or exercise patterns.

Further reading

The sociology of health and illness is an extensive subject and this brief introduction can only indicate some of the central concerns, trends and debates in sociological research. The following list includes general texts on the sociology of health and illness as well as writings on specific topics that are well worth the effort of reading.

Annandale, E. (1998) *The Sociology of Health and Medicine*. Cambridge: Polity Press.
This text provides an excellent account of the relationship between critical social theory and medical sociology. It is quite wide ranging and has particularly useful sections on health status, social stratification and inequalities in health.

Bartley, M. (2004) *Health Inequality: An Introduction to Theories, Concepts and Methods*. Cambridge: Polity Press.
This book is a useful resource for understanding key theories of health inequality and the methods employed by researchers in this field of study. It seeks to bridge some of the disciplinary divides that lie between sociology, psychology and biology – and show how all can contribute to the study of health inequalities.

Blaxter, M. (2004) *Health*. Cambridge: Polity Press.
This book discusses how health is defined, constructed, experienced and acted out, drawing upon a range of empirical data and theoretical approaches for Western countries.

Daykin, N. and Doyal, L. (eds) (1999) *Work and Health: Critical Perspectives*. Basingstoke: Macmillan – now Palgrave Macmillan.
This text is an edited collection of articles that set out to redefine the traditional boundaries of occupational health and work. It shows how a sociological approach can broaden commonsense understandings of what we mean by 'work' and 'health'.

Doyal, L. (1995) What Makes Women Sick? Gender and the Political Economy of Women's Health. Basingstoke: Macmillan – now Palgrave Macmillan.
This book is a key text devoted to sociology and gender issues. Doyal explores the structuralist and materialist perspectives on gender inequalities in society, with a particular focus on why women report more ill health than men, despite their greater longevity.

Frank, A. (1995) *The Wounded Storyteller: Body, Illness and Ethics*. Chicago: University of Chicago Press.
Frank suggests that ill people are more than victims of disease or patients of medicine; they are wounded storytellers. This book uses a biographical approach to show how people tell stories to make sense of their suffering and argues that, when they turn their diseases into stories, they find healing.

Gabe J., Bury M. and Elston M.A (2004) *Key Concepts in Medical Sociology*. London: Sage.
This is an excellent and authoritative resource that provides a good reference point for central concepts. Each section provides links to key literature.

Gabe, J., Kelleher, D. and Williams, G. (eds) (2006) *Challenging Medicine* (2nd edn). London: Routledge.
This text is an appraisal of the current changes to the health service and their effects upon the status and practice of health professionals. It draws upon debates around the expertise of medical professionals in the context of a rapidly changing social environment.

Lupton, D. and Tulloch, J. (2003) *Risk and Everyday Life*. London: Sage.
The study of risk has become closely connected to health studies. This book explores how people respond to, experience and think about risk as part of their everyday lives. It shows how sociological theory can provide a bridge between private and wider public concerns.

Nettleton, S. (2006) *The Sociology of Health and Illness* (2nd edn) Cambridge: Polity Press.
This is an accessible text that provides a wide ranging overview of the field. As a solid introduction Nettleton's book gives a clear explanation of concepts, theories and debates. Good use is made of contemporary research evidence.

Finally, it is important to remember that sociological research often appears in journals before it is described in books. Relevant journals include the *Sociology of Health and Illness, Social Science and Medicine, Women's Studies International Forum, Health Promotion International* and the *International Journal of Health Services*.

References

Acheson, D. (1998) *Independent Inquiry into Inequalities in Health Report*. London: Stationery Office.

Adler, N., Boyce, T., Chesney, M. et al. (1994) 'Socioeconomic status and health: the challenge of the gradient'. *American Psychologist* **49**: 15–24.

Ahmad, W.I.U. (1993) Making black people sick: 'race', ideology and health research, in W.I.U. Ahmad (ed.) *'Race' and Health in Contemporary Britain*. Milton Keynes: Open University Press, pp. 11–13.

Annandale, E. and Hunt, K. (1990) 'Masculinity, femininity and sex: an exploration of their relative contribution to explaining gender differences in health'. *Sociology of Health and Illness* **12**: 24–46.

Arber, S. (1998) Health, ageing and older women, in L. Doyal (ed.) *Women and Health Services: An Agenda for Change*. Buckingham: Open University Press, pp. 54–68.

Arber, S., and Khlat, M. (2002) 'Introduction to social and economic patterning of women's health in a changing world'. *Social Science and Medicine* **54**: 643–7.

Arber, S. and Thomas, H. (2001) From women's health to gender analysis of health, in W.C. Cockerham (ed.) *The Blackwell Companion to Medical Sociology*. Oxford: Blackwell, pp. 94–113.

Armstrong, D. (1995) 'The rise of surveillance medicine'. *Sociology of Health and Illness* **17**(3): 39–404.

Backett-Milburn, K., Wills, W., Gregory, S. and Lawton, J. (2006) 'Making sense of eating, weight and risk in the early teenage years: views and concerns of parents in poorer socioeconomic circumstances'. *Social Science and Medicine* **63**(3): 624–35.

Bartley, M. (2004) *Health Inequality: An Introduction to Theories, Concepts and Methods*. Cambridge: Polity Press.

Bartley, M., Blane, D. and Davey Smith, G. (1998) 'Introduction: beyond the Black Report'. *Sociology of Health and Illness* 20(5): 563–77.

Bartley, M., Sacker, A. and Clarke, P. (2004) 'Employment status, employment conditions, and limiting illness: prospective evidence from the British household panel survey 1991–2001'. *Journal of Epidemiology and Community Health* 58(6): 501–6.

Baum, F. (1999) 'Social capital: is it good for your health? Issues for a public health agenda'. *Journal of Epidemiology and Community Health* 53: 195–6.

Beck, U. (1992) *Risk Society: Towards a New Modernity*. London: Sage.

Bhui, K., Stansfeld, S., Mckenzie, K. et al. (2005) 'Racial/ethnic discrimination and common mental disorders among workers: findings from the empiric study of ethnic minority groups in the United Kingdom'. *American Journal of Public Health* 95: 496–501.

Bloomfield, K., Grittner, U., Kramer, S. and Gmel, G. (2006) 'Social inequalities in alcohol consumption and alcohol-related problems in the study countries of the EU concerted action "gender, culture and alcohol problems: a multinational study"'. *Alcohol and Alcoholism* 41: I26–36, Suppl. 1.

Bourdieu, P. (1984) *Distinction: A Social Critique of the Judgement of Taste*. London: Routledge.

Bury, M. (1982) 'Chronic illness as biographical disruption'. *Sociology of Health and Illness* 4(2): 167–82.

Bury, M. (2001) 'Illness narratives: fact or fiction?' *Sociology of Health and Illness* 23(3): 263–85.

Cameron, E. and Bernades, J. (1998) 'Gender and disadvantage in health: men's health for a change'. *Sociology of Health and Illness* 20(5): 673–93.

Caraher, M. and Coveney, J. (2004) 'Public health nutrition and food policy'. *Public Health Nutrition* 7(5): 591–8.

Courtenay, W.H. (2000) 'Constructions of masculinity and their influence on men's well-being: a theory of gender and health'. *Social Science and Medicine* 50: 1385–401.

Crossley, M. (1998) '"Sick role" or "empowerment": the ambiguities of life with an HIV positive diagnosis'. *Sociology of Health and Illness* 20(4): 507–31.

Cummins, S. and Macintyre, S. (2002) 'A systematic study of an urban landscape: the price and availability of food in Greater Glasgow'. *Urban Studies* 39(21): 195–7.

Cummins, S. and Macintyre, S. (2006) 'Food environments and obesity: neighbourhood or nation?' *International Journal of Epidemiology* 35: 100–4.

Cummins, S., McKay, L. and MacIntyre, S. (2005) 'McDonald's restaurants and neighborhood deprivation in Scotland and England'. *American Journal of Preventive Medicine* 29(4): 308–10.

Davey Smith, G. (2003) *Health Inequalities: Lifecourse Approaches*. Policy Press, Cambridge.

Davies, C. (1995) *Gender and the Professional Predicament in Nursing*. Buckingham: Open University Press.

Daykin, N. and Clarke, B. (2000) '"They'll still get the bodily care". Discourses of care and relationships between nurses and healthcare assistants in the NHS'. *Sociology of Health and Illness* 22(3): 349–63.

DeVisser, R. and Smith, J.A. (2006) 'Mister in-between: a case study of masculine identity and health-related behaviour'. *Journal of Health Psychology* 11: 685–95.

DoH (Department of Health) (1992) *The Health of the Nation*. London: HMSO.

DoH (Department of Health) (1999) *Saving Lives: Our Healthier Nation*. London: Stationery Office.

Doyal, L. (1995) *What Makes Women Sick? Gender and the Political Economy of Health*. Basingstoke: Macmillan – now Palgrave Macmillan.

Doyal, L. (ed.) (1998) *Women and Health Services: An Agenda for Change*. Buckingham: Open University Press.

Doyal, L. (2001) 'Sex, gender and health: the need for a new approach'. *British Medical Journal* 323: 1061–3.

Drever, F. and Bunting, J. (1997) Patterns and trends in male mortality, in F. Drever and M. Whitehead (eds) *Health Inequalities*. Decennial Supplement. Office for National Statistics, Series DS No. 15. London: Stationery Office, pp. 95–107.

Drever, F. and Whitehead, M. (eds) (1997) *Health Inequalities*. Decennial Supplement. Office for National Statistics, Series DS No. 15. London: Stationery Office.

Dundas, R., Morgan, M., Redfern, J. et al. (2001) 'Ethnic differences in behavioural risk factors for stroke: implications for health promotion'. *Ethnicity and Health* 6(2): 95–103.

Durkheim, E. (1952) *Suicide*. London: Routledge & Kegan Paul.

Everingham, C. (2001) 'Reconstituting community: social justice, social order and the politics of community'. *Australian Journal of Social Issues* 36(2): 105–22.

Foster, P. (1995) *Women and the Healthcare Industry: An Unhealthy Relationship?* Buckingham: Open University Press.

Foucault, M. (1976) *The Birth of the Clinic: An Archaelogy of Medical Perception*. London: Tavistock.

Foucault, M. (1979a) *The History of Sexuality*, vol. 1. London: Allen Lane.

Foucault, M. (1979b) *Discipline and Punish: The Birth of the Prison*. New York: Vintage.

Frank, A.W. (1991) For a sociology of the body: an analytical review, in M. Featherstone, M. Hepworth and B.S. Turner (eds) *The Body: Social Process, Cultural Theory*. London: Sage.

Frank, R. (2001) 'A reconceptualization of the role of biology in contributing to race/ethnic disparities in health outcomes'. *Population Research and Policy Review* 20: 441–55.

Freidson, E. (1970) *Professional Dominance*. New York: Atherton Press.

Frost, L. (2003) 'Doing bodies differently? Gender, youth, appearance and damage'. *Journal of Youth Studies* 6(1): 55–70.

Giddens, A. (1991) *Modernity and Self-identity: A Study of Comparative Sociology*. London: Polity Press.

Goffman, E. (1963) *Stigma*. London: Penguin.

Gough, B. and Conner, M.T. (2006) 'Barriers to healthy eating amongst men: a qualitative analysis'. *Social Science and Medicine* 62: 387–95.

Graham, H. (1987) 'Women's smoking and family health'. *Social Science and Medicine* 25(1): 47–56.

Graham, H. (1998) Health at risk: poverty and national health strategies, in L. Doyal (ed.) *Women and Health Services: An Agenda for Change*. Buckingham: Open University Press, pp. 22–38.

Green, J., Draper, A. and Dowler, E. (2003) 'Short cuts to safety: risk and "rules of thumb" in accounts of food choice'. *Health, Risk & Society* 5(1): 33–52.

Harding, S. and Rosato, M. (1999) 'Cancer incidence among first generation Scottish, Irish, West Indian and South Asian migrants living in England and Wales'. *Ethnicity and Health* 4(1–2): 83–92.

Healthcare Commission (2006) *The State of Healthcare 2006*. London: Commission for Healthcare Audit and Inspection.

Hitchman, C., Christie, I., Harrison, M. and Lang, T. (2002) *Inconvenience Food: the Struggle to Eat Well on a Low Income*. London: Demos.

Illich, I. (1977) *The Limits to Medicine*. Harmondsworth: Penguin.

Illsley, R. (1986) 'Occupational class, selection and the production of inequalities in health'. *Quarterly Journal of Social Affairs* 2(2): 151–65.

Johnson, T. (1993) Expertise and the state, in M. Gane and T. Johnson (eds) *Foucault's New Domains*. London: Routledge.

Johnson, T. (1995) Governmentality and the institutionalisation of expertise, in T. Johnson, G. Larkin and M. Saks (eds) *Professions and the State in Europe*. London: Routledge.

Jones, M. (2004) 'Anxiety and containment in the risk society: theorising young people's drugs policy'. *International Journal of Drug Policy* 15: 367–76.

Kamphuis, C., Giskes, K., de Bruijn, G. et al. (2006) 'Environmental determinants of fruit and vegetable consumption among adults: a systematic review'. *British Journal of Nutrition* 96(4): 620–35.

Kawachi, I., Kennedy, B.P., Lochner, K. et al. (1997) 'Social capital, income inequality, and mortality'. *American Journal of Public Health* 87: 1491–9.

Kunst, A.E., Feikje, G., Mackenbach, J.P. et al. (1998) 'Mortality by occupational class among men 30–64 years in 11 European countries'. *Social Science and Medicine* 46(11): 1459–76.

Lang, T. (2005) 'Food control or food democracy? Re-engaging nutrition with society and the environment'. *Public Health Nutrition* 8(1): 730–7.

Lang, T. and Heasman, M. (2004) *Food Wars: The Global Battle for Mouths, Minds and Markets*. London: Earthscan.

Lantz, P., Lynch, J., House, J. et al. (2001) 'Socio-economic disparities in health change in a longitudinal study of US adults: the role of health-risk behaviours'. *Social Science and Medicine* **53**(1): 29–40.

Lawlor, D.A., Ebrahim, S. and Davey Smith, G. (2001) 'Sex matters: secular and geographical trends in sex differences in coronary heart disease mortality'. *British Medical Journal* **323**: 541–5.

Lloyd, L. (1999) The wellbeing of carers: an occupational health concert, in N. Daykin and L. Doyal (eds) *Health and Work: Critical Perspectives*. Basingstoke: Macmillan – now Palgrave Macmillan, pp. 54–70.

Lupton, D. (1995) *The Imperative of Health: Public Health and the Regulated Body*. London: Sage.

Lupton, D. (2000) Food, risk and subjectivity, in S. Williams, J. Gabe, and M. Calnan (eds) *Health, Medicine and Society: Key Theories, Future Agendas*. London: Routledge, pp. 425–35.

Lupton, D. (2005) 'Lay discourses and beliefs related to food risks: an Australian perspective'. *Sociology of Health and Illness* **27**(4): 448–67.

Lynch, J., Due, P., Muntaner, C. and Davey Smith, G. (2000) 'Social capital: is it a good investment strategy for public health?' *Journal of Epidemiology and Community Health* **54**: 404–8.

Mackenbach, J.P., Kunst, A.E., Cavelaars, A.E. et al. (1997) Socioeconomic inequalities in morbidity and mortality in Western Europe. *Lancet* **349**: 1655–9.

Marmot, M. (2004) *Status Syndrome: How your Social Standing Directly Affects your Health and your Life Expectancy*. London: Bloomsbury.

Manly, J.J. (2006) 'Deconstructing race and ethnicity: implications for measurement of health outcomes'. *Medical Care* **44**: S10–S16.

McTaggart, L. (1996) *What Doctors Don't Tell You: The Truth about the Dangers of Modern Medicine*. London: Thorsons.

Mead, G.H. (1934) *Mind, Self and Society from the Standpoint of Social Behaviourism*. Chicago: Chicago University Press.

Millstone, E. and Lang, T. (2003) *The Atlas of Food: Who Eats What, Where and Why*. Brighton: Earthscan.

Moss, N.E. (2002) 'Gender equity and socioeconomic inequality: a framework for the patterning of women's health'. *Social Science and Medicine* **54**: 649–61.

Navarro, V. (1979) *Medicine under Capitalism*. London: Croom Helm.

Navarro, V. (2004) 'The politics of health inequalities research in the United States'. *International Journal of Health Services* **34**(1): 87–99.

Nazroo, J.Y. (1997) *The Health of Britain's Ethnic Minorities: Findings from a National Survey*. London: Policy Studies Institute.

Nazroo, J.Y. (2001) *Ethnicity, Class and Health*. London: Policy Studies Institute.

ONS (2007) *National Statistics Online*, www.statistics.gov.uk.

Parsons, T. (1951) *The Social System*. London: Routledge & Kegan Paul.

Parsons, T. (1975) 'The sick role and the role of the physician reconsidered'. *Millbank Memorial Fund Quarterly* summer: 257–78.

Payne, S. (1998) Hit and miss: the success and failure of psychiatric services for women, in L. Doyal (ed.) *Women and Health Services: An Agenda for Change*. Buckingham: Open University Press, pp. 83–99.

Porter, S. (1992) 'The poverty of professionalisation: a critical analysis of strategies for the occuaptional advancement of nursing'. *Journal of Advanced Nursing* 17: 720–6.

Porter, S. (1999) *Social Theory and Nursing Practice*. Basingstoke: Macmillan – now Palgrave Macmillan.

Portes, A. (1998) 'Social capital: its origins and applications in modern sociology'. *Annual Review of Sociology* 24: 1–24.

Putnam, R.D. (1995) 'Bowling alone: America's declining social capital. *Journal of Democracy* 6(1): 65–78.

Roberts, I. and Power, C. (1996) 'Does the decline in child injury mortality vary by social class? A comparison of class specific mortality in 1981 and 1991'. *British Medical Journal* 313(7060): 784–6.

Robertson, S. (2006) '"Not living life in too much of an excess": lay men understanding health and well-being'. *Health* 10: 175–89.

Shaw, A. (2004) 'Discourses of risk in lay accounts of microbiological safety and BSE: a qualitative interview study'. *Health, Risk & Society* 6(2): 151–71.

Shaw, A., McMunn, A. and Field, J. (eds) (2000) *The Scottish Health Survey 1998*. London: Stationery Office.

Shaw-Taylor, Y. (2002) 'Culturally and linguistically appropriate healthcare for racial or ethnic minorities: analysis of the US Office of Minority Health's recommended standards'. *Health Policy* 62: 211–21.

Stacey, M. (1988) *The Sociology of Health and Healing*. London: Unwin Hyman.

Thomson, R. and Holland, J. (1994) Young women and safer (hetero) sex: context, constraints and strategies, in S. Wilkinson and C. Kitzinger (eds) *Women and Health: Feminist Perspectives*. London: Taylor & Francis, pp. 13–32.

Townsend, P. and Davidson, N. (1982) *Inequalities in Health: The Black Report*. London: Penguin.

Türmen, T. (2003) 'Gender and HIV/AIDS'. *International Journal of Gynecology and Obstetrics* 82(3): 411–18.

Van Rossum, C., Shipley, M., Van de Mheen, H. et al. (2000) 'Employment grade differences in cause specific mortality. A 25 year follow up of civil servants from the first Whitehall study'. *Journal of Epidemiology and Community Health* 54: 178–84.

Weich, S., Nazroo, J., Sproston, K. et al. (2004) 'Common mental disorders and ethnicity in England: the empiric study'. *Psychological Medicine* 34: 1543–51.

WHO (World Health Organization) (2007) Mortality Statistics, www.who.int/whosis/whostat2007_1mortality.pdf.

Wicks, D. (1998) *Doctors and Nurses at Work: Rethinking Professional Boundaries*. Buckingham: Open University Press.

Wilkinson, R.G. (1996) *Unhealthy Societies: The Afflictions of Inequality*. London: Routledge.

Williams, G.H. (2003) 'The determinants of health: structure, context and agency'. *Sociology of Health and Illness* 25: 131–54.

Wilsnack, R.W., Kristianson, A.F., Wilsnack, S.C., and Crosby, R.D. (2006) 'Are US women drinking less (or more)? Historical and aging trends, 1981–2001'. *Journal of Studies on Alcohol* 67(3): 341–8.

Witz, A. (1992) *Professions and Patriarchy*. London: Routledge.

Zola, I. (1972) 'Medicine as an institution of social control'. *Sociological Review* 20(4): 487–504.

Health psychology

Outline of chapter

LEARNING OUTCOMES

This chapter will enable readers to:

- Understand and describe the basic principles of health psychology and how it differs from biomedicine

- Understand why the study of health behaviours is important

- Show an understanding of the role of health beliefs in predicting and potentially changing health behaviours, and how they relate to people's coping mechanisms when ill

- Illustrate the ways in which health professionals' beliefs may influence their interactions with patients

- Illustrate the role of psychology in the experience of illness, drawing upon theories of pain and pain management

Overview

Psychology focuses on what people believe and how they behave; health psychology explores how these beliefs and behaviours relate to health and illness. This chapter focuses on the beliefs that individuals have relating to health and illness and how these beliefs relate to their health behaviours and subsequently to their health status. This chapter is divided into three parts. The first part explores the contribution of psychology to studying health and illness, describing the background to psychology and highlighting the importance of beliefs concerning both health and illness on the part of both lay people and health professionals. Pain is used as an example of the role of psychology in the experience of illness. The second part describes the models that have been developed within health psychology, in particular focusing on the structured models of health beliefs and the self-regulatory model of illness behaviour. Finally, the case study on diet, eating habits and obesity explores in depth how psychological theories can be applied to a topical health issue.

Introduction

The roots of psychology date from the beginning of the twentieth century and the work of psychoanalysts such as Freud and Jung, as well as behaviourists such as Pavlov and Skinner. The psychoanalysts worked as therapists and developed theories based upon the patients whom they saw. In contrast, the behaviourists used strict experimental approaches and carried out laboratory studies, mostly on animals such as rats and pigeons. The two perspectives appear to be extremely different, but they were based upon the same fundamental questions that remain at the centre of modern-day psychology. Psychologists then and now ask:

- How do people think?
- What causes how people think?
- What changes how people think?
- How do people behave?
- What causes people's behaviour?
- What changes people's behaviour?

These questions form the basis of all the different branches of psychology from biological psychology, with its emphasis on brain chemicals and neurones, through social psychology and its emphasis on individuals and their social world, to cognitive psychology, with its focus on information-processing, problem-solving and language. Health psychology is a relatively new branch of psychology and draws upon the theories and research of its predecessors. Furthermore, although it asks similar questions, it applies these to the study of health and illness. In particular, health psychology asks:

- How do people think about their health and illness?

- How do people behave with regard to their health and illness?

- What impact do such beliefs and behaviours have upon their health and illness?

- What impact do health and illness have upon their beliefs and behaviours?

Health psychology places itself alongside other branches of psychology. However, as it is concerned with health and illness, it is also important to understand its relationship to biomedicine. The biomedical model of medicine was developed in the nineteenth century and emphasized that man was a part of nature and could therefore be studied in the same way that nature was studied. Health psychology has developed out of the biomedical model but differs in terms of the questions it asks and the answers it gives.

According to the biomedical model of medicine, disease either came from outside the body, invaded the body and caused physical changes within the body, or originated as internal involuntary physical changes. Such diseases may be caused by several factors, such as chemical imbalances, bacteria, viruses and genetic predisposition. Within the biomedical model, health and illness are seen as qualitatively different – you are either healthy or ill, there is no continuum between the two. Because illness is seen as arising from biological changes beyond their control, individuals are not seen as being responsible for their illness. The biomedical model seeks to address the manifestations of illness through surgery or drug treatments that aim to change the physical state of the body. According to the biomedical model of medicine, the mind and body function independently of each other, this perspective being comparable to a traditional dualistic model of the mind/body split.

CONNECTIONS

Chapter 1 discusses the biomedical model of health and illness in greater detail.

The contribution of psychology to health studies

During the twentieth century, the emergence of psychosomatic medicine, behavioural health, behavioural medicine and, most recently, health psychology has posed challenges for the biomedical model. Health psychology suggests that human beings should be seen as complex systems and that illness is caused by a multitude of interacting factors rather than a single causative factor. Health psychology claims that illness can result from a combination of biological (for example a virus), psychological (for example behaviours and beliefs) and social (for example employment) factors. This approach reflects the biopsychosocial model of health and illness (Engel, 1977, 1980; see Figure 5.1).

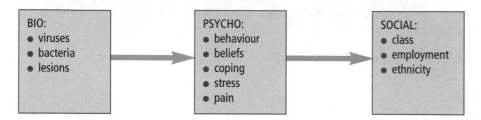

Figure 5.1 The biopsychosocial model of health and illness
Source: Engel, 1980

Health psychology therefore differs from the biomedical model in several important respects:

- Individuals may be held more responsible, through their behaviours and beliefs, for both the onset of illness and its management and cure

- Psychological factors are not solely a consequence of illness but may also contribute to its onset

- Treatment must be directed to the whole person rather than just his or her physical symptoms.

Health psychology emphasizes the role of psychological factors in the cause, progression and consequences of health and illness. Some of the key questions that health psychology tries to explore are:

- What is the role of psychology in the onset and development of illness?

- Should behaviour then be targeted for intervention?

- Can the study of beliefs predict unhealthy behaviour?

- Is it possible to change beliefs?

Health psychologists study the role of psychology in all areas of health and illness, including what people think about health and illness, the role of beliefs and behaviours in becoming ill, the experience of being ill in terms of adaptation to illness, contact with health professionals, coping with illness and compliance with a range of interventions, and the role of psychology in recovery from illness, quality of life and longevity. Health psychology therefore represents the study of the complex processes involved in the aetiology, impact and progression of illness.

Health beliefs and behaviours

It has been suggested that 50% of mortality from the 10 leading causes of death results from individual behaviour. This indicates that behaviour and lifestyle have a potentially major effect on longevity. In particular, Doll and Peto (1981) estimated the contribution of different factors as a cause of all cancer deaths and concluded that tobacco consumption accounts for 30% of all cancer deaths, alcohol for 3%, diet for 35% and reproductive and sexual behaviour for 7%. From this estimate, approximately 75% of all deaths from cancer can be attributed to behaviour. More specifically, lung cancer, which is the most common form, accounts for 36% of all cancer deaths in men and 15% in women in the UK. It has been calculated that 90% of all lung cancer mortality is attributable to cigarette smoking, which is also linked to other illnesses such as cancer of the bladder, pancreas, mouth, larynx and oesophagus, and coronary heart disease. The relationship between mortality and behaviour is also illustrated by bowel cancer, which accounts for 11% of all cancer deaths in men and 14% in women. Research suggests that bowel cancer is linked to behaviours such as a diet high in total fat, high in meat and low in fibre.

Therefore, **health behaviours** in terms of smoking, drinking alcohol, diet and exercise seem to be important in predicting the mortality and longevity of individuals. Assuming that individuals behave in ways that are in line with their beliefs, health psychologists have therefore attempted to understand and predict health-related behaviours by studying **health beliefs**. For example, the belief that smoking is dangerous should be associated with non-smoking or smoking cessation; the belief that cervical cancer is preventable should be associated with attendance for cervical screening; and the belief that exercise is beneficial should be associated with increased physical activity. Health psychologists thus study what people believe and whether this relates to how they behave. In addition, they explore whether beliefs can be changed and whether any shifts in beliefs predict subsequent changes in behaviour. In particular, individuals have beliefs about:

- *causality and control:* what has contributed to their ill health and whether these factors are controllable
- *risk:* to what extent they feel susceptible to certain diseases or conditions
- *confidence:* whether they feel that there are actions they can take that might affect the condition
- *beliefs about the illness:* what may have caused the illness, how long it might last and what they can do about it.

Beliefs about causality and control

Much work exploring people's beliefs relating to causality and control is based upon Heider's **attribution theory** (Heider, 1958). Attribution theory states that people want to understand what causes events because this makes the world seem more predictable and controllable. Since its original formulation, attribution theory has been developed, differentiations having been made between self-attributions (attributions about one's own behaviour) and other attributions (those made about the behaviour of others). In addition, the dimensions of **attribution** have been defined as follows:

- *internal versus external:* 'My failure to give up smoking is due to my lack of willpower' versus 'Others persuade me to carry on smoking'

- *stable versus unstable:* 'The cause of my failure to give up smoking will always be around' versus 'Next time I might succeed in resisting or avoiding peer pressure'

- *global versus specific:* 'The cause of my failure to give up smoking reflects my lack of willpower generally' versus 'I lacked willpower at this specific time'

- *controllable versus uncontrollable:* 'The cause of my failure to stop smoking was controllable by me' versus 'It was uncontrollable by me.'

Over recent years, attribution theory has been applied to the study of health and health-related behaviour. King (1982) examined the relationship between the attribution of an illness and attendance at a screening clinic for hypertension. The results demonstrated that if the hypertension was seen as external but controllable by the individual, he or she was more likely to attend the screening clinic – 'I am not responsible for my hypertension but I can control it.' Bradley et al. (1987) found a relationship between diabetic patients' beliefs about attributions for the responsibility and control of their condition and their choice of treatment. Patients who showed decreased personal control over their diabetes and attributed increased control to doctors were more likely to choose an insulin pump (which provides a continuous dose of insulin) rather than daily injections or other forms of treatment.

The internal versus external dimension of attribution theory has been specifically applied to health in terms of the concept of a health **locus of control**. People differ in terms of the extent to which they can make changes in their lives. Some people believe that what they do and what happens to them is up to them and regard events as personally controllable – an internal locus of control. Others, however, believe that events are largely not controlled by them – an external locus of control. Wallston and Wallston (1982) developed a measure of the health locus of control that evaluates whether individuals:

- regard their health as controllable by them, for example 'I am directly responsible for my health'

- believe that their health cannot be controlled by them but lies in the hands of fate, for example 'Whether or not I am well is a matter of luck'

- regard their health as under the control of powerful others, for example 'I can only do what my doctor tells me to do.'

> **?** How might locus of control be related to an individual's willingness to adopt a more healthy lifestyle?

People who generally have an external locus of control are less likely to take protective action regarding their health. Part of the work of health professionals may be to encourage them to take more control and set their own targets for change: merely expecting them to follow recommendations from a health professional is unlikely to be effective.

Beliefs about risk

People hold beliefs about their own susceptibility to a given problem and make judgements concerning the extent to which they are 'at risk'. Smokers, for example, may continue to smoke because although they understand that smoking is unhealthy, they do not consider themselves to be at risk of lung cancer. Likewise, a woman may not attend for a cervical smear because she believes that cervical cancer only happens to women who are not like her. People have ways of assessing their susceptibility to particular conditions, and this is not always a rational process. It has been suggested that individuals consistently estimate their risk of getting a health problem as less than that of others. Weinstein (1984) asked subjects to examine a list of health problems and to state 'compared to other people of your age and sex, are your chances of getting [the problem] greater than, about the same, or less than theirs?' The results of this study showed that most subjects believed that they were less likely than others to get the health problem. Weinstein called this phenomenon 'unrealistic optimism'; not everyone can be less likely to contract an illness. Weinstein (1987) suggested that people are likely to dismiss their risk and be unrealistically optimistic if:

- they have a lack of personal experience with the problem

- they believe that the problem is preventable by individual action

- they believe that if the problem has not yet appeared, it will not appear in the future

- the problem is infrequent.

Weinstein (1984) argued that individuals show selective focus by ignoring their own risk-increasing behaviour ('I may drink too much') and focusing primarily upon their risk-reducing behaviour ('but at least I don't drink and drive'). He also argues that individuals tend to ignore others' risk-decreasing behaviour ('My friends all drink sensibly but that's irrelevant'). Individuals may therefore be unrealistically optimistic if they focus on the times when they drink in moderation when assessing their own risk and ignore the times when they do not, in addition focusing on the times when others around them drink to excess and ignoring the times when they are more sensible.

Example 5.1

THE IMPACT OF BELIEFS AND BEHAVIOURS ON HEALTH – THE EXAMPLE OF STRESS

One of the reasons why stress has been studied so consistently is because of its potential effect on the health of the individual. Stress can affect health through either a behavioural or a physiological pathway. Most of the research into the stress–illness link has studied the physiological effects of stress. However, in support of the suggested behavioural pathway (Krantz et al., 1981) and in line with a psychological perspective, some recent research has examined the effect of stress on both specific health-related behaviours and more general behavioural change. Research, for example, suggests a link between stress and smoking behaviour in terms of smoking initiation, relapse and the amount smoked. Furthermore, not being able to smoke in a social situation can make the situation more stressful.

Contemporary definitions of stress regard the external environmental stress (for example problems at work) as a stressor, the response to the stressor (for example the feeling of tension) as stress or distress, and the concept of stress as something that involves biochemical, physiological, behavioural and psychological changes. Researchers have also differentiated between stress that is harmful and damaging (distress) and stress that is positive and beneficial (eustress). The most commonly used definition of stress is that of a transactional model stating that stress involves an interaction between the stressor and distress and therefore between people and their

environment (Lazarus and Launier, 1978). This approach to stress provides a role for an individual's psychological state and is a departure from more medical perspectives, with their focus on physiology.

Over recent years, theories of stress have emphasized forms of self-control as important in understanding stress. This is illustrated in theories of self-efficacy, hardiness and feelings of mastery. In 1987, Lazarus and Folkman suggested that self-efficacy was a powerful factor for mediating the stress response. Self-efficacy refers to individuals' feelings of confidence that they can perform a desired action. Research indicates that self-efficacy may have a role in mediating stress-induced immunosuppression and physiological changes such as those of blood pressure, heart rate and stress hormone levels. For example, the belief 'I am confident that I can succeed in this exam' may result in physiological changes that reduce the stress response. A belief in the ability to control one's behaviour may therefore relate to whether or not a potentially stressful event results in a stress response.

This shift towards emphasizing self-control is also illustrated by the concept of 'hardiness' (Maddi and Kobasa, 1984). Hardiness has been described as reflecting:

- personal feelings of control
- a desire to accept challenges
- commitment.

It has been argued that the degree of hardiness influences an individual's appraisal of potential stressors and the resulting stress response. The term 'feelings of mastery' (Karasek and Theorell, 1990) reflects individuals' control over their stress response. It has been argued that the degree of mastery may be related to the stress response. According to these recent developments, stress is conceptualized as a product of the individual's capacity for self-control. Successful coping and self-management eradicate stress, failed self-regulation results in a stress response, and stress-related illness is considered to be a consequence of prolonged failed self-management.

The relationship between stress and illness is not straightforward, and there is much evidence to suggest that several factors may mediate the stress–illness link. The way in which an individual copes with stress, for example, may reduce stress and subsequently decrease the chance of illness. In addition, increased social support has been related to a decreased stress response and a subsequent reduction in illness. Finally, the degree to which an individual feels in control of the stressor can influence the degree of stress experienced.

Therefore, from a psychological perspective, individuals' states of mind relate to stress and the stress response in terms of their appraisal of the external stressor ('Is it stressful?'), the degree of the stress response to this stressor ('Do I feel stressed?'), their ability to cope with and reduce this response ('It's OK, I can talk this over with my friends') and the degree of any subsequent changes in behaviour ('I think I'll have a cigarette'). Accordingly, each of these factors will in turn determine the extent of any resulting ill health.

THINKING
ABOUT

Smoking is a stimulant, yet people use smoking to calm them down when under stress. Why might this be? Do doctors have the right to try and take away a behaviour that helps people to cope with their lives?

Beliefs about confidence

Individuals also hold beliefs about their ability to carry out certain behaviours. Bandura (1977) has termed this **self-efficacy** to reflect the extent to which people feel confident that they can do whatever it is they wish to do. A smoker, for example, may feel that she should stop smoking but have very little confidence that she will be able to do so. Likewise, an overweight man may be convinced that he should do more exercise but think that this goal is unlikely to be achievable. These two examples would be said to have low self-efficacy. In contrast, a woman who was motivated to attend for a health check, and felt confident that she could, would be said to have high self-efficacy. Self-efficacy is defined not to reflect a personality trait, that is, this person always has high self-efficacy, but to describe a belief about a particular behaviour at a particular time, that is, this person shows high self-efficacy now in terms of changing this behaviour.

Beliefs about illness

Illness beliefs have been defined as 'a patient's own implicit common-sense beliefs about their illness' (Leventhal et al., 1980, 1997). Such beliefs provide individuals with a framework for coping with and understanding their illness, and for telling them what to look out for if they are becoming ill. There are five cognitive dimensions to these beliefs:

- *Identity:* what label is given to the illness (the medical diagnosis) and the symptoms experienced, for example 'I have a chest infection (diagnosis) with a cough (symptoms)'

- *The perceived cause of the illness:* causes may be biological or psychosocial. People may explain their illness as reflecting different causal models. One person, for example, may believe that 'My chest infection was caused by a virus', whereas another may believe, 'My chest infection was caused by stress and being run down'

- *Time line:* beliefs about how long the illness will last, that is, whether it is acute (short term) or chronic (long term), for example 'My chest infection will be over in a few days'

- *Consequences:* perceptions of the possible effects of the illness on an individual's life. The consequences may be physical, such as pain and a lack of mobility, emotional, such as a loss of social contact or loneliness, or a combination of the two, for example 'My chest infection will prevent me going to college, which will prevent me seeing my friends'

- *Curability and controllability:* individuals also represent illnesses in terms of whether they believe that the illness can be treated and cured, and the extent to which the outcome of their illness is controllable either by themselves or by powerful others, for example 'If I rest, my chest infection will go away' or 'If I take my medication, my chest infection will go away.'

There is some evidence for a similar structure of illness representation in other cultures. Weller (1984) examined models of illness in English-speaking Americans and Spanish-speaking Guatamalans. The results indicated that illness was predominantly conceptualized in terms of contagion and severity. Lau (1997) argued that contagion is a version of the cause dimension, that is, the illness is caused by a virus, and that severity is a combination of the magnitude of the perceived consequences and beliefs about the time line, that is, how will the illness affect my life and how long will it last?, dimensions that support those described by Leventhal and his colleagues.

Researchers in New Zealand and the UK have developed the illness perception questionnaire (Weinman et al., 1996). This asks subjects to rate a series of statements about their illness that reflect the dimensions identified by

Leventhal et al. (1997). The questionnaire has been used to examine beliefs about illnesses such as chronic fatigue syndrome, diabetes and arthritis, and provides further support for the dimensions of illness beliefs.

Individuals have beliefs related to both their health and illness. These beliefs influence their behaviours, which may in turn impact on how healthy they are. The decisions people make are not, however, wholly a product of their beliefs. It is also not only lay people who have such beliefs. Being healthy or ill can bring individuals into contact with a range of health professionals, including GPs, nurses, midwives, hospital doctors and alternative practitioners. These health professionals also have their own beliefs and behaviours.

Communication in health settings

The study of health professionals' beliefs developed from the examination of doctor–patient communication and the original focus on compliance. Haynes et al. (1979) defined **compliance** as 'the extent to which the patient's behaviour (in terms of taking medications, following diets or other lifestyle changes) coincides with medical or health advice'. Compliance has excited an enormous amount of clinical and academic interest over the past few decades, and it has been calculated that 3,200 English articles on compliance have been listed between 1979 and 1985 (Trostle, 1988). Nowadays, people tend to prefer the term 'adherence' to compliance, as compliance is considered to describe the patient in a passive role. This chapter, however, will use the term compliance as this is what is still often used in the literature.

Compliance is regarded as important primarily because following the recommendations of health professionals is considered to be essential to patient recovery. Studies estimate, however, that about half the patients with a chronic illness such as diabetes or hypertension are non-compliant with their medication regimens, and that even compliance for a behaviour as apparently simple as using an inhaler for asthma is poor. Compliance also has financial implications: recent figures obtained from a patient compliance survey conducted in 2004 estimated the annual cost of non-compliance to be £60 billion (www.datamonitor.com).

? What factors might contribute to a patient's compliance with a medical regimen?

Ley (1988) developed the cognitive hypothesis model of compliance. This claims that compliance can be predicted by a combination of:

● patient satisfaction with the process of the consultation

● understanding the information given

● recall of this information.

Several studies have been carried out to examine each element of the cognitive hypothesis model, which is illustrated in Figure 5.2.

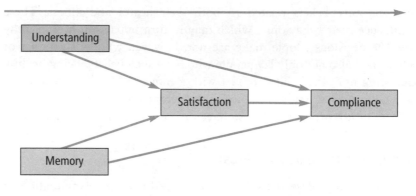

Figure 5.2 Ley's model of compliance

HEALTH CONSULTATIONS

Numerous studies have looked at patients' understanding of what they have been told in a consultation, the extent to which they remember it and whether they feel satisfied with the consultation. Ley (1988) examined the extent of patient satisfaction with the consultation. He reviewed 21 studies of hospital patients and found that 41% of patients were dissatisfied with their treatment and 28% of general practice patients were similarly dissatisfied. Studies show that the level of patient satisfaction stems from various components of the consultation, in particular the affective aspects (for example emotional support and understanding), the behavioural aspects (for example prescribing and adequate explanation) and the competence (for example appropriateness of referral, and diagnosis) of the health professional. Ley (1988) has also reported that satisfaction is determined by the content of the consultation and that patients want to know as much information as possible, even if it is bad news. In studies looking at cancer diagnosis, for example, patients showed improved satisfaction if they were given a diagnosis of cancer rather than if they were protected from this information.

Several studies have also examined the extent to which patients understand the content of the consultation. One study by Boyle (1970) examined patients' definitions of different illnesses and reported that, when given a checklist, only 85% correctly defined arthritis, 77% jaundice, 52% palpitations and 80% bronchitis. Boyle further examined patients' perceptions of the location of organs and found that only 42% correctly located the heart, 20% the stomach and 49% the liver. This suggests that the understanding of the content of the consultation may well be low.

Further studies have examined the understanding of illness in terms of causality and seriousness. Roth (1979) asked what patients thought caused peptic ulcers and found a variety of responses, such as problems with the teeth and gums, food, digestive problems or excessive stomach acid. He also examined what individuals thought caused lung cancer and found that although the understanding of the causality of lung cancer was high in terms of smoking behaviour, 50% of individuals thought that lung cancer caused by smoking had a good prognosis.

Researchers have also examined the process of recall of the information given during the consultation. A study by Bain (1977) examined the recall from a sample of patients who had attended a GP consultation and found that 37% could not recall the name of the drug, 23% could not recall the frequency of the dose and 25% could not recall the duration of the treatment. A further study by Crichton et al. (1978) found that 22% of patients had forgotten the treatment regimen recommended by their doctors.

In a meta-analysis of the research into the recall of consultation information, Ley (1988) found that recall is influenced by a multitude of factors. Ley argued, for example, that anxiety, medical knowledge, intellectual level, the importance of the statement, the primacy effect and the number of statements affect recall. He concluded, however, that recall is not influenced by the age of the patient, which is contrary to some predictions of the effect of ageing on memory and some of the myths and counter-myths of the ageing process.

? What do these studies suggest about how patient compliance might be improved?

Traditional models of the communication between health professionals and patients have emphasized the transfer of knowledge from expert to lay person. There are, however, several problems with this educational approach, which can be summarized as follows:

● It assumes that the communication from the health professional is from an expert whose knowledge base is one of objective knowledge and does not involve the health beliefs of that individual health professional

● Patient compliance is seen as positive and unproblematic

● Improved knowledge is predicted to improve the communication process

● The approach does not include a role for patient health beliefs.

Doctors are traditionally regarded as having an objective knowledge set that comes from their extensive medical education. If this were the case, it could be predicted that doctors with a similar level of knowledge and training would behave in a similar way. In addition, if doctors' behaviour were objective, it would also be consistent. Considerable variability has, however, been found among doctors in terms of different aspects of their practice. In particular, health professionals have been shown to vary in terms of their diagnosis of asthma, their prescribing behaviour (ranging between 15% and 90% of patients being prescribed drugs), the methods used by doctors to measure blood pressure, and their treatment of diabetes (see Marteau and Johnston, 1990).

According to a traditional educational model of doctor–patient communication, this variability could be understood in terms of a differing level of knowledge and expertise: some individuals know more or less than others, and there is a correct way of behaving and a correct diagnosis that experts make successfully, whereas novices make errors. This variability can, however, also be understood by examining health professionals' own health beliefs.

Patients are described as having **lay health beliefs** that are individual and variable, whereas health professionals are usually described as having professional beliefs that are often assumed to be consistent and predictable. If, however, health professionals vary in the diagnoses they make, the conclusions they reach and the treatments they prescribe, this suggests a role for the health professionals' own health beliefs, which may vary as much as the patient's. In particular, these beliefs appear to play a central role in the development of the health professionals' original hypothesis, for example 'This patient looks as if she has a chest infection', 'This patient is anxious but not physically ill', 'This patient wants to tell me something but is embarrassed' or 'This patient could have cancer.'

Health professionals have their own beliefs concerning health and illness, which influence their choice of hypothesis. Some may believe that health and illness are determined by biomedical factors, whereas others may view health and illness as relating to psychosocial factors. A patient suffering from tiredness may be seen by the former as anaemic and by the latter as suffering from stress. Health professionals will also hold beliefs about the prevalence and incidence of any given health problem. For example, whereas one doctor may regard appendicitis as a common childhood complaint and hypothesize that a child presenting with acute abdominal pain has appendicitis, another may consider appendicitis to be rare and not consider this hypothesis.

Health professionals also have beliefs about the seriousness and treatability of a disease and are particularly motivated to reach a correct diagnosis for serious but treatable conditions. A health professional may, for example, diagnose appendicitis in a child presenting with abdominal pain because appendicitis is both a serious and a treatable condition. There is a high 'payoff' for a correct diagnosis of such conditions. Health professionals' existing knowledge of the patient will also influence their original hypothesis. Such knowledge may include the patient's medical history, their psychological state, an understanding of their psychosocial environment and a belief about why the patient uses the medical services. In addition, the development of the original hypothesis may be influenced by the health professional's stereotyped views concerning the class, ethnicity or physical appearance of a patient. Furthermore, health professionals' mood, their profile characteristics (such as age and sex), their geographical location and their previous experience may all affect the decision-making process. Therefore, the variability in health professionals' behaviour can be understood in terms of the many pre-existing factors involved in the decision-making process.

In summary, lay people have beliefs about their health and illness. These can take the form of beliefs about cause and control, risk, confidence and the illness in question. However, it is not only lay people who hold such beliefs. Research exploring health professionals' behaviour indicates that their beliefs are just as complex, particularly in areas related to decision-making and diagnosis. Beliefs are therefore central to the experience of being ill in terms of health-related behaviours, beliefs about illness and the beliefs of health professionals. The role of such psychological factors in the experience of illness is illustrated in the research on pain and the role of beliefs and behaviours in both its increase and decrease.

The experience of being ill and the example of pain

Early models of pain described pain within a biomedical framework as an automatic response to an external factor. From this perspective, pain was seen as a response to a painful stimulus involving a direct pathway connecting the source of pain (for example a burnt finger) to the area of the brain that detected the painful sensation. Although psychological changes ('I feel anxious') were described as resulting from the pain, there was no room in these models for psychology in either the cause or the moderation of pain ('My pain feels better when I think about something else'). Psychology began, however, to play an important part in understanding pain throughout the twentieth century. This was based upon several observations:

- It was observed that medical treatments for pain, for example drugs and surgery, were, in the main, useful only for treating acute pain, that is, pain of short duration. Such treatments were fairly ineffective for treating chronic pain, that is, pain which lasts for a long time. This suggested that there must be something else involved in the pain sensation that was not included in the simple stimulus–response models.

- It was also observed that individuals with the same degree of tissue damage differed in their reporting of the painful sensation and/or of a pain response. Beecher (1956) observed soldiers' and civilians' requests for pain relief in a hospital during the Second World War. He reported that, although soldiers and civilians often showed the same degree of injury, the soldiers requested less medication than the civilians. He found that whereas 80% of the civilians requested medication, only 25% of the soldiers did. Beecher suggested that this reflected a role for the meaning of the injury in the experience of pain: for the soldiers, the injury had a positive meaning as it indicated that their time at war was over. This meaning mediated the pain experience.

- The third observation was phantom limb pain. Between 5% and 10% of amputees tend to feel pain in an absent limb. Their pain can actually get worse after the amputation and continue even after complete healing. Sometimes the pain can feel as if it is spreading at the site, often being described as that of a hand being clenched with the nails digging into the palm. Phantom limb pain has no physical basis because the limb is obviously missing. In addition, not everybody feels phantom limb pain, and those who do, do not experience it to the same extent.

Example 5.3

THE GATE CONTROL THEORY OF PAIN

Melzack and Wall (1965) developed the gate control theory of pain, which represented an attempt to introduce psychology into the understanding of pain. This model is illustrated in Figure 5.3. It suggested that although pain still could be understood in terms of a stimulus–response pathway, this pathway was complex and mediated by a network of interacting processes. The gate control theory thus integrated psychology into the traditional biomedical model of pain, not only describing a role for physiological causes and interventions, but also allowing for psychological causes and interventions.

Melzack and Wall suggested that there was a gate existing at spinal cord level, which received input from the peripheral nerve fibres, that is, the site of injury, descending central influences from the brain relating to the psychological state of the individual – in terms of, for example, attention, mood and previous experiences – and the large and small fibres that constitute part of the physiological input to pain perception. They argued that the gate integrates all the information

from these different sources and produces an output. This output then sends information to an action system, which results in the perception of pain, the degree of pain relating to how open or closed the gate is. Melzack and Wall suggested that several factors open the gate:

● physical factors, such as injury or activation of the large fibres
● emotional factors, such as anxiety, worry, tension and depression
● behavioural factors, such as focusing on the pain or boredom.

The gate control theory also suggests that certain factors close the gate:

● physical factors, such as medication or stimulation of the small fibres
● emotional factors, such as happiness, optimism or relaxation
● behavioural factors, such as concentration, distraction or an involvement in other activities.

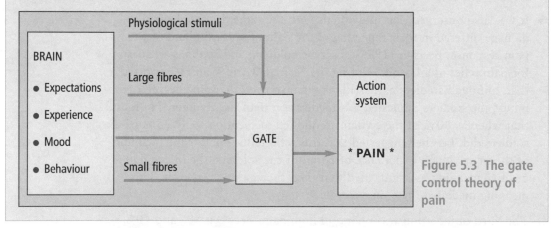

Figure 5.3 The gate control theory of pain

The gate control theory was a development from previous theories, in that it allowed for the existence of mediating variables and emphasized active perception rather than passive sensation (Melzack and Wall, 1965). The gate control theory and the subsequent attempts at evaluating the different components of pain perception reflect a three-process model of pain. The components of this model are:

- physiological processes such as tissue damage

- the release of endorphins and changes in heart rate

- subjective-affective-cognitive and behavioural processes.

The latter two sets of process indicate a central role for psychological factors in pain perception and have been studied as follows.

Subjective-affective-cognitive processes

Learning processes

- *Classical conditioning*: research suggests that classical conditioning may have an effect on the perception of pain. As described by theories of associative learning, an individual may associate a particular environment with the experience of pain. For example, if an individual, because of past experience, associates the dentist with pain, pain perception may be enhanced as a result of this expectation when attending the dentist. In addition, because of the association between these two factors, the individual may experience increased anxiety when attending the dentist, which may also increase pain.

- *Operant conditioning*: research suggests that there is also a role for operant conditioning in pain perception. Individuals may respond to pain by showing pain behaviour, for example resting, grimacing, limping or staying off work. Such pain behaviour may be positively reinforced by, for example, sympathy, attention and time off work, which may itself increase pain perception (see the section on Behavioural processes below).

Anxiety

Anxiety also appears to influence pain perception. Fordyce and Steger (1979) have examined the relationship between anxiety and acute and chronic pain, reporting that anxiety has a different relationship to these two types of pain. In terms of acute pain, pain increases anxiety, the successful treatment of the pain then decreasing the pain, which subsequently decreases the anxiety. This can then cause a further decrease in the pain level. Therefore, with acute pain, because of the relative ease with which it can be treated, anxiety relates to this pain perception in terms of a cycle of pain reduction.

The pattern is, however, different for chronic pain. With chronic pain, pain increases anxiety, but the treatment of chronic pain is often not very effective, the pain then further increasing anxiety, which further increases the pain. In terms of the relationship between anxiety and chronic pain, there is thus a cycle of pain increase.

Neurosis

It has also been suggested that personality, in particular neurosis, may be related to pain perception. Hysteria, hypochondriasis and depression have been labelled the 'neurotic triad'. Sternbach et al. (1973) reported that an increase in the neurotic triad is related to an increase in chronic pain and can be related to less sleep, reduced social and work life and feelings of exhaustion. In addition, an increased preoccupation with pain may be associated with increased pain.

Cognitive states

One of the most important factors that influences pain is the cognitive state of the individual. Beecher (1956), in his study of soldiers' and civilians' requests for medication, was one of the first people to examine this and ask the question 'What does pain mean to the individual?' Beecher argued that differences in pain perception were related to the *meaning* of pain for the individual. In Beecher's study, the soldiers benefited from their pain. This has been described in terms of 'secondary gain', whereby the pain may have a positive reward for the individual.

Behavioural processes

The way in which an individual responds to the pain can itself increase or decrease the perception of the pain. In particular, research has looked at pain behaviours, which have been defined by Turk and colleagues (Turk and Rennert, 1981; Turk et al., 1985) as facial or audible expressions, for example clenched teeth and moaning, distorted posture or movement, for example limping or protecting the painful area, negative affect, for example irritability and depression, and the avoidance of activity, for example not going to work or lying down. It has been suggested that pain behaviours are reinforced by attention, the acknowledgement they receive, and through secondary gains such as not having to go to work. Positively reinforcing pain behaviour may increase pain perception. Pain behaviour can also cause a lack of activity, muscle wastage, a lack of social contact and a dearth of distraction, leading to the adoption of a sick role, which can also increase pain perception.

Pain treatment: a role for psychology?

If psychology is involved in the perception of pain, recent research has suggested that psychology can also be involved in the treatment of pain. There are several methods of pain treatment that reflect an interaction between psychology and physiological factors:

- *Biofeedback* has been used to enable individuals to exert voluntary control over their bodily functions. The technique aims to decrease anxiety and tension and therefore decrease pain.

- *Relaxation* methods are also used. These aim to decrease anxiety and stress, and consequently decrease pain.

- *Operant conditioning* is related to an increased pain perception. It can therefore also be used in pain treatment to reduce pain. Some aspects of pain treatment aim positively to reinforce compliance as a means to reduce pain and discourage pain behaviour such as not walking or standing in ways that avoid pain. By doing so, it is hoped that people will avoid the secondary gains of pain such as being let off normal duties or staying in bed, which in turn could make the pain worse.

- A *cognitive approach* to pain treatment involves factors such as attention diversion – encouraging the individual not to focus on the pain – and imagery – encouraging the individual to have positive, pleasant thoughts. Both these factors appear to decrease pain.

- *Hypnosis* has also been shown to reduce pain. However, whether or not this is simply an effect of attention diversion is unclear.

Multidisciplinary pain clinics

Over recent years, multidisciplinary pain clinics have been set up to treat pain and attempt to challenge the factors that cause or exacerbate pain. The goals set by these clinics include factors such as:

- *improving physical and lifestyle functioning:* this involves improving muscle tone, self-esteem, self-efficacy and distraction, and decreasing boredom, pain behaviour and secondary gains

- *a decreasing reliance on drugs and medical services:* this involves improving personal control, decreasing the sick role and increasing self-efficacy

- *increasing social support and family life:* this aims to increase optimism and distraction, and decrease boredom, anxiety, sick role behaviour and secondary gains.

Theoretical and methodological perspectives

Health psychology draws upon a range of **models** in its approach. These models help us to understand:

- people's views about the causes of ill health

- the extent to which people feel that they can control their life and make changes

- how people explain their health and ill health, which is crucial to making sense of the strategies they adopt to promote health, prevent ill health and manage illness.

The health belief model

The health belief model (see Figure 5.4) was initially formulated by Rosenstock in 1966, being developed by Becker and colleagues throughout the 1970s and 80s. The health belief model is used to predict people's adoption of preventive health behaviours and in the behavioural response to medical treatment for illness.

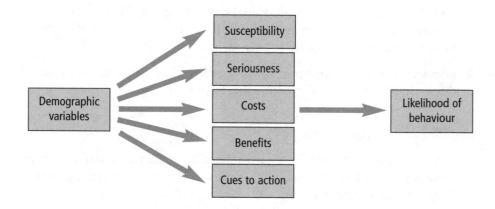

Figure 5.4 The health belief model

The health belief model predicts that behaviour is a result of a set of stable, core beliefs concerning:

- *susceptibility* to illness, for example 'My chances of having a heart attack are low'

- the *seriousness* of the illness, for example 'Heart disease is a serious illness'

- the *costs* involved in carrying out the behaviour, for example 'Eating less will be stressful and boring'

- the *benefits* involved in carrying out the behaviour, for example 'Eating more healthily will make me feel better'

- *cues to action*, which may be internal, such as the symptom of breathlessness, or external, such as information in the form of health education leaflets.

Becker and Rosenstock's (1987) revised health belief model includes:

- an assessment of sufficient motivation to make health issues salient or relevant
- the belief that change following a health recommendation will be beneficial to the individual at a level of acceptable cost.

> **?** How might the health belief model be used to predict the likelihood of a smoker giving up? What are the strengths and weaknesses of this model of behaviour change?

The health belief model would predict smoking cessation if an individual perceived that she was highly susceptible to lung cancer, lung cancer was a serious health threat, the benefits of stopping smoking, for example more money and less odour, were high and the costs of such action, for example potential weight gain or isolation in the peer group, were comparatively low. Furthermore, she is more likely to give up if she is subjected to external cues to action, such as a leaflet in the doctor's waiting room, or internal cues to action, such as the symptom of breathlessness perceived (correctly or otherwise) to be related to lung cancer.

The protection motivation theory

As a result of some of the criticisms of the health belief model and the emerging focus on self-efficacy (see above), Rogers (1983) developed the protection motivation theory (see Figure 5.5), which expanded the health belief model to include additional factors. The protection motivation theory claims that health-related behaviours are a product of five components:

- *self-efficacy*, for example 'I am confident that I can attend for a cervical smear'
- *response effectiveness*, for example 'Having a smear will enable abnormalities to be detected early'
- *severity*, for example 'Cervical cancer is a serious illness'
- *vulnerability*, for example 'My chances of getting cervical cancer are high'
- *fear*, for example an emotional response, in response to education or information.

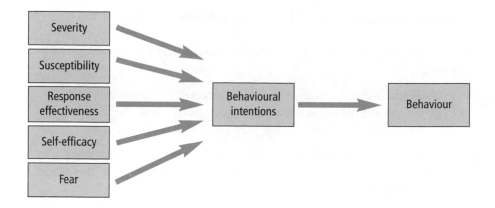

Figure 5.5 The protection motivation theory

These components predict behavioural intentions, for example 'I intend to change my behaviour', which are related to behaviour. Response effectiveness and self-efficacy relate to coping appraisal, that is, individual self-appraisal, whereas severity, vulnerability and fear relate to threat appraisal, that is, assessing the outside threat. Information, which can be either environmental, such as verbal persuasion or observational learning, or intrapersonal, such as prior experience, influences the five components of the protection motivation theory, giving rise to either an adaptive coping response, that is, behavioural intention, or a maladaptive coping response, for example avoidance or denial.

? How might the protection motivation theory be applied to those thinking about taking up exercise?

Information on the contributory role of a poor fitness level to coronary heart disease would increase individuals' anxiety and their perception of how serious coronary heart disease was (perceived severity) and might also increase their belief that they were likely to have a heart attack (perceived vulnerability/susceptibility). If the individuals also felt confident that they could change their level of physical activity (self-efficacy) and that this change would have a beneficial outcome (response effectiveness) such as weight loss, they would be more likely to change their behaviour (behavioural intentions). This would be seen as an adaptive coping response to the information. Alternatively, they might not perceive themselves to be unfit and might therefore deny that the information had any relevance to them. This would be seen as a maladaptive coping response.

The theory of planned behaviour

The theory of reasoned action (Fishbein and Ajzen, 1975) suggests that people's beliefs relate to their social world, and that the expectations of others who are important to them will affect their behaviour. The theory of reasoned action therefore sees the individual within a social context and, in contrast to the traditional approach in which behaviour is seen as rational, includes a role for values.

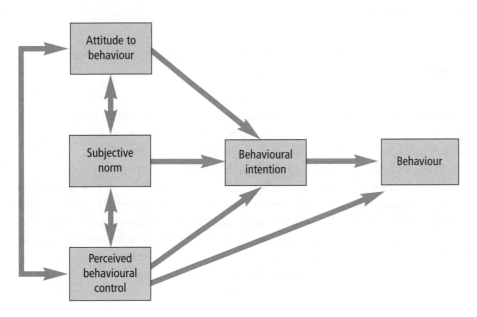

Figure 5.6 The theory of planned behaviour

The theory of planned behaviour (see Figure 5.6) was developed by Ajzen (1988) and represented a progression from the theory of reasoned action. This theory views intentions as 'plans of action in pursuit of behavioural goals'. These intentions are the result of the following beliefs:

● **Attitude** *towards a behaviour:* this is composed of a positive or a negative evaluation of a particular behaviour and the beliefs about the outcome of the behaviour, for example 'Dieting is boring but will improve my health.'

● *Subjective norm:* this includes both the perception of social norms and pressures to perform a behaviour, and an evaluation of the individual's motivation to comply with this pressure, for example 'People who are important to me will approve if I stop smoking and I want their approval.'

● *Perceived behavioural control:* this reflects individuals' beliefs that they can carry out a particular behaviour. It is derived from internal control factors (for example skills, abilities and information) and external control factors (for example obstacles such as a lack of time, money or opportunity), both relating to past behaviour.

According to the theory of planned behaviour, these three factors predict behavioural intentions, which are then linked to behaviour. The theory of planned behaviour also states that perceived behavioural control could have a direct effect on behaviour without the mediating effect of behavioural intentions.

> **?** How might the theory of planned behaviour be applied to someone who wanted to reduce their drinking?

The theory of planned behaviour would make the following predictions. If an individual believed that cutting down on drinking would make their life more productive and would be beneficial to their health (the attitude to the behaviour), and believed that the important people in their life wanted them to stop (subjective norm), as well as believing that they were capable of reducing or stopping drinking because of their past behaviour and an evaluation of internal and external control factors (high behavioural control), this would predict a high intention to stop drinking (behavioural intention). The model also predicts that perceived behavioural control could predict behaviour without the influence of intentions. For example, if someone believed that they could not stop drinking because they were dependent on alcohol, this would be a better predictor of their behaviour than would their intention to stop drinking.

The stages of change model

The stages of change model (also known as the transtheoretical model of behaviour) was originally developed by Prochaska and DiClemente (1982). Unlike other models of beliefs and behaviours, this model does not try to explain what contributes to a decision to change but describes how the change might take place.

Prochaska and DiClemente's model of behaviour change is based on the following stages:

1. *precontemplation:* not intending to make any changes

2. *contemplation:* considering a change

3. *preparation:* making small changes

4. *action:* actively engaging in a new behaviour

5. *maintenance:* sustaining the change over time.

The model is cyclic and bidirectional. In other words, an individual may move to the preparation stage and then back to the contemplation stage several times before progressing to the action stage. Furthermore, even when an individual has reached the maintenance stage, he or she may slip back to the contemplation stage over time. Many smokers, for example, contemplate stopping smoking, stop smoking for a while, start smoking again with no intention to stop and then start contemplating cessation again.

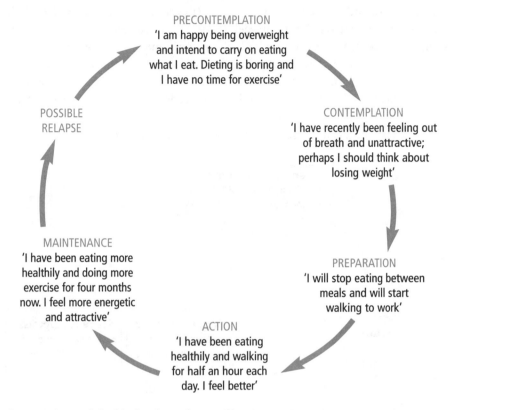

PRECONTEMPLATION
'I am happy being overweight and intend to carry on eating what I eat. Dieting is boring and I have no time for exercise'

POSSIBLE RELAPSE

CONTEMPLATION
'I have recently been feeling out of breath and unattractive; perhaps I should think about losing weight'

MAINTENANCE
'I have been eating more healthily and doing more exercise for four months now. I feel more energetic and attractive'

PREPARATION
'I will stop eating between meals and will start walking to work'

ACTION
'I have been eating healthily and walking for half an hour each day. I feel better'

Figure 5.7 Model of behaviour change

An individual may not have an awareness of contemplating, actioning and maintaining change but will at different stages focus on either the costs of a behaviour, for example 'Taking up exercise will mean that I have less time with my children', or the benefits of the behaviour, for example 'Exercise will make me feel fitter.'

The stages of change model has been applied to several health-related behaviours, such as smoking, alcohol use, exercise and screening behaviour.

THINKING ABOUT

Imagine that you were trying to convince a friend to stop smoking. What beliefs do you think you would have to change in order to be successful? How would you go about doing this? Consider this, bearing in mind the models described above.

The self-regulatory model

The above models tend to be used to explore the predictors of health-related behaviours. In contrast, the self-regulatory model is commonly used to examine how individuals adjust to illness (Leventhal et al., 1985, 1997). In particular, the self-regulatory model (Figure 5.8) suggests that illness and symptoms are dealt with by individuals in the same way as other problems. Thus, if an individual is usually healthy, any onset of illness will be interpreted as a problem, and the individual will be motivated to re-establish their state of health. To do this, an individual needs first to make sense of the problem and then to cope with it.

The three stages of the self-regulatory model are described below.

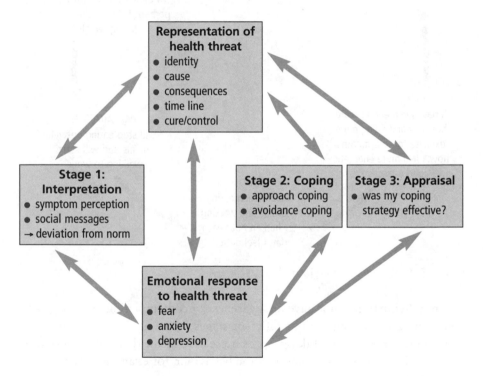

Figure 5.8 Self-regulatory model of illness behaviour

Stage 1: interpretation

An individual may be confronted with the problem of a potential illness through two channels: symptom perception and social messages.

Symptom perception

Symptom perception ('I am feeling breathless') is not a straightforward process but is influenced by individual differences, moods and cognitions.

Pennebaker (1982) argues that individuals vary in the amount of attention they pay to their internal state. In addition, being more internally focused does not necessarily mean being more accurate in terms of symptom perception. In a study evaluating the accuracy of detecting changes in heart rate, Pennebaker (1982) reported that individuals who were more focused on their internal state tended to overestimate any changes in their heart rate compared with subjects who were externally focused. Being internally focused has also been shown to relate to a perception of a slower recovery from illness. Being internally focused may result in an exaggerated perception of symptom change rather than a more accurate one.

An individual's cognitive state may also influence his or her symptom perception. Ruble (1977) carried out a study in which she manipulated women's expectations of when they were due to start menstruating. She gave subjects an 'accurate physiological test' and told women either that their period was due very shortly or it was at least a week away. The women were then asked to report any premenstrual symptoms. The results showed that believing that they were about to start menstruating (even though they were not) increased the number of reported premenstrual symptoms. This indicates an association between cognitive state and symptom perception.

The factors contributing to symptom perception can be illustrated by a condition known as 'medical students' disease', described by Mechanic (1962). A large component of the medical curriculum involves learning about the symptoms associated with a multitude of different illnesses. More than two-thirds of medical students incorrectly report that at some time they have had the symptoms they are being taught about. This phenomenon can perhaps be understood in terms of mood, cognition and social norms. Medical students become quite anxious as a result of their workload, which may heighten their awareness of any physiological changes, making them more internally focused. In addition, medical students are thinking about symptoms as part of their course, which may result in a focus on their own internal state. Furthermore, once one student starts to perceive symptoms, others may model themselves on this behaviour. Therefore, symptom perception influences how an individual interprets the problem of illness.

Social messages

Information about illness also comes from other people, in the form of a formal diagnosis from a health professional ('The doctor has diagnosed this breathlessness as asthma'), or a positive test result from a routine health check. Such messages may or may not be a consequence of symptom perception. In addition, information about illness may come from lay individuals who are not health professionals. Before (and often after) consulting a health professional, people often access their social network – their 'lay referral system' (colleagues, friends and family) – and seek their information and advice. For example, someone with a sore throat may speak to another friend who had a similar condition or may take up a suggestion of a favoured home remedy. Such social messages will influence how the individual interprets the 'problem' of illness.

Individuals may therefore receive information about the possibility of illness through either symptom perception or social messages. This information influences how an individual makes sense of the problem and the development of illness cognitions that will be constructed according to the dimensions of identity, cause, consequences, time line and cure/control (see above). These cognitive representations of the 'problem' will give the problem meaning and will enable the individual to develop and consider suitable coping strategies.

Stage 2: coping

People cope with illness in many different ways, but, broadly speaking, coping can be considered in terms of two main categories:

- *approach coping*, such as taking pills, going to the doctor, resting and talking to friends about emotions
- *avoidance coping*, which involves denial and wishful thinking.

Taylor (1983) examined the ways in which individuals adjust to threatening events including illness and rape. Taylor suggested that coping consists of:

- a search for meaning – 'Why did it happen to me?'
- a search for mastery – 'How can I prevent it happening again?'
- a process of self-enhancement – 'I am better off than a lot of people.'

Taylor argued that these three processes are central to developing and maintaining illusions that constitute a process of cognitive adaptation.

Stage 3: appraisal

Appraisal involves individuals evaluating the effectiveness of the coping strategy to determine whether to continue with this strategy or try an alternative one.

The model is self-regulatory because its three components (interpretation, coping and appraisal) interrelate in order to maintain the status quo, that is, they regulate the self. Therefore, if the individual's normal state (health) is disrupted (by illness), the model proposes that the individual is motivated to return the balance to normality. This self-regulation involves the three processes interrelating in an ongoing and dynamic fashion.

THINKING
ABOUT

Some people are always seriously ill and frequently visit their GP ('I have bronchitis', 'I have tonsilitis', 'I have a migraine'), whereas others only have mild complaints ('I have a cough', 'I have a sore throat', 'I have a headache'). How might this relate to the way in which they make sense of their symptoms?

Developing interventions to change health-related behaviour

Health psychology theory provides a framework for understanding behaviour and beliefs and exploring how these factors may relate to illnesses. These theories have drawn on social cognition models, implementation intentions and the self-regulatory model to inform interventions aiming to change behaviours and beliefs.

Using social cognition models

Social cognition models have been developed to describe and predict health behaviours such as smoking, attending health screening, eating and exercise. In recent years, there has been a call towards using these models to inform and develop interventions to change behaviours. This has been based upon two observations. First, it was observed that many interventions designed to change behaviour were only minimally effective. For example, reviews of early interventions to change sexual behaviour concluded that these interventions had only small effects (for example, Oakley et al., 1995) and dietary interventions for weight loss may result in weight loss in the short term but the majority show a return to baseline by follow-up (for example, NHS Centre for Reviews and Dissemination, 1997). Second, it was observed that many interventions were not based upon any theoretical framework nor were they drawing upon research that had identified which factors were correlated with the particular behaviour. Some researchers have therefore outlined how theory can be translated into interventions. In particular, Sutton (2002) describes a series of steps that can be followed to develop an intervention:

● identify target behaviour and target population

● identify the most salient beliefs about the target behaviour in the target population using open-ended questions

● conduct a study involving closed questions to determine which beliefs are the best predictors of behavioural intention. Choose the best predictor as the target belief

● analyse the data to determine the beliefs which best discriminate between intenders and non-intenders. These are further target beliefs

- develop an intervention to change these target beliefs.

Over recent years, an increasing number of behavioural interventions have drawn upon a theory of behaviour change to change behaviours such as condom use, sun cream use and cervical cancer screening. For example, Quine et al. (2001) followed the steps outlined above to identify salient beliefs about safety helmet wearing for children. They then developed an intervention based upon persuasion to change these salient beliefs. The results showed that after the intervention, the children showed more positive beliefs about safety helmet wearing than the control group and were more likely to wear a helmet at five months follow-up.

Using implementation intentions

Social cognition models emphasize the relationship between the intention to behave in a certain way and actual behaviour. Research indicates, however, that intentions do not always translate into behaviour. Gollwitzer's (1993) notion of implementation intentions have been employed to strengthen this association. Gollwitzer regards carrying out an intention as involving the development of specific plans as to what an individual will do, given a specific set of environmental factors. Implementation intentions therefore describe the 'what' and the 'when' of a particular behaviour. For example, the intention 'I intend to stop smoking' will be more likely to be translated into 'I have stopped smoking' if the individual makes the implementation intention 'I intend to stop smoking tomorrow at 12.00 when I have finished my last packet.' Some experimental research has shown that encouraging individuals to make implementation intentions can actually increase the correlation between intentions and behaviour for behaviours such as reducing dietary fat. Gollwitzer and Sheeran (2006) carried out a meta-analysis of 94 independent tests of the impact of implementation intentions on a range of behavioural goals including eating a low-fat diet, using public transport, exercise and a range of personal goals. The results from this analysis indicated that implementation intentions had a medium to large effect on goal attainment. By tapping into variables such as implementation intentions, it is argued that the models may become better predictors of actual behaviour.

Using the self-regulatory model

Research indicates that patients' beliefs about their illness may relate to a range of health outcomes in terms of adherence to medication, attendance at rehabilitation, return to work and adjustment. Interventions have therefore been developed to change beliefs and promote more positive outcomes. For example, Petrie et al. (2002) aimed to change illness cognitions and examined the subsequent impact upon a range of patient outcomes. The intervention consisted of three sessions of about 40 minutes with a psychologist and was designed to address and change patients' beliefs about their myocardial infarction (MI). Throughout the intervention, the information and discussion were targeted to the specific beliefs and concerns of the patient. The results showed that patients who had received the intervention reported more positive views about their MI at follow-up in terms of beliefs about consequences, time line, control/cure and symptom distress. They were also better prepared to leave hospital, returned to work at a faster rate and reported a lower rate of angina symptoms. The intervention therefore appeared to change cognitions and improve patients' functional outcome after MI. The study of beliefs and behaviour related to food and diet is illustrated in the following case study.

CASE STUDY The impact of beliefs on behaviour: the example of obesity and diet

The increase in both adult and child obesity has been well documented. As a means to explain this increase, researchers have focused their attention on the role of the obesogenic environment and have highlighted the importance of factors such as the food industry, food advertising, food labelling, the availability of energy-dense foods and an environment that has been increasingly designed to encourage a sedentary lifestyle through the use of cars, computers and television. Central to this change is a shift in two key behaviours; eating behaviour and physical activity. We will focus on the links between obesity and diet and explore why people eat what they eat and how this relates to obesity onset and maintenance.

Research exploring how much and what obese people eat is problematic due to the difficulty in measuring diet without changing it. However, there is evidence that obese people eat relatively more fat than non-obese people, while the very process of weight gain indicates that they are eating more than their body requires (see Ogden, 2003).

Within psychological research, there are three main theories of eating behaviour that can help us to understand why some people eat differently and more than others, and why some may become overweight and obese. These are the cognitive approach, the developmental model and the impact of dieting on eating behaviour.

A cognitive approach to diet

Most research using a cognitive approach has drawn upon social cognition models to predict eating behaviour. For example, attitudes have been found to predict fat intake, table salt use, eating in fast-food restaurants, consuming low-fat milk and healthy eating conceptualized as high levels of fibre and fruit and vegetables and low levels of fat (for example, Povey et al., 2000). A cognitive approach to eating behaviour therefore emphasizes the role of cognitions and explores how these cognitions predict what we eat. From this perspective, we eat food because we have positive thoughts about it. The obese may overeat because they have more positive thoughts about foods that are then translated into behaviour.

CONNECTIONS

Chapter 1 discusses the biological processes involved in weight gain.

A developmental approach

In contrast, a developmental approach to eating behaviour emphasizes the importance of learning in terms of both operant and classical conditioning and focuses on the development of food preferences in childhood. Social learning describes the impact of observing other people's behaviour on one's own behaviour and is sometimes referred to as 'modelling' or 'observational learning'. In one study, peer modelling was used to change children's preference for vegetables (Birch, 1980). The target children were placed at lunch for four consecutive days next to other children who preferred a different vegetable to themselves (peas versus carrots). By the end of the study, the children showed a shift in their vegetable preference that persisted at a follow-up assessment several weeks later. The impact of social learning has also been shown in an intervention study designed to change children's eating behaviour using video-based peer modelling (Lowe et al., 1998). Food preferences therefore change through watching others eat. In terms of obesity, some people may overeat or eat more unhealthily because they have watched others close to them doing so.

Parental attitudes to food and eating behaviours are also central to the process of social learning. For example, Olivera et al. (1992) reported a correlation between mothers' and children's food intakes for most nutrients in preschool children. Contento et al. (1993) found a relationship between mothers' health motivation and the quality of children's diets and Brown and Ogden (2004) reported consistent correlations between parents and their children in terms of reported snack food intake and eating motivation. Obesity clearly runs in families. This may reflect the transmission of eating-related attitudes and behaviours from parent to child.

Associative learning refers to the impact of contingent factors on behaviour. Some research has examined the effect of rewarding eating behaviour, as in 'If you eat your vegetables, I will be pleased with you.' For example, Birch et al. (1980) showed that if food was given to children in association with positive adult attention, the preference for the food increased. Rewarding eating behaviour seems to improve food preferences. Other research has explored the impact of using food as a reward. For these studies, gaining access to the food is contingent upon another behaviour, as in 'If you are well behaved, you can have a biscuit.' Birch et al. (1980) presented children with foods either as a reward, as a snack or in a non-social situation (the control). The results showed that food acceptance increased if the foods were presented as a reward but that the more neutral conditions had no effect. This suggests that using food as a reward increases the preference for that food. The relationship between food and rewards, however, appears to be more complicated than this. In an early study, Lepper et al. (1982) told children stories about children eating imaginary foods called 'hupe' and 'hule', in which the child in the story could only eat one if he or she had finished the other. This is analogous to saying 'If you eat your vegetables, you can eat your pudding.' Although parents use this approach to encourage their children to eat vegetables, the evidence indicates that this may be increasing their children's preference for pudding even further, as pairing two foods results in the 'reward' food being seen as more positive than the 'access' food. In terms of obesity, people may overeat and become obese because they have learned that higher fat, unhealthier foods are more rewarding than others and/or because their parents used unhealthier foods as rewards for eating the healthier foods.

The role of dieting

The final theoretical perspective that may illuminate why some people become obese is the focus on dieting and restraint theory (see Ogden, 2003). Dieting is the conscious attempt to cognitively control food intake. Many people who are already obese diet as a means to lose weight. Dieting, however, may be not only a consequence of obesity but also a cause, as there is evidence that dieting is often characterized by periods of overeating which is precipitated by factors such as lowered mood and eating a high-calorie food. From this perspective, it has been argued that attempting to eat less paradoxically causes overeating, as the process of denial and self-control makes food more attractive and creates a situation whereby the individual becomes increasingly preoccupied with eating. There is also some evidence that overeating is reflected in weight gain, particularly in women. For example, French et al. (1994) reported the results from a cross-sectional and longitudinal study of 1,639 men and 1,913 women who were involved in a worksite intervention study for smoking cessation and weight control. The cross-sectional analysis showed that a history of dieting, current dieting and previous involvement in a formal weight loss programme were related to a higher body weight in both men and women. Similarly, the prospective analysis showed that baseline measures of involvement in a formal weight loss programme and dieting predicted increases

in body weight at follow-up. However, this was for women only. In particular, women who were dieting or who had been involved in a formal weight loss programme at baseline gained nearly 0.9 kg more than those who had not. Klesges and colleagues (1992) reported similar results in their study of 141 men and 146 women who were followed up after one year. This showed that both the dieting men and women were heavier than their non-dieting counterparts at baseline. Higher baseline weight and higher restraint scores at baseline also predicted greater weight gain at follow-up in women. If dieters perceive themselves to be overweight, but are not necessarily obese, and if dieting causes overeating and subsequent weight gain, then dieting could predictably play a causal role in the development of obesity. It is possible that dieting also results in the relative overconsumption of high-fat foods as these are the foods that dieters try to avoid.

Obesity is on the increase in both adults and children and research suggests a clear role for changes in behaviour, particularly diet. Psychological theories focusing on cognitions, learning and the role of dieting suggest that overeating may be a result of their beliefs about food, how and what they have seen others eat, how food was presented to them in their childhood and their subsequent attempts to diet and reduce their food intake.

Summary

- Health psychologists are interested in how people think about their health and their health-related attitudes and beliefs

- Health psychologists have developed various models to explain the relationship between attitudes, beliefs and behaviours, as well as to predict the decisions that people make

- The study of individual beliefs provides an insight into people's health-related behaviour and how unhealthy behaviours can be changed

- Health psychologists study how people make sense of illness and how these beliefs may contribute to the onset, progression and possible treatment of illness

- Understanding the role of psychological factors may help people to adopt preventive health beliefs and behaviours and reduce the impact of being ill

Questions for further discussion

1. Why do people continue to behave in unhealthy ways? Discuss with reference to smoking, diet, exercise or alcohol.

2. There is no such thing as physical illness: all illnesses have a psychological component. Discuss.

3. Why is patient adherence to medical treatment regimes so low? How might it be increased?

Further reading

Bowling, A. (2001) *Measuring Disease* (2nd edn). Buckingham: Open University Press.
Provides a useful overview of the theory behind measuring quality of life and a clear review of the existing scales for assessing health status.

Connor, M. and Norman, P. (eds) (2005) *Predicting Health Behaviours* (2nd edn). Buckingham: Open University Press.
Provides a thorough description of the social cognition models and the extent to which they predict health-related behaviour.

Ogden, J. (2007) *Health Psychology: A Textbook* (4th edn). Buckingham: Open University Press.
A comprehensive overview of health psychology covering a range of health psychology areas of research and theory. The current chapter was based on this book.

References

Ajzen, I. (1988) *Attitudes. Personality and Behaviour*. Chicago: Dorsey Press.

Bain, D.J.G. (1977) 'Patient knowledge and the content of the consultation in general practice'. *Medical Education* 11: 347–50.

Bandura, A. (1977) 'Self efficacy: toward a unifying theory of behavior change'. *Psychological Review* 84: 191–215.

Becker, M.H. and Rosenstock, I.M. (1987) Comparing social learning theory and the health belief model, in W.B. Ward (ed.) *Advances in Health Education and Promotion*. Greenwich, CT: JAI Press, pp. 245–9.

Beecher, H.K. (1956) 'Relationship of significance of wound to the pain experienced'. *Journal of the American Medical Association* **161**: 1609–13.

Birch, L.L. (1980) 'Effects of peer models' food choices and eating behaviors on preschoolers' food preferences'. *Child Development* **51**: 489–96.

Boyle, C.M. (1970) 'Differences between patients' and doctors' interpretations of common medical terms'. *British Medical Journal* **2**: 286–9.

Bradley, C., Gamsu, D.S., Moses, J.L. et al. (1987) 'The use of diabetes-specific perceived control and health belief measures to predict treatment choice and efficacy in a feasibility study of continuous subcutaneous insulin infusion pumps'. *Psychology and Health* **1**: 133–46.

Brown, R. and Ogden, J. (2004) 'Children's eating attitudes and behaviour: a study of the modelling and control theories of parental influence'. *Health Education and Research* **19**(3): 261–71.

Contento, I.R., Basch, C., Shea, S. et al. (1993) 'Relationship of mothers' food choice criteria to food intake of pre-school children: identification of family subgroups'. *Health Education Quarterly* **20**: 243–59.

Crichton, E.F., Smith, D.L. and Demanuele, F. (1978) 'Patients' recall of medication information'. *Drug Intelligence and Clinical Pharmacy* **12**: 591–9.

Doll, R. and Peto, R. (1981) *The Causes of Cancer*. New York: Oxford University Press.

Engel, G.L. (1977) 'The need for a new medical model: a challenge for biomedicine'. *Science* **196**: 129–35.

Engel, G.L. (1980) 'The clinical application of the biopsychosocial model'. *American Journal of Psychiatry* **137**: 535–44.

Fishbein, M. and Ajzen, I. (1975) *Belief, Attitude, Intentional Behaviour: An Introduction to Theory and Research*. Reading, MA: Addison-Wesley.

Fordyce, W.E. and Steger, J.C. (1979) Chronic pain, in O.F. Pomerleau and J.P. Brady (eds) *Behavioural Medicine: Theory and Practice*. Baltimore: Williams and Wilkins, pp. 125–53.

French, S.A., Jeffery, R.W., Forster, J.L. et al. (1994) 'Predictors of weight change over two years among a population of working adults: the healthy worker project'. *International Journal of Obesity* **18**: 145–54.

Gollwitzer, P.M. (1993) Goal achievement: the role of intentions, in W. Stroebe and M. Hewstone (eds) *European Review of Social Psychology* **4**: 141–85.

Gollwitzer, P.M. and Sheeran, P. (2006) 'Implementation intentions and goal achievement: a meta-analysis of effects and processes'. *Advances in Experimental Social Psychology* **38**: 69–119.

Haynes, R.B., Sackett, D.L. and Taylor, D.W. (eds) (1979) *Compliance in Healthcare*. Baltimore, MD: Johns Hopkins University Press.

Heider, F. (1958) *The Psychology of Interpersonal Relations*. New York: John Wiley & Sons.

Karasek, R. and Theorell, T. (1990) *Healthy Work: Stress, Productivity and the Reconstruction of Working Life*. New York: Basic Books.

King, J.B. (1982) 'The impact of patients' perceptions of high blood pressure on attendance at screening: an attributional extension of the health belief model'. *Social Science and Medicine* 16: 1079–92.

Klesges, R.C., Isbell, T.R. and Klesges, L.M. (1992) 'Relationship between dietary restraint, energy intake, physical activity, and body weight: a prospective analysis'. *Journal of Abnormal Psychology* 101: 668–74.

Krantz, D.S., Glass, D.C., Contrada, R. and Miller, N.E. (1981) *Behavior and Health. National Science Foundations Second Five Year Outlook on Science and Technology*. Washington, DC: US Government Printing Office.

Lau, R.R. (1997) Cognitive representations of health and illness, in D. Gochman (ed.) *Handbook of Health Behaviour Research*, vol. I. New York: Plenum Press, pp. 51–70.

Lazarus, R.S. and Folkman, S. (1987) 'Transactional theory and research on emotions and coping'. *European Journal of Personality*, 1: 141–70.

Lazarus, R.S. and Launier, R. (1978) Stress related transactions between person and environment, in L.A. Pervin and M. Lewis (eds) *Perspectives in International Psychology*. New York: Plenum Press, pp. 287–327.

Lepper, M., Sagotsky, G., Dafoe, J.L. and Greene, D. (1982) 'Consequences of superfluous social constraints: effects on young children's social inferences and subsequent intrinsic interest'. *Journal of Personality and Social Psychology* 42: 51–65.

Leventhal, H., Meyer, D. and Nerenz, D. (1980) The common sense representation of illness danger, in Rachman, S. (ed.) *Medical Psychology* 2: 7–30.

Leventhal, H., Prohaska, T.R. and Hirschman, R.S. (1985) Preventive health behaviour across the life span, in J.C. Rosen and L.J. Solomon (eds) *Prevention in Health Psychology*. Hanover, NH: University Press of New England.

Leventhal, H., Benyamini, Y., Brownlee, S. et al. (1997) Illness representations: theoretical foundations, in K.J. Petrie and J.A. Weinman (eds) *Perceptions of Health and Illness: Current Research and Applications*. Harwood Academic: Amsterdam, pp. 19–45.

Ley, P. (1988) *Communicating with Patients*. London: Croom Helm.

Lowe, C.F., Dowey, A. and Horne, P. (1998) Changing what children eat, in A. Murcott (ed.) *The Nation's Diet: The Social Science of Food Choice*. Harlow: Addison Wesley Longman, pp. 57–80.

Maddi, S. and Kobasa, S.G. (1984) *The Hardy Executive: Health Under Stress*. Homewood, IL: Dow Jones-Irwin.

Marteau, T.M. and Johnston, M. (1990) 'Health professionals: a source of variance in health outcomes'. *Psychology and Health* 5: 47–58.

Mechanic, D. (1962) *Students under Stress: A Study in the Social Psychology of Adaptation*. Glencoe, IL: Free Press.

Melzack, R. and Wall, P.D. (1965) 'Pain mechanisms: a new theory'. *Science* **150**: 971–9.

NHS Centre for Reviews and Dissemination (1997) *Systematic Review of Interventions in the Treatment and Prevention of Obesity.* York: University of York.

Oakley, A., Fullerton, D., Holland, J. et al. (1995) 'Sexual health education interventions for young people: a methodological review'. *British Medical Journal* **310**: 158–62.

Ogden, J. (2003) *The Psychology of Eating: From Healthy to Disordered Behaviour.* Oxford: Blackwell.

Olivera, S.A., Ellison, R.C., Moore, L.L. et al. (1992) 'Parent–child relationships in nutrient intake: the Framingham children's study'. *American Journal of Clinical Nutrition* **56**: 593–8.

Pennebaker, J. (1982) *The Psychology of Physical Symptoms.* New York: Springer Verlag.

Petrie, K.J., Cameron, L.D., Ellis, C.J. et al. (2002) 'Changing illness perceptions after myocardial infraction: an early intervention randomized controlled trial'. *Psychosomatic Medicine* **64**: 580–6.

Povey, R., Conner, M., Sparks, P. et al. (2000) 'The theory of planned behaviour and healthy eating: examining additive and moderating effects of social influence variables'. *Psychology and Health* **14**: 991–1006.

Prochaska, J.O. and DiClemente, C.C.D. (1982) 'Transtheoretical therapy: toward a more integrative model of change'. *Psychotherapy: Theory Research and Practice* **19**: 276–88.

Quine, L., Rutter, D.R. and Arnold, L. (2001) 'Persuading school-age cyclist to use safety helmets: effectiveness of an intervention based on the theory of planned behaviour'. *British Journal of Health Psychology* **6**: 327–45.

Rogers, R.W. (1983) Cognitive and physiological processes in fear appeals and attitude change: a revised theory of protection motivation, in J.R. Cacioppo and I.M. Rosenstock (1966) 'Why people use health services'. *Millbank Memorial Fund Ouarterly* **44**: 94–124.

Roth, H.P. (1979) Problems in conducting a study of the effects of patient compliance of teaching the rationale for antacid therapy, in S.J. Cohen (ed.) *New Directions in Patient Compliance.* Lexington, MA: Lexington Books, pp. 111–26.

Ruble, D.N. (1977) 'Premenstrual symptoms: a reinterpretation'. *Science* **197**: 291–2.

Sternbach, R.A., Wolf, S.R., Murphy, R.W. and Akeson, W.H. (1973) 'Traits of pain patients: the low back "loser"'. *Psychosomatics* **14**: 226–9.

Sutton, S. (2002) Using social cognition models to develop health behaviour interventions: problems and assumptions, in D. Rutter and L. Quine (eds) *Changing Health Behaviour: Intervention and Research with Social Cognition Models.* Buckingham: Open University Press, pp. 193–208.

Taylor, S.E. (1983) 'Adjustment to threatening events: a theory of cognitive adaptation'. *American Psychologist* **38**: 1161–73.

Trostle, J.A. (1988) 'Medical compliance as an ideology'. *Social Science and Medicine* 27: 1299–308.

Turk, D. and Rennert, K. (1981) Pain and the terminally ill cancer patient: a cognitive social learning perspective, in H. Sobel (ed.) *Behaviour Therapy in Terminal Care*. Cambridge, MA: Ballinger.

Turk, D.C., Wack, J.T. and Kerns, R.D. (1985) 'An empirical examination of the 'pain-behaviour' construct'. *Journal of Behavioral Medicine* 8: 119–30.

Wallston, K.A. and Wallston, B.S. (1982) Who is responsible for your health? The construct of health locus of control, in G.S. Sanders and J. Suls (eds) *Social Psychology of Health and Illness*. Hillsdale, NJ: Laurence Erlbaum, pp. 65–95.

Weinman, J., Petrie, K.J., Moss-Morris, R. and Horne, R. (1996) 'The Illness Perception Questionnaire: a new method for assessing the cognitive representation of illness'. *Psychology and Health* 11: 431–46.

Weinstein, N. (1984) 'Why it won't happen to me: perceptions of risk factors and susceptibility'. *Health Psychology* 3: 431–57.

Weinstein, N. (1987) 'Unrealistic optimism about illness susceptibility: conclusions from a community-wide sample'. *Journal of Behavioural Medicine* 10: 481–500.

Weller, S.S. (1984) 'Cross cultural concepts of illness: variables and validation'. *American Anthropologist* 86: 341–51.

Cultural and anthropological studies

LEARNING OUTCOMES

This chapter will enable readers to:

- Understand what is meant by culture and how it can be applied to health

- Gain an overview of the discipline and development of cultural studies, including its theoretical and methodological approaches

- Reflect upon the insights that cultural studies can give to our understanding of health, illness and healthcare

Overview

Health and illness are commonly defined in biological terms but can also be seen as being shaped by culture – a system of shared meanings, experiences and practices. Culture is reflected in the customs and areas of knowledge of social life, including religion, ethnicity, diet and dress. Cultural studies is a relatively new field that adopts a multidisciplinary approach to the study of culture, drawing on insights from anthropology, sociology, communication studies, literature and the visual arts among others. This chapter illustrates how cultural studies can be applied to health practices and illness behaviours. Ethnic beliefs, customs and traditions relating to health are explored. Lay knowledge and beliefs regarding health and illness, and their relationship to medical discourses, are used to illustrate the complexity and diversity of cultural concepts of health and illness. Official and unofficial representations of health in the media are compared and contrasted. The contribution to cultural studies of different methodological approaches, including ethnography, discourse analysis and semiotics, is discussed. The chapter concludes with a case study exploring the cultural significance of different forms of infant feeding.

Introduction

Culture is a central concept of cultural studies, yet also one of the most contested. Ideas of culture derive from a range of disciplines and perspectives. Perhaps the most familiar concept comes to us from the arts and literature, in which culture is seen as representing an elite form of knowledge and artistry. Within cultural studies, however, it is the social dimension of culture that is often seen as most significant. Cultures are systems of shared meanings, representations and practices that comprise the whole of social life. Thus, cultural manifestations may be found in religious beliefs, ethnic identity, diet, dress, leisure, codes of behaviour and systems of knowledge. Culture is the way in which we make sense of the world:

> To some extent, culture can be seen as an inherited 'lens', through which the individual perceives and understands the world ... and learns how to live within it. Growing up within any society is a form of enculturation, whereby the individual slowly acquires the cultural 'lens' of that society. (Helman, 2000, p. 2)

Every object, action and person is assigned a meaning by us as we try to interpret our encounters and fit them into a unifying framework. The study of culture is thus the study of signification: we examine and deconstruct what certain cultural practices or objects signify.

Certain ideas and representations can become dominant in society, particularly if they are disseminated through the mass media. It would, however, be far too simplistic to portray cultural ideals as being unanimously held: culture should not be understood as a homogeneous entity.

The contribution of cultural studies and anthropology to health studies

Cultural studies is a relatively new discipline. However, the study of culture is also the principal focus of anthropology, which has a much longer history. In the past, anthropology tended to be associated with nineteenth-century colonialism and a somewhat voyeuristic focus on other cultures. As Russell and Edgar (1998, p. 3) describe, it was traditionally 'the study of "exotic" peoples in "other" places'. Contemporary anthropology is a more wide-ranging and reflexive discipline, which studies culture in many settings, from the unusual to the familiar. While the general meaning of anthropology is the study of humanity, it has several specialisms. Medical anthropology in particular has made an important contribution to understandings of health. The main focus of medical anthropology is seeking to explain people's ideas and behaviour in relation to health by examining the influence of their culture. It does so by exploring the relationship between the biological and the social. However, ideas about health and illness inevitably are linked to wider cultural beliefs and influences. As such, the anthropological approach is holistic. It also stresses understanding cultures from within, that is, studying them in their own terms as opposed to measuring them against a different cultural standard.

If culture shapes how we interpret the world, then health and illness are part of this process of finding meaning. Adopting this approach to health makes certain issues of interest:

● who is classed as healthy and who is classed as ill

● how we feel and describe symptoms

● how we seek help and from whom

● whether an illness is seen as stigmatizing

● how identity is linked to health

● how illness is treated

● how people adapt to changed bodies or circumstances as a result of illness.

These forms of knowledge may be hierarchical. One way of understanding health and illness may be considered less legitimate within one group than another. For example, lay people's ideas of what counts as healthy eating may have less authority than the views of health professionals, who have taken on the beliefs of a distinctive culture of learning and practice in the course of their medical training. Culture can thus be seen as linked to power. This is also evident in the fact that lay people's ideas, across a range of cultures within a society, are likely to reflect dominant ideas to some extent. The cultural ideas of specific groups seldom constitute a wholly separate system, but take elements of the dominant culture and interweave them with alternate beliefs. An example of this could be someone who combines the use of complementary medicine with mainstream treatments.

Dominant ideas of health and healthcare are that they are scientific and primarily rooted in biological fact; medicine and healthcare have tended not to be seen as culturally determined. The exception is research into the health and cultural beliefs of ethnic minority groups in which minority cultures have been represented as faulty for supporting health practices not in keeping with Western norms (Ahmad, 1996).

Yet culture embraces the whole of our social life and systems of knowledge, including knowledge relating to health and healthcare. Information on health comes to us via numerous sources apart from the medical profession, such as our families and friends, literature, the media, self-help groups and the internet. Health is not only a property of our bodies, but also an item of **consumption**. Many products, from sportswear and slimming aids to organic foods and water filters, are marketed as 'healthy' or 'healthier'. These products not only reflect our current conceptions of health, but also help to create new beliefs and ideas. Our health, illnesses and lifestyles cannot be divorced from the culture within which we live.

Cultural studies focuses on the importance of culture in defining ourselves, our bodies and our identities. In contrast to Marxist perspectives, which state that culture is produced from economic structures, some cultural studies' theorists argue that culture should be seen more as autonomous and dynamic. **Structuralists** such as de Saussure (1960) and Lévi-Strauss (1970) focus on the ways in which meaning is socially created, especially through language. From de Saussure's perspective, different languages share the essential quality of ordering the world into interrelated categories. Thus, language orders our conceptual understanding of the world. Lévi-Strauss applied this idea of conceptual structure to all cultural practices, such as kinship networks, cooking and myths:

> All cultures make sense of the world, and while the meanings that they make of it may be specific to them, the ways by which they make those meanings are not; they are universal. Meanings are culture-specific, but the ways of making them are universal to all human beings. (Fiske, 1990, p. 116)

For Lévi-Strauss, the fundamental contribution of language was the construction of binary oppositions: the division of the world into two categories that are mutually dependent on one another for their meaning, for example hot and cold. Health and disease can also be understood as binary oppositions. Concepts that defy being placed into oppositional categories, possessing characteristics that blur the boundary, are termed 'anomalous categories'. When these categories are seen as being too disturbing to established social knowledge, they become the subject of taboos. Thus, Lévi-Strauss argued that homosexuality was seen as taboo because it undermined gender identity. The category in which someone is placed, such as mentally ill/physically ill or able bodied/disabled, may have profound consequences for how people perceive themselves and how they are treated. Transitions between one category and another, such as deciding when someone is officially well, are also socially significant and culturally specific (Helman, 2000, p. 2).

Postmodernists argue that, in our postindustrial world, identities and ideas proliferate to create a pluralistic society. Pluralism means that there is a variety of subcultures and groups, each of which is valid. **Postmodernism** rejects the grand narratives of perspectives such as Marxism that seek to explain society by reference to a unifying underlying set of ideas (Doyle, 1995). The modernist concept of linear progress is dismissed, as is the search for an ultimate objective truth such as economic determinism. Within a postmodern world, traditional sources of solidarity and **identity** become dislocated. As family and working structures fragment, we are left without easy certainties. Geographic or social class location, for example, will not be sufficient to give us a central, lifelong identity. In this context, the **body** can act as a source of identity, giving a stability that we lack from other sources. The pursuit of a certain look, level of fitness or lifestyle can all be ways for us to define ourselves; they are not simply reflections of whether we are ill or healthy.

CONNECTIONS

Chapter 4 also discusses structuralist and postmodern perspectives on society and social roles. It explains contemporary critiques in sociology including the focus on embodiment and the meanings attached to our corporeal selves.

Postmodernity is characterized by a plurality of **discourses**. An extreme form of this view is very relativist, and any boundaries between high and low, good or bad are rejected. No forms of knowledge or belief are superior, they are simply different. So a doctor's knowledge of a medical condition is not intrinsically more valid than a lay person's, and biomedicine is not more grounded in 'reality' than homeopathy. All knowledge and practice must be understood within discourse and culture: there is no external or absolute reality that can be known. There are also less extreme forms of postmodernist perspectives, for example the acknowledgement that there are incontrovertible biological aspects of health and illness, but that these are mediated and made meaningful through social processes.

Cultural practices in relation to health

Contemporary concerns are particularly focused on the relationship between lifestyles and health, and lifestyles derive – at least in part – from cultural beliefs. In order to understand why individuals eat certain foods, take exercise or drink too much, we need to see these activities as everyday cultural practices and look at their meanings.

Usually people are not consciously aware of carrying out cultural practices. Activities and behaviour simply feel normal or 'common sense'. While many everyday activities have a bearing on health, individuals may not interpret them in this way or have thoughts of health uppermost in their minds. As Bury (2005, p. 8) notes: 'Health risks vie with the routine nature of daily life, with its own pressures and pleasures, constraints and potentialities.'

Putting extra blankets on a baby may not be just to stop the baby getting cold, but because it is an outward show of our caring, and loving parenting is an important cultural value. However, this practice may put babies at higher risk of sudden infant death syndrome (SIDS), and runs counter to official advice (Directgov, 2007). Practices such as sunbathing or using tanning equipment are carried out because of a cultural preference for tanned skin, although this may have damaging implications for health in the form of promoting melanoma.

Cultural practices can be deeply embedded in social groups and are a vital part of the expression of identity. They can also be highly resistant to change. Health promotion activities, either at the individual or collective level, are unlikely to be successful if they simply exhort people to live more healthily and fail to engage with the meanings behind cultural practices. For example, the food choices that people make are often circumscribed not only by material factors such as cost and accessibility, but also by ideas of tradition or emotional significance.

Example 6.1

FOOD AS CULTURE

Food is never 'just food' and its significance can never be purely nutritional. Furthermore, it is intimately bound up with social relations, including those of power, of inclusion and exclusion, as well as cultural ideas about classification (including food and non-food, the edible and the inedible), the human body and the meaning of health. (Caplan, 1997, p. 3)

One of the most powerful ways in which food is intertwined with culture is through the family. The rise in family diversity, brought about by factors such as a higher divorce rate, cohabitation, lone parenthood and same-sex relationships, has led many to decry the demise of the 'traditional' nuclear, patriarchal family, This social anxiety is exemplified in the concern that the family meal, when the whole family sits down to eat together, is under threat. The supposed downfall of this ritual has been linked to a rise in the consumption of unhealthy food. Murcott (1997) argues that the notion that families always ate together in the past is an idealized one: upper-class families, for example, tended to separate adults and children, so that children would eat either in the nursery or at boarding schools away from home. Murcott traces concerns about the decline in the family meal to the earlier part of the twentieth century, arguing that this is a recurrent metaphor for the state of the family.

The shared meal has come to signify the ideal family. Symbolic meals, such as Sunday dinner, acquire great importance. The roles that family members take within this meal communicate their position. In the UK, the husband traditionally carves the meat, displaying his authority and role as provider. The woman is placed in the subject position of wife and mother by cooking a meal, while the children are placed as dependants, the grateful recipients of their parents' care. This family ideal remains the dominant model, although it faces continual challenges from the growth in family diversity.

Food has traditionally been used as a marker of cultural identity: 'Simple equations such as 'we eat meat, they don't' ... affirm, in shared patterns of consumption and shared notions of edibility, our difference from others' (James, 1997). James (2004) studied the food choices of African-Americans, a group who are at particularly high risk of conditions such as obesity and diabetes. Aspects of poor diet among this group include consuming foods high in fat, calories and sodium, while eating insufficient quantities of fruit, vegetables and high-fibre foods (DHHS, 2000 in James, 2004). However, these choices are not simply made in wilful disregard of healthy eating messages. Food is an essential part of a cultural identity. In the case of African-Americans, diet reflects the history of a group who were shaped by slavery and segregation. Food is also a large part of family gatherings, where providing or asking for 'healthy' as opposed to more traditional food could be seen as rude. James (2004, p. 357) illustrates this with a quote from one of her participants:

I tried to tell my dad that if we have beans and rice, we don't need to eat meat because the beans already have the protein. He didn't like that and I still had to get up and fix him some meat.

Participants in James's study felt that relinquishing their customary foods was also relinquishing their cultural heritage and acquiescing to the dominant culture. There was thus considerable reluctance to give up food choices, coupled with difficulties such as the expense of healthier alternatives.

Notions of what comprises British food can be seen as ways of identifying and placing oneself in the world, just as we may categorize ourselves as members of communities or workplaces. However, just as some of these traditional sources of identity begin to break down into multiple possibilities, so British food has become subject to tremendous diversity. James points out that a new trend is occurring in British eating habits, namely 'food Creolization', in which hybrid dishes evolve. However, class differences in the type of food eaten persist, the middle and upper classes tending to shun Creolization in favour of authentic cooking, either British or foreign. Similarly, the British preoccupation with food as an easily prepared necessity continues.

Sources: Caplan, 1997; James, 1997, 2004; Murcott, 1997

Food is intimately related to identity and social relations rather than purely nutrition. Strategies to promote healthier diets are therefore directly attempting to refashion cultural practices. Success is more likely if the context of these practices is understood and acknowledged than if it is denied. Adapting a diet to maximize its positive elements and minimize negative ones is more likely to result in change rather than pursuing a prescriptive and culturally insensitive approach.

Health and illness across cultures

One of the clearest ways of demonstrating the importance of the relationship between health, illness and culture is to examine variations in beliefs across groups. The dominance of biomedicine within Western societies tends to suggest that health and illness are natural, universal phenomena and the body simply a biological entity. Yet understandings can vary both across and within cultures and societies. Health and illness are culturally specific concepts and experiences, so must be understood from *within* cultures.

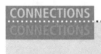

CONNECTIONS

Chapters 1 and 2 explain the nature and development of the Cartesisan dualism separating mind and body within Western science and philosophy.

There are many cultures within the boundaries of a wider society; these may gain their cultural identity from a number of factors, such as class, region, gender or ethnicity. Ethnicity has most commonly been associated with cultural beliefs and practices but it is not the only basis for the identification of a cultural grouping.

CONNECTIONS

Chapter 4 discusses the ways in which ethnicity and race have been used to classify populations and examines the reasons why ethnicity is strongly associated with poor health status and access to health services.

The relationships between ethnicity and culture are seldom straightforward or simplistic:

- Members of an ethnic group will not necessarily share a single culture

- Not all members will adhere strictly to specific cultural or religious beliefs, for example some Muslims drink alcohol

- Cultural beliefs may not necessarily be the overriding factor in decisions and understandings about health

- What a person believes may not always dictate what they do in practice.

? Ahmad (1996, p. 215) argues that culture needs to be treated as a set of 'flexible guidelines' that influence behaviour rather than as something that determines actions and outlook. Why might this be the case and what are the implications for professional practice?

There are numerous ways in which ethnicity may influence belief and practice in relation to health and illness. For example, different ethnic groups may have different forms of self-care activity and use different remedies if ill. A variety of herbal or other forms of traditional remedies may be used, either in conjunction with Western medicine or instead of it. Treatment of illness is often dependent on assumptions about its causes. Very different explanatory models may be used, linking illness to a variety of internal, external or social factors. Many cultures would attribute forms of illness not to disease agents, but to the evil eye, in various manifestations. In Italy, for example, amulets may be worn to combat the evil eye (Spector, 2004, p. 79). Illness attributable to such forces, including witchcraft or voodoo, is avoided by certain forms of behaviour, such as taking care not to antagonize practitioners.

Illnesses may not be defined and understood in the same way as Western conceptualizations that are rooted in biology. Kaur (1996 in Dein, 2006) notes that there are several languages that do not contain a word for cancer. Cancer may be classified as another kind of illness or as separate illnesses, depending on their site of occurrence.

Example 6.2

CULTURAL PERCEPTIONS OF MENTAL HEALTH

Mental illnesses are conceptualized differently across cultures. Pote and Orrell (2002) have explored perceptions in relation to schizophrenia, a diagnosis that is frequently open to dispute and contestation. They asked their sample, taken from 13 broad categories of ethnicity, to rate different symptoms in terms of how indicative they were of mental illness. Significant differences were that hallucinatory behaviour and suspiciousness were less likely to be seen as signs of being mentally ill by Bangladeshis, whereas Afro-Caribbeans were less likely to see unusual thought content in these terms. Ethnicity emerged as the most significant predictor of these differences between perceptions, but other factors such as religion, education, sex and contact with people with mental health problems were also influential.

Source: Pote and Orrell, 2002

Reactions to illness or disability may also vary in terms of fatalism or emotional response. Katbamna et al.'s (2000) research involving people from British south Asian communities identified both similarities and differences in attitudes to disability between the communities and in relation to white groups. For example, while stigmatizing disability is widespread, they found that female carers who were Pakistani Muslim or Gujurati Hindu were most likely to feel that they were being blamed for producing a disabled child. A common preoccupation was that disclosing disability would negatively affect marriage prospects, particularly in the case of arranged marriages. Hindus and Sikhs were more likely to perceive disability as karma and hence to struggle with the notion of being punished. Caring responsibilities were even more heavily gendered than among most white ethnic groups in Britain.

Medical practitioners therefore need to be sensitive to the various ways in which health and illness are interpreted by different ethnic groups, without separating culture from the wider social framework.

Example 6.3

MEANINGS OF HYPERTENSION

A study was carried out largely in response to concerns expressed by a GP relating to difficulties he experienced in communicating information about hypertension and its treatment regimen to his Afro-Caribbean patients, a group with a higher than average incidence of the condition.

Morgan (1996) found that Afro-Caribbean patients had a greater tendency not to take prescribed medication, often preferring to use familiar herbal remedies. This group found the commonness of this condition among family and friends to be a reassuring indication of normality, rather than seeing a high incidence as being illustrative of elevated risk. Among both groups, there was a relatively low level of awareness that hypertension and high blood pressure were one and the same thing. Several respondents understood hypertension to be a nervous condition relating to stress. This reiterates the fact that different groups may understand diseases differently. Medical discourse provides forms of knowledge and language that are not universally shared by lay groups.

One factor that did vary between ethnic groups was that Afro-Caribbeans were more likely to identify strokes as a dangerous outcome, whereas white males highlighted heart conditions. Each group thus correctly identified the risk to which it was most likely to be exposed. Afro-Caribbeans, however, tended to take a more fatalistic approach, which appeared to increase acceptance and reduce anxiety. Thus, whereas Morgan identifies some differences in perception relating to hypertension between white and Afro-Caribbean people, she also draws out a number of similarities that characterize lay understanding as opposed to medical interpretation.

Source: Morgan, 1996

While cultural studies as a discipline has only recently focused specifically on health, there are many studies of health and culture that have sought to explain 'bad' health and health behaviours in a simplistic manner as a result of culture. What cultural studies can contribute to this debate is a challenge to such notions, highlighting the interplay between culture, resistance, power and inequality within society.

The role of traditional healers illustrates what can be a negative response by a biomedical healthcare system to aspects of traditional cultures. Traditional healing includes many different approaches. For example, Catholics associate different saints with different ailments, such as St Vitus (epilepsy), or may undertake pilgrimages to holy sites such as Lourdes to pray for healing. The phrase 'traditional healer' (TH) is commonly used to describe someone who seeks to heal the sick using methods and a belief system outside Western biomedicine.

Healers may have different origins. They may be religious figures, have undergone special training or be regarded as wise women, for example. They may be purely secular technicians skilled in a particular aspect of care, like childbirth, or they may draw on sacred knowledge. Often their approach is characterized as much by a different relationship with the person seeking help as by the belief system under which they practise. This is indicated in Table 6.1, which compares the role of a medical professional in the US to that of a traditional healer.

Table 6.1 Traditional homeopathic healer compared with modern allopathic physician

Healer	Physician
Maintains informal, friendly, affective relationship with the entire family	Businesslike, formal relationship; deals only with the patient
Comes to the house day or night	Patient must go to the physician's office or clinic, and only during the day; may have to wait for hours to be seen; home visits are rarely, if ever, made
For diagnosis, consults with head of house, creates a mood of awe, talks to all family members, is not authoritarian, has social rapport, builds expectation of cure	Rest of family usually ignored; deals solely with the ill person and may deal only with the sick part of the person; authoritarian manner creates fear
Generally less expensive than the physician	More expensive than the healer
Has ties to the 'world of the sacred'; has rapport with the symbolic, spiritual, creative or holy force	Secular; pays little attention to the religious beliefs or meaning of a given illness
Shares the world view of the patient, that is, speaks the same language, lives in the same neighbourhood, or in some similar socioeconomic conditions; may know the same people; understands the lifestyle of the patient	Generally does not share the world view of the patient, that is, may not speak the same language, live in the same neighbourhood, or understand the socioeconomic conditions; may not understand the lifestyle of the patient

Source: Spector, 2004, p. 118

CONNECTIONS

Chapter 1 describes the features of biomedicine and its scientific processes of investigation in contrast to these forms of care that do not separate mind from body.

These properties of THs can also be seen in societies where there is little access to Western-style healthcare. In sub-Saharan Africa, for example, the majority of the rural population are excluded from healthcare provision due to travel, costs and lack of services. In these circumstances, the role of THs is crucial. Baskind and Birbeck (2005) studied how THs provide care for people with epilepsy (PWE) in Zambia. In this area, epilepsy is a highly stigmatizing condition that can undermine social networks and employability, leading to great disadvantage. THs are usually the main source of care. A notable feature of their involvement is that they focus on the PWE's individual and social circumstances, contextualizing the disease, and providing causal explanations. Taking a detailed personal and medical history is a central part of their approach, and underscores the fact that they share a conceptual and social framework with the person consulting them. Baskind and Birbeck found that there is a high correlation between the THs' accounts of the symptoms of epilepsy and those recognized by modern medicine. However, there is divergence over causality. THs see witchcraft as the underlying cause of epilepsy, although this may operate alongside other factors. Treatment involves providing an antidote, often using ingredients thought to have been used in the original witchcraft. There is also a role for 'immunizing' family members, as the seizures are thought to be contagious via bodily fluids. If treatment fails, PWEs might be referred to other, more powerful healers, or to hospitals, which are seen as able to mobilize specific treatments effectively. Baskind and Birbeck point out that there can be harmful consequences of care from THs. Treatment may be ineffective or dangerous, and fees can be expensive. Nevertheless, there can be significant benefits:

> If a healer's treatment allows the family members of a PWE no longer to fear contagion, perhaps the family is more willing to assist the PWE when they experience seizures … In addition, after a first seizure, some individuals worry constantly about the possibility of another seizure. Many will never have a second seizure, or the next seizure will not occur for months or years … Perhaps the TH's ritual treatment alleviates this worry and allows the person to return to the social fold as 'normal'. At times, the THs seem to function as the community's moral conscience – pointing out broken taboos and violated norms. (Baskind and Birbeck, 2005, p. 1125)

? **Should traditional healers be included in the management and treatment of conditions such as HIV/AIDS?**

THs can retain a powerful role in contemporary healthcare, either because there is no readily accessible alternative or because they offer a personalized service that is compatible with the patient's conceptual framework. Medical professionals need to acknowledge the role that THs play in different societies, as they may well be involved in shared care.

Lay knowledge and beliefs

There are three sectors of knowledge and belief about health (Kleinman, 1980):

- The professional sector refers to orthodox Western medicine
- The alternative sector refers to beliefs about health that stem from other medical traditions, such as folk medicine or complementary therapies
- The lay sector represents the general public or patients, notably someone who is not a professional.

There has often been a tendency to devalue lay understandings as being an inaccurate version of medical expertise.

THINKING
ABOUT

Think about someone you know with a long-standing condition. Do you think they have expert knowledge about it?

In recent years, people with long-standing conditions or disabilities have come to be seen as experts on their experiences, in a way that medical professionals, lacking personal knowledge, can never hope to emulate. The terms 'lay knowledge' and 'lay expert' have been used to denote authority. Prior (2003), however, claims that it is misleading to use the idea of the lay expert. He argues that lay people may have a highly developed awareness of living with and managing illness, but they lack the technical medical knowledge that is acquired through professional education and training. Nevertheless, there is an increased emphasis on harnessing lay experiences within orthodox medicine; this is one way in which a blurring of the boundaries between the different sectors identified by Kleinman (1980) is occurring.

CONNECTIONS

Chapter 3 discusses the emergence of a 'lay epidemiology' in which the information collected by members of the public has been used to profile diseases or conditions.

Evidence of the recognition now afforded to lay understandings is provided in initiatives such as the expert patient programme (DoH, 2001). This approach seeks to encourage self-management programmes among patients who experience chronic, long-term conditions. It recognizes that living with conditions such as rheumatoid arthritis, diabetes or epilepsy involves the development of day-to-day strategies to cope with issues such as pain, fatigue and poor sleep. The illness may also have adverse consequences, such as disruption to employment prospects or an impact on other family members. In the absence of a cure, often the best approach is developing coping strategies to minimize the problems associated with the illness. This may entail identifying effective ways of dealing with diet, exercise, energy levels or social situations.

Approaches such as the expert patient programme seek to capitalize on the growth of lay self-help groups. Kelleher (1994) identifies various ways in which such groups operate, from being focused on members to heightening public awareness, fund-raising and repositioning specific medical conditions or social groups higher on the political agenda. Self-help groups also vary in their relationship to medical professionals: some operate hand in hand, others occupy a complementary role, and others are more directly challenging.

One recurring feature of self-help groups is their emphasis on the emotional experience of illness, which is often ignored by medical professionals, who focus purely on clinical factors. This represents differing interpretations of the *meaning* of illness.

THINKING ABOUT

Have you been part of a self-help group? What support did you hope it would provide?

There has been extensive research into lay constructions of health and illness. Blaxter's (1990) study found five common concepts of health:

1. *Health as not ill:* health as the absence of symptoms or medical input. This concept meant that some people with ongoing conditions were still able to define themselves as healthy. It was more commonly used by people in good health than those in bad health.

2. *Health as physical fitness:* usually associated with having energy and being fit; most used by younger men.

3. *Health as social relationships:* associated with maintaining one's social role and network; used more frequently by women than men.

4. *Health as function:* being able to carry out tasks and activities: often employed by older people of both sexes.

5. *Health as psychosocial wellbeing:* health as a mental state of wellbeing. While it was the commonest definition, it was less used by young men and most used by those from higher occupational groups.

What is evident from these concepts is that their use is shaped, although not dictated, by membership of different social groups stratified by a range of factors. Whether someone considers themselves to be healthy, and what this idea of healthy means, is thus variable.

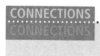

CONNECTIONS

Chapter 5 explores the attributions that people have for the causes of their illness.

Medical professionals and lay people may therefore:

● Define health differently

● Have different causal explanations for illness

● Have different understandings of risk

● Have different priorities when controlling illness – perhaps not rating medical compliance as foremost over social obligations or employment (Kelleher, 1994).

Example 6.4

THE MENOPAUSE AND HORMONE REPLACEMENT THERAPY: UNDERSTANDINGS OF RISK

Women's attitudes to risk are shaped by a number of factors, including:

- personal experiences and histories
- core beliefs about illness
- construct of being a woman
- ideas about concepts such as fatalism and control.

Risks were given meaning by placing knowledge, context and presentation against personal experience and core beliefs. The patient's perspective thus varies markedly from the medical perspective which views risk in terms of numerical descriptions. (Walter and Britten, 2002, p. 584)

Medical assessment of risks in relation to treatments like HRT need to be communicated to patients in ways that are meaningful. For example, risks could be related to other familiar processes such as antenatal care or the use of contraceptives. Risk assessment in antenatal care is often individualized, for example a woman will be given her own risk of having a child with Down syndrome. Walter and Britten's (2002) study suggests that general risk information is less easy for people to relate to. They recommend that medical practitioners ask patients about their attitudes to and experiences of risk, as well as about their symptoms. This would enable them to personalize and communicate information more effectively.

CONNECTIONS

Chapter 5 discusses the ways in which patients experience pain, showing that its physiological cause may be mediated by psychological elements such as anxiety or distraction.

Communication of pain between patient and medical professional is not a simple exchange of information. It is mediated by many factors, including the cultural repertoire of understandings available to each, the explanatory models used, the expectations of how they think the other party is behaving or interpreting behaviour, and personal responses to pain. There can be differences in reactions to and expressions of pain, emotion or stoicism across different ethnic groups (Davidhizar and Giger, 2004).

Example 6.5

ACCOUNTS OF PAIN

While there are many aspects of illness that can be observed or measured, this is not always the case. Even aspects that can be rendered visible to the medical gaze require interpretation. In addition, there are symptoms and experiences associated with illness that cannot easily be quantified by an observer and medical practitioners rely on patients' accounts. One example of this is pain. It is possible to observe physical trauma that would be assumed to cause pain, such as

injuries, but some episodes of pain may be unexplained. This means that practitioners may judge a person's pain on several levels:

- as part of a diagnostic process
- in terms of whether it seems a plausible reflection of their physical condition
- whether it is being expressed at a level they consider reasonable in view of their expectations.

One important issue that shapes the communication of pain is the fact that pain can be perceived in moral terms; to express too much pain, particularly if it does not match a medical professional's assessment of symptoms, can lead to assumptions of malingering, deceit or exaggeration. May et al. (1999) discuss attitudes surrounding chronic lower back pain (CLBP), a widely experienced condition that is often difficult to attribute to a specific observable cause. This has led to suspicion regarding the integrity of patients complaining of CLBP. The authors discuss various historical shifts in perceptions, from the construction of 'railway spine' in the nineteenth century (when it was assumed that damage to the back was claimed in order to receive compensation from the railway companies), to the notion of hysteria, which was linked to Freud's theories among others, and established the idea that back pain could be a neurotic and somatic symptom rather than a physical problem. May et al. comment that a divide began to be constructed between 'real', that is, organic, pain and 'untrustworthy' pain that could not as easily be explained. This divide has continued to be reflected in contemporary attitudes to CLBP, as demonstrated by the extract below:

- The patient expresses symptoms of pain and fatigue; these are formulated in terms of biomechanical degeneration or exhaustion of functional performance and are undoubtedly *real* experiences. The patient interprets these within a strict 'biomedical' model of organic cause and expects the clinician to act upon this basis.

- The clinician investigates potential organic cause, discounts the presence of sinister pathological signs and interprets expressed symptoms in the context of a psychosocial model. The patient understands this as casting doubt upon the *reality* of embodied experiences and is demoralized and dissatisfied. Both parties are ultimately pessimistic about the extent to which the other is 'willing' to hear their interpretation of expressed symptoms. (May et al., 1999, p. 530)

Representations of health

One of the most important arenas in which we can observe the cultural properties of health is that of the media. Cultural studies makes a valuable contribution to our analysis of how messages on health are formulated, interpreted and exchanged. The mass media helps us to make sense of the world by shaping our common-sense, cultural ideas and interpretation of the world. Russell and Edgar (1998, p. 4) state: 'Representations, linguistically and symbolically codified, are seen as creating social reality rather than just reflecting it.'

Ideas about health are conveyed through two channels:

- official channels, which refer to the sphere of public health and health information

- non-official channels, which refer to discourses concerning health within popular culture.

These channels are not discrete but overlap.

Public health and health promotion

This broad field includes concepts of health and illness contained within policy documents, public health initiatives, health promotion initiatives and publicity campaigns by charities. In many ways, public health campaigns resemble advertising: they are designed to sell us an idea of good health and the means of achieving it.

 Why is it more difficult to 'sell' health in a public information campaign than to advertise a commercial product?

The differences between selling health in a public information campaign and advertising a commercial product are summarized in Table 6.2.

Table 6.2 Selling health in a public information campaign and advertising a commercial product

Public information campaign	Commercial marketing of a product
The aim is to effect fundamental behavioural changes among a large section of the population	The aim is to effect a small change in behaviour, such as brand-switching, among a section of the market
The budget is likely to be limited	The budget may be considerable
Market research is likely to be limited	Market research is likely to be detailed
It may be perceived as unethical to oversell potential gains from following advice	Exaggerated claims may be made, albeit within legal standards
The rewards for acquiescence may not be immediate	The rewards of consumption are perceived as being immediate

Health and popular culture

Health issues appear in popular culture in different ways, including:

- press reports, which may be based on official government pronouncements
- medical advisory columns
- television dramas.

The media act as gatekeepers of the public's awareness, reporting material that is deemed to be most interesting, most important or likely to increase circulation or viewing figures. Oinas (1998) presents an analysis of how medical advisory columns promote a medicalized construction of menstrua-

internet use is linked to specific conditions and complements more traditional sources, such as medical professionals, rather than representing an alternative perspective. Their research indicates that people who use internet health sites are aware of the potential for risk in terms of the trustworthiness of information. However, they tended to see this as a general risk and one to which they themselves would not fall prey. Nettleton et al. (2005) see the convergence of information as representing a form of third way between the idea of the internet as liberating people from the constraints of medical discourse and the idea that it conveys damaging and incorrect messages.

Reporting of diseases in the media tends to draw on a familiar stock of metaphors and imagery. Often these involve military language, in which diseases are characterized as invaders, while people with illnesses are portrayed as battling them bravely. Another common image is that of plague.

Example 6.7

SARS IN THE MEDIA

An example of a disease that has received a high degree of coverage in recent years is severe acute respiratory syndrome (SARS). SARS attracted widespread attention and reporting in 2003 after the World Health Organization (WHO) sent out an international alert. Most cases were in China, although a number of other locations were affected. In the UK, newspaper coverage tended to vary between portraying the disease as a major threat or dismissing fears as an alarmist panic. The focus was strongly on any perceived threat to the UK. Two sets of metaphors were used: 'SARS as killer', with its brutal properties represented in terms like 'hit' and 'attack'; and 'Control', represented in terms like 'contain' and 'tackle', and institutional and bureaucratic responses (Wallis and Nerlich, 2005, p. 2632). The lack of war metaphors contrasts with reporting in countries where the threat was more immediate, where they continued to feature heavily. War metaphors failed to gain ground as there was no sole country that could be identified as the prime site, the threat was distant, therefore the prime aim was to avoid panic, and there was no clear expectation of victory. In addition, the fact that the UK was involved in war in Iraq may have made militaristic metaphors less palatable.

Eichelberger (2007) identified a high level of blame and stigma directed at the

community of New York's Chinatown in 2003, despite the fact that there were no reported cases of SARS there. Media speculation on the likelihood of an epidemic led to a consequent drop in both tourism and business in Chinatown. Eichelberger argues that there was a high degree of 'othering' in media coverage. 'China was defined as a diseased threat to the modern healthy world' (Eichelberger, 2007). The remedy was for China to effect cultural change. Reportage in the US was heavily racialized, with frequent images of Asians wearing face masks, portraying Asians as a source of infection. Eichelberger notes that in the May 2003 edition of *Time* magazine, the only photos of Asians were included in the context of SARS stories.

In China where the majority of cases occurred, Zhang (2006) outlines how media coverage ranged from restrictive, in the early days of SARS cases, to overwhelming, when the number of cases rose dramatically. He notes that this has been credited with having a permanent impact on the nature of the media in China, which has traditionally been very secretive and subject to strong central control. In relation to TV coverage, he argues that while the frequency of reports increased, the content still reflected the continuing political status quo rather than signifying any wholesale shift in dominant discourses. The key current affairs programme in China concentrated on praising government officials for their handling of the situation. This contrasted with the alarmist tone of reporting in other countries far less affected by the disease, as in the UK's press use of 'killer' metaphors discussed above. Language used in the Chinese media was more moderate, and drew on military imagery to invoke feelings of solidarity and heroic struggle.

The differences in the representation of SARS show that even when dealing with a contagious disease that has the potential to cross boundaries swiftly, the meaning of the disease is still demonstrably a cultural product. As such, it is fluid and open to different interpretation in different contexts. Reporting of the disease was shaped by a number of factors:

- the previous cultural repertoire of disease imagery
- the political and international context
- ideas of blame or compassion for people with the disease
- the perceived level of risk
- a managerial approach to global problems.

Theoretical and methodological approaches

Cultural studies is interdisciplinary and draws on a vast framework of knowledge and approaches, including sociology, media studies, philosophy, literature, anthropology and the visual arts. Its outlook is above all that of a critical perspective. Cultural studies challenges the boundaries, status and concerns of many more rigidly defined fields of study. Thus, cultural studies can perhaps best be thought of as a 'cross-disciplinary and anti-disciplinary field as well as an intellectual movement' (Alasuutari et al., 1998). It is in some ways perhaps most easily characterized by its preoccupations, which centre around culture and meaning, and the complex power relations that shape them.

Many writers make a different claim for the origins of cultural studies. It has been variously traced back to Victorian observers such as Booth and Mayhew, to early US sociologists (Jenks, 1993) or, less traditionally, to the work in the 1970s of the Kamiriithu Community Education and Cultural Centre in Kenya (Wright, 1998). However, most accounts of the development of cultural studies cite the influence of three seminal figures and their works: Raymond Williams' *Culture and Society* (1961), E.P. Thompson's *The Making of the English Working Class* (1978/1963) and Richard Hoggart's *The Uses of Literacy* (1958) (Hall, 1980).

These authors, while divergent in their approaches and concerns, were notable for identifying and celebrating working-class culture. Hoggart became the first director of the Birmingham Centre for Contemporary

Cultural Studies, which is often credited as the academic grouping that consolidated the identity of cultural studies and provided the impetus for growth and expansion within universities across the world.

In theoretical terms, the key concept articulated by these authors was that culture began to be seen as a social feature that could not be reduced solely to a materialist base. This signalled a theoretical shift away from classical Marxism, which saw the whole of social life, and hence culture, as a product of the economic structure, designed to maintain and legitimate the status quo. It is here that the concept of **ideology** becomes central. From the classical Marxist perspective, ideological beliefs are often false: they serve to obscure the realization that society ultimately works in the best interests of the dominant classes.

Marxist analyses of the social structure remain a strong, if contested, influence within cultural studies. Few, however, now subscribe to the idea that all the features, beliefs and ideologies of a society are determined by its mode of production or economic organization. This shift away from reductionism is in part derived from the influence of the work of writers such as Althusser and Gramsci.

Althusser (1971) theorized that ideologies and cultures could be seen as having relative autonomy from the economic superstructure, and that all classes participated in the promotion and processes of ideology, rather than the dominant class imposing beliefs upon others. Ideological apparatuses, such as education, religion or the family, shape our cultural practices by means of rituals. One of the most pervasive mechanisms of ideology is that of 'interpellation', also referred to as 'hailing'. This concept refers to the fact that we are continuously placed in our subject positions, such as mothers, older people or patients, by the way in which we are addressed within different forms of communication.

? In what ways are people hailed or reaffirmed as patients within the healthcare system?

Doctor–patient relationships serve to reinforce the power of the medical professional over the lay person. The use of professional titles, coupled with the use of symbolic clothing such as white coats, serves to confirm the power of the expert. Thus, while this form of ideological practice and perpetuation is more subtle than Marx's concept of oppression, it still involves the collusion of all subjects in ideological dominance.

Gramsci (1971) suggests that for ideologies to become dominant (or hegemonic), they must continually struggle to reassert themselves through winning the consent of both individuals and institutions. When a system of beliefs becomes dominant, this is often achieved by such a high degree of consent that the beliefs become naturalized. The most powerful set of ideas are those which deny their ideological quality by portraying themselves as natural and 'true'. Thus, the biomedical model of health could be described as hegemonic in that it has become so firmly established that we see it as objective and rooted in the natural realm of biology.

Across a range of disciplines that explore the interface of culture and health, a variety of approaches that could be termed 'social constructionist' have taken hold, reflecting the influence of postmodernism discussed earlier in this chapter. Social constructionism (or social constructivism, as it is sometimes called) looks at ways in which our understanding of the world is shaped within specific societies. At one extreme, there are 'strong' versions of social constructionism that are very relativistic. At this end of the spectrum, nothing has any objective reality, not even the physical world; everything must be understood as a social construction. At the other end of the spectrum, 'weak' approaches acknowledge a physical, material reality but see social issues as being constructed. Between these two extremes, many writers take an approach that acknowledges the biological and the social. This recognizes objective phenomena, but states that they are only given meaning through social processes. As Blaxter (2004) notes, this means that processes such as disease, pathogens and pain are acknowledged, but the way they are responded to and conceptualized is socially constructed. She states that:

> *What counts* as disease or abnormality is not 'given' in the same sense as biological fact is given. It depends on cultural norms and culturally shared rules of interpretation. (Blaxter, 2004, p. 28)

Given the eclectic, multidisciplinary nature of cultural studies, it inevitably makes use of a wide range of methodologies that originate in a range of different academic fields. Alasuutari (1995, p. 2) states that:

> Cultural studies methodology has often been described by the concept of *bricolage*: one is pragmatic and strategic in choosing and applying different methods and practices.

In theory, then, all methodologies are appropriate for use. However, given the emphasis that cultural studies places on *meaning*, it tends, maybe unsurprisingly, to focus primarily on qualitative approaches. These approaches can best be conceived as forming a broad spectrum, ranging from those which focus on people as the direct source of information to those which study texts.

Methods that centre around people may include or combine different forms of observational studies, types of direct questioning such as semi-structured interviewing or less formal means such as the use of narratives or life histories. At the other end of the spectrum, there is the direct study of cultural artefacts or texts. A text is any cultural product – television, film, newspapers, broadcasts, advertisements, pictures or architecture – that can be analysed for the meanings it contains. Along the spectrum lie a variety of methodologies that incorporate a range of techniques.

Ethnography

The use of ethnography in cultural studies derives principally from anthropology. It stems from the fieldwork tradition in which researchers immerse themselves in the group or community being studied in order to understand its culture from within. Many methods may be employed in the search for understanding, including interviewing, observation and informal conversations. Data may be noted in a number of ways, such as tape-recordings, but the principal method of collection is through the use of the researcher's notes and observations recorded in a fieldwork diary. One of the aims of ethnography is often termed, following Geertz's (1973) influential work, 'thick description'.

Two issues immediately become apparent with this method of research. First, there is an ethical question. Observation may be overt or covert. The latter approach seeks to avoid 'contaminating' findings, which may occur if the research subjects know that they are being observed. This method can, however, be characterized as exploitative. Given the time-consuming nature of an extended period of fieldwork, there is also the danger that the findings may in practice be based on sketchy or sporadic observations, a tendency characterized by Murdock (1997) as 'thin descriptions'.

Second, however fully the researchers immerse themselves within the group, there will inevitably be an element of subjective interpretation. In attempting to understand any culture and its practices, the researchers' interpretation will be shaped by their own cultural location. Many critiques of an earlier, more confident and authoritative ethnography have come from feminist writers who have challenged the notion of the traditional research hierarchy by which subjects become objectified (Atkinson and Coffey, 1995). Feminist researchers have been at the forefront of the cultural studies' goal of enabling the voice of marginalized groups to be heard; ethnography can be a valuable method in this cause.

Example 6.8

CULTURAL CONCEPTS OF HEALTH

Adelson's study of health beliefs among the Cree of Whapmagoostui in northern Quebec clearly illustrates the fact that concepts of health must be understood as cultural. She characterizes her research as participant observation, including interviews with over 20% of the adults in the community, which took place over a two-year period. Adelson found that there was no direct translation of the term 'health'; the term used by the Cree translates most closely as 'being alive well'. This concept is closely bound to the Cree's specific sociocultural context:

'being alive well' is defined through local beliefs and practices, simultaneously incorporating references to an idealized past and consolidating issues of cultural identity. 'Being alive well' is inseparable from community, history, identity, and ultimately resistance. (Adelson, 1998)

The history of the Cree village studied is one of contact with prospectors, hunters and traders. As for many indigenous people exposed to outside groups, this contact both altered the traditional way of life and introduced new diseases. The community was transformed by contact, modernization and cultural exchange. In 1989, the community was mobilized by its opposition to a proposal by the Quebec provincial government to initiate a hydroelectric project that would have had an immense impact on the local environment. Although successful in their opposition, they face continual challenges in the face of sovereignty disputes. The specific history and conditions of the Cree form a vital context in understanding concepts of health.

The concept of 'being alive well' is distinct from Western biomedical constructions of health and is not rooted in physiology. It is possible to be unwell in the Western sense of the word yet still be in a state of 'being alive well'. 'Being alive well' relates more to a way of life associated with practices such as carrying out physical activity, keeping warm and eating traditional Cree foods, which reflects the people's strong relationship with the land and its preservation. The vigour of the land and the Cree themselves is associated with an idealized past that existed before the 'white man' came. The customs and conditions introduced by the 'white man' are seen as weakening the sense in which the Cree can 'be alive well'. This study illustrates the ways in which groups can be studied by ethnographic methods in order to bring cultural practices and beliefs alive. Health in this example is both a product of sociocultural conditions and a marker of cultural identity.

Source: Adelson, 1998

Discourse and conversation analysis

Broadly speaking, a discourse is a series of terms, values, symbols and words that gather about a topic or group. Discourses are permeated and shaped by cultural and ideological connotations. Discourse analysis in the linguistic sense involves analysing patterns and structures of talk in order to reveal the forms and constraints of social interaction. Within this broad approach, the term 'conversation analysis' is often used more narrowly to describe a specific methodology for analysing how language shapes the discussion of two or more parties.

Conversation analysis permits us to go beyond an examination of the content of a conversation or interview in order to examine how both parties interact and construct their subject positions. Any conversation can be analysed for the incidence of patterned regularities of speech that allow the participants to position themselves in relation to one another. We can, for example, examine how men and women talk to one another, how couples structure a narrative when they are relating an event, and how medical consultations establish the relative social positions of doctor and patient. A crucial element of this approach is that it is only the conversation that is subjected to analysis: all other forms of context or background must be excluded. Transcriptions of conversations for the purposes of analysis therefore follow very detailed rules. All speech must be reproduced verbatim, pauses timed to within a tenth of a second, and the points at which interruptions and responses occur precisely noted.

At the heart of conversation analysis is the recognition that conversations tend to follow certain rules. At a basic level, this comprises turn-taking, that is, the way in which participants negotiate the order of utterances. One important feature is that of pairs of utterances, for example question – answer, invitation – acceptance/refusal. Subverting these implicit rules may result in a call for justification or explanation (Alasuutari, 1995). There can also be a significant difference between the types of conversation. An everyday discussion may have different properties from 'institutional talk' such as meetings or lay person–expert interactions. Conversation analysis, then, reveals how structures of power within society operate through the formal, if often unacknowledged, rules of speech engagement. While conversation analysis is a rigorous approach with a carefully detailed focus, it is also possible to combine its insights with knowledge of broader cultural patterns and relationships.

Ten Have (1991) argues that such talk is asymmetrical and reflects a hierarchical organization of speech interaction. This is in part the result of inherent power imbalances between the lay person and medical expert. In addition, the talk itself actively produces asymmetry. First, the patient's, rather than the doctor's, problems are the focus. Second, the carrying out of the tasks of the encounter (complaint presentation, examination, diagnosis and treatment) is dominated by the doctor. Ten Have discusses a number of ways in which this asymmetry becomes manifest in talk. For example, how doctors elicit information frames patients' replies, and is often designed to produce brief answers. Patients are not encouraged simply to narrate an account of their illness. Doctors also display control by questioning without context or justification: they are not required to explain the reasoning behind their questions. Doctors' non-committal replies reveal nothing of their reaction to responses. Thus, Ten Have states that asymmetry is produced by the doctors' role as initiators and their control of the information they divulge.

An interesting example of discourse analysis, a broader approach than conversation analysis, is found in Blumenreich and Siegel's (2006) study of the imagery used in children's books about HIV/AIDS. They examine the way in which children's understandings become shaped by dominant discourses. One text is shown to reproduce messages of social stigma, even though its explicit aim appears to be to generate understanding for HIV-positive children. The child with HIV is depicted as naturally an outcast, for whom sympathy is required as befitting his victim status. The child's mother, who is shown as a drug user, does not receive much compassion. The author makes frequent use of war metaphors in discussing how the AIDS virus operates. In an overview of children's novels, Blumenreich and Siegel (2006) found that common themes were a tendency to use outdated information, a neglect of new treatments that help people to live with HIV, a lack of ethnic diversity among characters and the use of stereotypical views of people with HIV/AIDS.

Blumenreich and Siegel (2006) identify three principal discourses:

- *a public service discourse:* this has a health education approach and deals with themes of transmission and appropriate behaviour. Risk groups are portrayed as threats to the general population, who are somehow different. When members of the general population become infected, they are seen as innocent victims, with the unspoken inference being drawn that others are 'guilty' victims. The main aim of this discourse appears to be to reassure the general population.

● *a medical discourse:* much of medical scientific writing about AIDS uses war metaphors. Typical terminology is about fighting off invaders, defences and enemies. Children's texts draw heavily on this imagery, which again sets up divisions between good and bad, normal and abnormal.

● *a secrecy discourse:* characters often discuss secrets associated with diagnosis, or the fact that they have to lie about situations, or piece together facts by themselves rather than being told information directly. This secrecy is often echoed in plots that conceal characters' sexuality or personal circumstances.

Countering these discourses, however, were some texts that sought to convey oppositional discourses. A limited number show children who are HIV positive being healthy or misbehaving like other children. Sometimes HIV-positive children are shown as being good friends and as having something to offer rather than just people who require kindness. Only a couple of books include direct treatment of the topic of death, although texts that feature children's own discussions of living with HIV/AIDS show that this is an issue uppermost in their minds.

Most of the books studied engage with common cultural concerns about HIV and AIDS. In doing so, their intent is often to reassure and inform children, helping them to deal with difficult situations. However, in the process they draw on dominant imagery and reinforce constructions of disease, which shapes children's understandings. In Althusser's language, children 'interpellate' these images and messages and take them on as their own.

Semiotics

Semiotics (or semiology) focuses on the study of signs contained within texts. Signs are comprised of two components:

● signifiers, which are sounds, words or images

● the signified, which are the concepts represented by signifiers.

Thus a photograph of someone with a stethoscope around her neck (the signifier) would suggest the concept of medical power (the signified). Meaning emerges from the relationship between the signifier and the signified.

? Consider well-known advertisements such as that for Marlboro cigarettes. The Marlboro man was depicted as a cowboy riding a horse in open country. What is signified by this image?

The Marlboro man immediately brings forth ideas of the Wild West, freedom, masculinity and independence. These images successfully made consumers and potential consumers perceive Marlboro to be a man's cigarette. By contrast, cigarettes such as Silk Cut, aimed at female consumers, emphasized the 'lightness' or mildness of the cigarette.

When we are part of a culture, we learn and internalize complex and shifting patterns of associations, which can be termed 'codes'. Thus, we develop a way of making sense of the world in which we learn to read off meanings and associations from signs within everyday life. This is not necessarily something we carry out consciously: the process may become instinctive and automatic. However, as these relationships and associations are dynamic and changing, not everyone will work with the same system of codes or understand codes in the same way. This can lead to what has been termed 'aberrant coding': a mismatch of meaning between those who produce cultural artefacts and those who receive them. Thus, a public health message, for example, may fail because its makers use terms or images that do not conjure up the same pattern of associations in the minds of its target group.

CASE STUDY Infant feeding across cultures

The ability to breastfeed is in many respects universal, although there will always be women who find it difficult or impossible. However, the meaning and value which is afforded to breastfeeding, its duration, the way in which difficulties are perceived and responded to, and the transition to weaning are all subject to tremendous cultural variation.

Currently, the dominant wisdom regarding breastfeeding in the West is that it is demonstrably best for babies. In recent years, there have been numerous studies showing that breastfeeding is a superior form of nutrition in comparison to formula feeding and that it has powerful health benefits for both mothers and infants (Stuart-Macadam, 1995). Despite this evidence, there exist considerable disparities in rates of breastfeeding between cultures.

Attitudes towards breastfeeding among mothers, families and potential support networks, the general public, medical professionals and policy-makers all contribute to the cultural milieu in which breastfeeding either does or does not take place.

One way to identify how breastfeeding is mediated by cultural factors is to explore changes in practices over time. Formula milk, a heavily modified version of cow's milk that is safe for babies to drink, is a comparatively recent invention. Its introduction opened up a new range of possibilities for infant nutrition, as well as associated shifts in the discourse surrounding the desirability of breastfeeding. Prior to this, although many of the concerns of breastfeeding were familiar, such as insufficient milk, the dilemmas, values and strategies often differed. Fildes (1986) has conducted extensive research on the history of infant feeding and identifies a wealth of associated practices. For example, in ancient India, newborn babies would be given a mix of ghee and honey until the mother's milk came in some three to four days later. She states that colostrum is still commonly regarded as a harmful or taboo substance in certain developing societies, in spite of current medical evidence suggesting that it is a vital source of antibodies and proteins for the newborn baby. Fikree et al. (2005), for example, identified 'risky traditional newborn care practices', such as giving babies honey, water or tea as their first feed, in their study of neonatal care in Pakistan.

Such practices are not confined to developing countries. Bentley et al.'s (1999) study of young African-American mothers from low-income backgrounds found that semi-solids, such as cereals, were introduced as early as within the first two weeks. Introducing solids too early has been associated with allergies and obesity (Skinner, 1997 in Bentley et al., 1999). The babies' grandmothers often played a valued and key role in childcare, so their views on infant feeding became part of the cultural 'common sense' on which the young mothers drew. Therefore, grandmothers' advice was often followed, even when it conflicted with that of health professionals. There was a strong sense that milk alone was inadequate and that babies who were seen as small or who cried or woke up frequently needed solids. Babies' behaviour was also frequently interpreted as signs that they were 'greedy'. Giving solids was therefore a way of responding positively to a hungry baby, and was constructed as a sign of good parenting. This study shows the importance of engaging with the social context when attempting to promote breastfeeding, in this case understanding why solids would be given and realizing that the mother is not the only significant carer.

In Senegal, Aubel et al. (2004) found that engaging grandmothers in a community health programme had a significant impact on raising awareness of optimal feeding practices. In Senegal, although breastfeeding is widespread, it is often supplemented by other foods and fluids rather than being exclusive, and it is not always immediate. In Aubel et al.'s study, involving grandmothers in education sessions increased their knowledge of nutrition, raised self-esteem and increased the respect shown for them within households and the wider community.

Throughout history, an inability to breastfeed is well documented. In the past, however, the recommended strategy was to use a wet nurse – another lactating woman who could nurse the baby instead of its mother. This practice ensures that a baby benefits from breast milk. Elements of this practice are still witnessed today when women donate excess milk to milk banks. In some periods and cultures, wet nurses could be of high standing. At other times, they were poor and seen as either exploited or as potentially dangerous and exploitative themselves.

Entwined with ideas about wet nurses and breastfeeding are concerns about the concept of motherhood and how women should behave. Fildes (1986, p. 27) discusses the views of Roman philosophers such as Pliny and Tacitus, who stressed the importance of maternal breastfeeding for nutrition and attachment. They also noted a class element, deploring the fact that poor women fed their own children while richer mothers employed wet nurses. Fildes highlights a contrast with medical writers of the time, who were keener that the most suitable person would breastfeed. This would not necessarily be the mother, especially if she were ill or became pregnant, as this was seen to spoil her milk and potentially damage the child. Nevertheless, debates about breastfeeding versus wet nursing continued in many societies, echoing contemporary debates concerning breast-feeding versus formula feeding. In relation to Europe in the late sixteenth and seventeenth century, Fildes (1986, p. 100) notes that:

> Wet nursing was an ancient, deeply-ingrained and widely-accepted social custom, and wealthy mothers who decided to nurse their own babies were sufficiently exceptional to attract comment (often adverse) both from close friends and from the wider social circle.

Women's objections to breastfeeding largely centred on the fear of losing their looks or becoming ill. Breastfeeding was thought to make women look older, produce sagging breasts and inhibit the range of fashionable clothing that could be worn. There is documentation of women enduring considerable damage to their breasts from feeding. Repeated cuts became infected, scar tissue resulted and sometimes children chewed through nipples. Here we see a dilemma for women – whether to conform to the role of good mother or the role of attractive, desirable woman.

The breast can be seen as a complex signifier. Its biological function is to provide breast milk to nurture a baby. However, this cannot be separated from the social value we attach to the process and to the woman who nurses. The breast is a signifier not just of motherhood, but also of sexuality and feminine identity. Promoting the advantages of breastfeeding currently takes place in a cultural context that sees breasts as primarily sexualized rather than nurturing. Because of these connotations, exposing the breast can also be seen as indecent, which can impose restrictions on mothers being able to feed in public places.

Among women who are keen to breastfeed, the inability to do so can provoke intense feelings of shame and grief. However, even successful feeding can be tremendously stressful. Flacking et al.'s (2007) study of mothers of premature infants in Sweden found that establishing a secure bond was sometimes difficult due to the need for their babies to receive specialist care, which often entailed physical separation, and the intense emotions and exhaustion associated with anxieties for their babies' wellbeing. Mothers felt under tremendous pressure to breastfeed, as its nutritional value was critical for their vulnerable babies. Sweden has a strong culture of breastfeeding, which is seen as a marker of good mothering. Being able to breastfeed was a vital aspect of these women's role of good mother. Unhappy experiences of breastfeeding or failing to find the experience enjoyable created feelings of anxiety in mothers about the nature of their bond with their child. Women who bottle-fed expressed feelings of shame about doing so in public.

In order to promote breastfeeding among mothers, health professionals have to understand the specific cultural factors that contribute to women's decisions. These can be very variable. A study of breastfeeding in Brazil, for example, found that an extremely high intention to breastfeed among pregnant women translated into a much lower rate of continuing breastfeeding – 29% at six months compared to rates of 50–63% in other Latin American countries (Scavenius et al., 2007). In poorer countries, the protective effect of breastfeeding is even more important, so the public health goal of exclusive breastfeeding for at least six months is crucial. As 98% of newborn deaths occur in developing countries, care practices are key to survival (WHO, 1996). Scavenius et al. (2007) trace the discrepancy between intent and breastfeeding practice in Brazil to features of the social context in recent years, including the promotion of formula milk via the US development programme in the 1970s, which contrasts with the strong health promotion emphasis on breastfeeding. They draw on Van Esterik's (1988 in Scavenius et al., 2007) distinction between breast milk as product and breastfeeding as process to characterize Brazil's cultural understanding. Cultures that focus on breast milk as a product are more likely to have beliefs about the quality or supply of milk, to use supplements and cease exclusive breastfeeding comparatively early. Cultures that see breastfeeding as a process perceive it as a complex social activity and have ways to facilitate this pattern of interaction between mother and child,

including overcoming difficulties. This results in longer exclusive breastfeeding. Scavenius et al. (2007) argue that their research demonstrates an important interaction between the biological and the social. In biological terms, milk is stimulated by frequent suckling. However, the frequency of suckling is linked to social factors, such as the value attached to mothers' breastfeeding, its acceptability in public, whether other roles such as employment constrain mothers, or the way in which identity is intertwined with nursing.

Summary

- Cultural studies usually focuses on the reflexive examination of one's own cultural norms and practices, whereas anthropology has traditionally centred on the examination of other societies' norms, values and practices

- Health and illness are cultural concepts that convey social and cultural meanings

- Lay knowledge and beliefs about health and the management of disease and illness are now recognized as an important resource

- The media plays an important role in the different cultural discourses around health and illness

- The example of infant feeding demonstrates how women balance competing biological and cultural discourses when making decisions, and how health practitioners need to engage with these different discourses if they are to be effective

- There is no one grand narrative such as biology that explains health and illness, but rather many competing discourses

Questions for further discussion

1. The term 'cultural competence' is widely used to describe organizations that recognize and address issues of diversity. What elements would you expect to be included?

2. Why should health professionals understand the cultural context of health decisions?

Fiske, J. (1990) *Introduction to Communication Studies* (2nd edn). London: Routledge.

Flacking, R., Ewald, U. and Starrin, B. (2007) '"I wanted to do a good job": experiences of "becoming a mother" and breastfeeding in mothers of very preterm infants after discharge from a neonatal unit'. *Social Science and Medicine* 64: 2405–16.

Geertz, C. (1973) *The Interpretation of Cultures: Selected Essays*. New York: Basic Books.

Gillett, J. (2003) 'Media activism and internet use by people with HIV/AIDS'. *Sociology of Health and Illness* 25(6): 608–24.

Gramsci, A. (1971) *Selections from Prison Notebooks*. London: Lawrence & Wishart.

Hall, S. (1980) 'Cultural studies: two paradigms'. *Media, Culture and Society* 2: 57–72.

Helman, C. (2000) *Culture, Health and Illness* (4th edn). Oxford: Butterworth Heinemann.

Hoggart, R. (1958) *The Uses of Literacy*. London: Penguin.

James, A. (1997) How British is British food?, in P. Caplan (ed.) *Food, Health and Identity*. London: Routledge, pp. 71–86.

James, D.J. (2004) 'Factors influencing food choices, dietary intake, and nutrition-related attitudes among African Americans: application of a culturally sensitive model'. *Ethnicity and Health* 9(4): 349–67.

Jenks, C. (1993) *Culture*. London: Routledge.

Karpf, A. (1988) *Doctoring the Media: The Reporting of Health and Medicine*. London: Routledge.

Katbamna, S., Bhaktra, P. and Parker, G. (2000) Perceptions of disability and care-giving relationships in South Asian communities, in W.I.U. Ahmand (ed.) *Ethnicity, Disability and Chronic Illness*. Buckingham: Open University Press.

Kelleher, D. (1994) Self-help groups and their relationship to medicine, in J. Gabe, D. Kelleher and G. Williams (eds) *Challenging Medicine*. London: Routledge, pp. 104–17.

Kleinman, A. (1980) *Patients and Healers in the Context of Culture: An Exploration of the Borderland between Anthropology, Medicine and Psychiatry*, Berkley: University of California Press.

Lévi-Strauss, C. (1970) *The Raw and the Cooked: Introduction to a Science of Mythology*, vol. I. London: Jonathan Cape.

May, C., Doyle, H. and Chew-Graham, C. (1999) 'Medical knowledge and the intractable patient: the case of chronic low back pain'. *Social Science and Medicine* 48(4): 523–34.

Moore, O. (1996) *PWA: Looking AIDS in the Face*. Basingstoke: Macmillan – now Palgrave Macmillan.

Morgan, M. (1996) The meanings of high blood pressure among Afro-Caribbean and white patients, in D. Kelleher and S. Hillier (eds) *Researching Cultural Differences in Health*. London: Routledge, pp. 11–37.

Murcott, A. (1997) 'Family meals – a thing of the past?', in P. Caplan (ed.) *Food, Health and Identity*. London: Routledge, pp. 32–49.

Murdock, G. (1997) Thin descriptions: questions of method in cultural analysis, in J. McGuigan (ed.) *Cultural Methodologies*. London: Sage, pp. 178–92.

Nettleton, S., Burrows, R. and O'Malley, L. (2005) 'The mundane realities of the everyday lay use of the internet for health, and their consequences for media convergence'. *Sociology of Health and Illness* 27(7): 972–92.

Oinas, E. (1998) 'Medicalisation by whom? Accounts of menstruation conveyed by young women and medical experts in medical advisory columns'. *Sociology of Health and Illness* 20(1): 52–70.

Picardie, R. (1998) *Before I Say Goodbye*. London: Penguin Books.

Pote, H. L. and Orrell, M. W. (2002). 'Perceptions of schizophrenia in multi-cultural Britain'. *Ethnicity and Health* 7(1): 7–20.

Prior, L. (2003) 'Belief, knowledge and expertise: the emergence of the lay expert in medical sociology'. *Sociology of Health and Illness* 25: 41–57.

Russell, A. and Edgar, I.R. (1998) Research and practice in the anthropology of welfare, in I.R. Edgar and A. Russell (eds) *The Anthropology of Welfare*. London: Routledge.

Scavenius, M., van Hulsel, L., Meijer, J. et al. (2007) 'In practice, the theory is different: a processual analysis of breastfeeding in northeast Brazil'. *Social Science and Medicine* 64: 676–88.

Seale, C. (2005) 'New directions for critical internet health studies: representing cancer experience on the web'. *Sociology of Health and Illness* 27(4): 515–40.

Spector, R. (2004) *Cultural Diversity in Health and Illness* (6th edn). Upper Saddle River, NJ: Pearson/Prentice Hall.

Stuart-Macadam, P. (1995) Biocultural perspectives on breastfeeding, in P. Stuart-Macadam and K.A. Dettwyler (eds) *Breastfeeding: Biocultural Perspectives*. New York: Aldine de Gruyter.

Ten Have, P. (1991) Talk and institution: a reconsideration of the 'asymmetry' of doctor–patient interaction, in D. Boden and D.H. Zimmerman (eds) *Talk and Social Structure*. Cambridge: Polity Press, pp. 138–63.

Thompson, E.P. (1978/1963) *The Making of the English Working Class*. London: Penguin.

Turner, B. (1992) *Regulating Bodies: Essays in Medical Sociology*. London: Routledge.

Turow, J. (1989) *Playing Doctor: Television Storytelling and Medical Power*. New York: Oxford University Press.

Wallis, P. and Nerlich, B. (2005) 'Disease metaphors in new epidemics: the UK media framing of the 2003 SARS epidemic'. *Social Science and Medicine* 60: 2629–39.

Walter, F.M. and Britten, N. (2002) 'Patients' understandings of risk: a qualitative study of decision-making about the menopause and hormone replacement therapy in general practice'. *Family Practice* 19(6): 579–86.

WHO (World Health Organization) (1996) *Perinatal Mortality: A Listing of Available Information*, FRH/MSM, 96.7. Geneva: WHO.

Williams, R. (1961) *Culture and Society (1780–1950)*. Harmondsworth: Penguin.

Wright, H.K. (1998) 'Dare we de-centre Birmingham? Troubling the "origin" and trajectories of cultural studies'. *European Journal of Cultural Studies* 1(1): 33–56.

Wurtzel, E. (1996) *Prozac Nation*. London: Quartet Books.

Zhang, X. (2006) 'Reading between the headlines: SARS, *Focus* and TV current affairs programmes in China'. *Media, Culture and Society* 28(5): 715–37.

Social policy and health

Outline of chapter

LEARNING OUTCOMES

This chapter will enable readers to:
- Understand the organization and development of social policies
- Examine the process of social policy-making
- Understand the role of social policies in influencing health
- Assess the contribution of social policy to health studies

Overview

The discipline of social policy examines how and why certain issues relating to people's welfare come to be seen as the legitimate focus of state intervention. Social policy also critically examines the consequences, both intended and unintended, of state intervention, regulation and legislation. The first part of the chapter considers the contribution of social policy to health studies. It looks at the historical development of social policies, including health policies, identifying key issues such as the extent of state involvement in the provision of welfare and the ways in which changing political ideologies have affected views on this. The second part considers the methods and analytical tools of the social policy discipline. It traces the development of social policy and examines some of the key theoretical and methodological approaches, with a particular focus on the relevance of these for health studies. It looks at the policy process, how certain issues become part of the policy agenda and how policies are negotiated, formulated and implemented. The third part is a case study on obesity that examines how this topical health issue has become a legitimate focus for policy development.

Introduction

Social policy is the study of how the **welfare** of individuals is organized in any society, in particular the role of the state in relation to the welfare of its citizens. The term 'social policy' is used in two senses. It sometimes refers to a particular kind of decision, such as that relating to education or health. It may also refer to the academic discipline that studies such policies. In order to avoid confusion, in this chapter the term 'social policy' will refer to the academic discipline; otherwise, the plural form, 'social policies' will be used.

The term 'social policies' is conventionally used to describe policy in relation to welfare benefits, unemployment, education, housing, health and social services. All these areas are related and also influenced by other government policies, such as those on transport and the environment, and particularly economic policy. For example, a study of state intervention in health might focus on transport policy and congestion charging, given concerns about poor air quality and rising rates of asthma.

The twentieth century saw the development of state welfare and the establishment of a National Health Service in the UK. This has raised certain core questions, which are still relevant today:

● What is the role of the state? When and how far should it be involved in people's lives?

● How should welfare be organized and funded?

● How are contemporary social problems identified?

- Who benefits from social policies?

- Whose values do social policies reflect?

- What are the broader functions of social policies?

- How efficient and effective are policies in providing welfare?

Social policy is informed by economics in relation to the allocation of resources for welfare and by politics through decision-making that determines the provision of welfare. Decisions about whether a primary care trust (PCT) should pay for treatment that has a low chance of success, whether NHS services should be based on users' views, and whether people should be forced through legislation and regulation to choose a healthier lifestyle are value judgements. The rising costs of the health service and the increasing needs and demands of an ageing population provide a challenge to policy-makers.

The contribution of social policy to health studies

Social policy is concerned not just with what the state provides, but also with broader issues of entitlement and responsibility in society. The provision of healthcare is based on considerations about who is entitled to receive state support and at what level. A core concept is that of **need**.

? How would you define need? Are different people or population groups more in need than others? How do you decide?

The concept of human need is basic to understanding human health and welfare, yet it is a problematic concept. Attempts to define human need have raised questions about whether need is, and should be, an objective, universal concept, or whether it is, and should be, determined by variable historical, geographical and cultural factors (Doyal and Gough, 1991).

How any society sets about meeting human needs raises further problematic concepts, such as those of **social justice** and **equity**. These refer to criteria of fairness – of who 'ought' to get what when resources are being allocated. Criteria of fairness may take into account the level of need or be based on some notion of merit.

This raises the question of whether welfare should be regarded as a right. Marshall (1950) identifies social rights as essential to **citizenship** and the full membership of any society. Social rights include economic security, a share in good living standards and cultural heritage. Access to welfare was, for Marshall, a matter of citizen rights. However, the degree of entitlements and how citizens' rights to welfare can be enforced remain the subject of political and ideological argument.

Where a welfare system embraces the idea of rights, then to what extent is meeting human needs the responsibility of families, communities or the state?

Margaret Thatcher, prime minister in the 1980s, referred to the UK as a 'nanny state', by which she meant the welfare state had taken over functions that were more properly carried out by families, and had encouraged people to neglect their responsibilities. The concept of 'welfare dependency' was coined to describe those who were perceived to be content to rely on state benefits instead of seeking to provide for themselves.

Welfare systems are capable of enhancing or diminishing individual autonomy. A basic principle of community care policies was that individual needs should be recognized and met in ways that enhanced the individuality and autonomy of service users, in contrast to institutionalized forms of care. For example, the introduction of direct payments for disabled people under the Community Care (Direct Payments) Act 1996 enables them to decide how their care is delivered once their needs have been assessed.

The organization of welfare

? What do you understand by the term 'welfare'? Whose responsibility is the welfare of others?

There are different views about responsibility for the provision of social welfare. Many people immediately think that the state should provide for those in need. The term 'welfare state' is something of a misnomer since there are many different providers of individual welfare. Welfare can be understood as a system that comprises five main spheres of activity: This **mixed economy of welfare** providers refers to:

- the state
- informal welfare
- the private sector
- the voluntary sector
- occupational welfare

Figure 7.1 shows how all five spheres contribute to welfare in the case of Alice James. Alice is 80 years old and lives alone. She has recently returned home after being discharged from hospital following treatment for a fractured hip. Her ability to remain at home is likely to depend on services being provided on a more long-term basis in order for her daughter to return to work. However, unless Alice has access to her own financial resources and is able to purchase these for herself, she will be dependent on the state (the local social services department) for help. Her daughter's financial security in old age is likely to be affected if she decides to give up work to care for Alice, as contributions to her occupational pension scheme will be stopped. Without the informal care provided by her daughter, Alice may not be able to remain at home and may have to sell her home to help pay towards residential care supplied by the private sector. The extent and importance of informal care, which is domestic and private, is often underestimated.

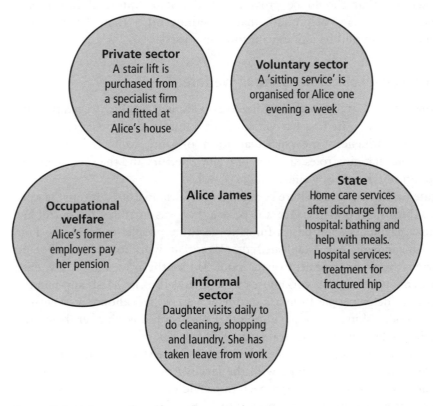

Figure 7.1 Spheres of welfare: the mixed economy

There are many obvious ways in which people benefit from welfare, for example through the receipt of benefits, education and NHS services. It is common to think that people living on the lowest incomes benefit the most from welfare, yet much welfare spending benefits better off people most.

The state has a fluctuating relationship with all other sectors in the organization and management of people's welfare. Take, for example, its regulatory role. In the private sector, it has taken on responsibility for regulating tobacco advertising, in the voluntary sector, it places controls on the way in which charities raise funds, while in the occupational sector, it imposes rules on health and safety at work. State intervention in the informal sector is a highly contentious area. In cases of neglect or violence, intervention is widely accepted and, indeed, expected. At other times, however, the state's role is questioned.

? Should the state provide financial recompense to carers?

Financial recompense would recognize the support provided by carers, but it might cloud the caring relationship and make it harder for carers to take on this role. The giving of time, money or expertise is a key element in the provision of welfare. While there is a concern that informal care provides core services that should be provided by the state, informal care is also promoted on the moral grounds that something other than the pursuit of financial gain should be a dominant force in society.

The changing role of the state in welfare

Although state activity in welfare involves planning, funding, regulating and providing services, its role has varied. Both values and organizational traditions have influenced the particular form of state welfare. This section outlines the changing roles of different welfare sectors and the socioeconomic and political context of welfare.

State involvement in welfare goes back centuries. In 1601, during the reign of Elizabeth I, a Poor Law Act was passed that was intended to control and organize payments from parish funds to destitute people. In 1834, the Poor Law Amendment Act established the Victorian workhouses that became notorious for their treatment of the poor. Under the principle of 'less eligibility', conditions in the workhouses were intended to be harsh and punitive in order to deter people from asking for help. The 'workhouse test' ensured that anybody asking for help had no other means of looking after themselves or their families and that the state was their last resort.

In the late nineteenth century, the workhouse system was under a great deal of strain, unable to cope with the level of need but also more widely regarded as an unacceptable approach to providing welfare. Problems such as poverty, unemployment, infant mortality, ill health and poor housing conditions led to pressure for state action. The realization that epidemic diseases, such as cholera, spread through inadequate water and sewage services and poor housing conditions to affect everyone was an important factor in promoting and legitimating state intervention.

Welfare services in the nineteenth century demonstrate how different values applied in practice. For example, the Charity Organization Society, which worked with families in poverty, maintained an individualistic approach. It was concerned with identifying the 'deserving poor', distinguishing between the 'helpable' and the 'unhelpable'. From a different perspective, campaigners such as Charles Booth and Joseph Rowntree argued that poverty was the outcome of the economic and industrial system rather than individual idleness or immorality and that social reforms were therefore needed.

In the early twentieth century, the liberal government of the British Prime Minister Lloyd George introduced a series of measures, including the first retirement pension in 1908 and a limited health insurance scheme in 1911. After the First World War, welfare schemes based on the principle of social insurance were developed. Individual contributions paid from wages into an insurance scheme entitled workers to claim benefits when they were unemployed, sick or retired.

Britain becomes a welfare state 1945–50

The postwar period (1945–50) saw the development of Britain's welfare system. The British model differs from that of most of Europe in its approach to social policy and is a distinctive example of a comprehensive and universal welfare system. It reflects the principles of the postwar period and the pragmatic influence of regeneration.

The basic principles underpinning the development of the welfare state in the 1940s were:

- **universalism**
- comprehensiveness
- **collectivism**.

In practice, these principles meant that every citizen should be included within the system of benefits and services, and that the range of services should cater for all their needs 'from cradle to grave'.

Collectivism, demonstrated through the taxation of those in work to pay for services, represented a major shift from the Victorian position on individual responsibility for welfare. Welfare services were established on the basis of rights rather than charity. The provision of free education and healthcare could be seen as a means of reducing social and economic inequality by compensating for low wages and raising the standard of living of poorer people. Because resources for the new system came from income tax, there was a redistribution of resources from the better off to the poorer, thus reducing the overall economic inequality.

Example 7.1

THE BEVERIDGE REPORT

William Beveridge was appointed by the wartime coalition government to review the range of insurance schemes that had developed since the turn of the century. The report he produced in 1942 was a plan for a comprehensive reform of social polices in which healthcare would be universally available and funded from taxation. He identified what he considered to be the major social problems of the day, which he termed the 'five giants stalking the land': want, ignorance, squalor, disease and idleness.

Beveridge's report formed the basis of the postwar Labour government's welfare state. Key policies included the Education Act 1944, the Family Allowances Act 1945, the National Health Service Act 1946, the National Insurance Act 1946 and the National Assistance Act 1948. These Acts established sickness and unemployment benefits, retirement pensions for men at 65 and women at 60, maternity benefits and widows' benefits. In addition, subsidies to local authorities enabled a programme of council house building, and full employment was made possible by the buoyant economy after the war. The five giants were tackled, though not destroyed.

Source: Beveridge, 1942

The state became the dominant player in the formal welfare system, with the private and voluntary sectors occupying a more peripheral position. Influenced by the ideas of Marshall (1950), there was a widespread consensus across the political parties that a welfare state was desirable in the development of a civilized society.

Established in 1948, the NHS was a classic example of the above principles. It was based on the following:

- Healthcare should be provided according to people's needs rather than their ability to pay. It should be free at the point of delivery to ensure that people seek help when they need it

- Healthcare should be collectively financed from general taxation

- Healthcare should be comprehensive to cover the whole range of people's health needs in one centrally planned service

- Healthcare should be universal and equally available to all sectors of the population and in all areas of the country

- The NHS should be concerned with reducing inequalities in health.

? In what ways have the principles of universalism, collectivism and comprehensiveness in the NHS been challenged?

The principle of universal provision has proved difficult to achieve and regional variations in mortality and morbidity rates remain a problem. An expanding system of welfare has had little impact on social and health inequalities. Many government and research reports testify to ongoing health inequalities (Townsend and Davidson, 1982; Acheson, 1998; Davey Smith et al., 2001, 2002).

The assumption that improved health would lead to a reduction in demand for healthcare was shown to be wrong in the context of medical advances and raised public expectations. There is concern that some areas and populations gain more from the NHS than others. For example, there is debate over 'postcode prescribing', whereby groups in some areas receive NHS treatment for conditions such as infertility, whereas others have to seek private treatment for the same conditions. The National Institute for Health and Clinical Excellence (NICE) provides advice and guidance on what should and should not be provided by the NHS.

The principle of comprehensiveness has not been put fully into practice in the NHS. There have always been contested areas, such as dentistry, optical services and chiropody that are neither fully incorporated into the NHS nor fully privatized. The 1990 reforms to the NHS presented a new approach to the allocation of resources. The aim of the internal market was to facilitate the flow of funds for treatment. NHS districts were encouraged to trade with each other on a contractual basis, through which the funds followed the patients. There was less emphasis on calculating the amount allocated to the regions and more on encouraging competition between providers so that money would be provided for services rendered.

Challenging welfare 1980–97

The 1970s saw the end of economic expansion and full employment. In 1979, the Conservatives, led by Margaret Thatcher, were elected to government. It was argued that welfare spending was too high, and that the near monopoly position of the state had stifled entrepreneurial activity in welfare and created inefficient and unresponsive bureaucracies. The Conservatives' programme was to 'roll back the state' and stimulate the private market. Conservative policies also sought to control professional groups such as doctors, social workers and teachers who were seen as responsible for driving up the cost of welfare as each sought to improve its status.

The challenge to state welfare from the political Right was both an economic argument and an ideological challenge. Welfare was characterized as having sapped the moral fibre of the nation and created a culture of dependency. The Conservatives viewed the NHS as a large and inefficient bureaucracy. Poor management systems had created funding problems, and professionals had too much power and autonomy.

CONNECTIONS

Chapter 9 discusses how the NHS has changed from an administered service to a managed one.

During the 1980s, NHS reforms focused on promoting efficiency and choice through, for example, the introduction of competitive tendering for ancillary services such as laundry and catering, and stimulating private healthcare provision. The Griffiths Report (DHSS, 1983) into management in the NHS resulted in attempts to create a more businesslike culture through recruiting general managers, clarifying lines of accountability and improving productivity. By the late 1980s, a fundamental restructuring of the welfare state was underway. A government review in 1988 led to the NHS and Community Care Act 1990, which resulted in a reorganization of the NHS and the separation of the functions of providing and purchasing healthcare to create an **internal market:**

- *Providers:* the large public hospitals became self-governing trusts, whose business was to provide healthcare services

- *Purchasers:* health authorities and fundholding GPs were given funds from the Department of Health to purchase healthcare from the providers on behalf of their patients.

Le Grand and Bartlett (1993) describe the NHS after 1990 as a 'quasi-market', because it was still financed from taxation, and remained in public ownership.

Parallel reforms in community care occurred after 1990. Local social services departments were designated as purchasers and required to develop a mixed economy of care from providers by stimulating competition in the private and voluntary sectors, as well as by encouraging unpaid care in the community. Care in the community had been a long-standing aim for many who wanted to see an end to institutional care for older and disabled people and those with mental health problems and learning disabilities. Community care was seen as both a means of restoring civil rights and dignity to marginalized groups and a means of cutting costs.

Alongside these reforms, two key policy documents were published on public health. *Promoting Better Health* (DoH, 1987) and *The Health of the Nation* (DoH, 1992) focused on prevention and wellness in contrast to the NHS provision of an illness service (Malin et al., 2002).

John Major became the Conservative prime minister in 1990. His administration promoted a consumerist approach, focusing on service users' rights and expectations with the introduction of the *Patient's Charter* (DoH, 1991). Policies introduced service standards, performance indicators, league tables and target-setting to reduce the length of hospital stays and the number of empty beds, and to provide quicker treatment in order to continue the drive for efficiency, choice and quality in healthcare.

In 1992, the government introduced the public finance initiative (PFI) to encourage the private sector to make capital investment in the NHS in return for a contract of usually 30 years to design, build and operate services. It is argued that as this introduces profits and returns for shareholders alongside the need to repay the initial investment from the NHS budget, funding is reduced.

Reforms to health services in the period 1980–97 encouraged a managerialist approach for reasons of greater efficiency and financial cost control. Private sector, self-help, consumerist and voluntary services were encouraged in order to improve choice and quality (Baggott, 2004).

Social policies from 1997

The election of the New Labour government and Prime Minister Tony Blair in 1997 introduced the notion of a 'third way', which draws on both the welfare system and the market approach (Giddens, 1998; Powell, 2000). New Labour stated its intention to modernize welfare provision as a service that was efficient, transparent, accountable, tailored to individual needs and making use of information technology (Miller, 2004). The mixed economy of welfare providers continues but there is an apparent difference in terms of the value base of welfare. New Labour has developed 'social inclusion' policies such as the New Deal for lone parents to address the status of excluded or marginalized people, particularly those not in paid employment. Initially, New Labour remained committed to strict limits on public spending introduced by the previous Conservative administration, until agreeing a 1% increase in national insurance contributions in the April 2002 budget to fund growth in the NHS.

? In what ways could it be said that the UK government is reintroducing the original principles of the NHS?

Two White Papers (DoH, 1997, 1999) signified a re-emergence of some of the original aims of the NHS, such as universal provision and a reduction in health inequalities. The idea of clinical excellence is also linked to equality. Clinical standards were established centrally so that regional inequalities could be addressed.

Example 7.2

KEY CHANGES IN HEALTH SINCE 1997

The New NHS: Modern, Dependable (DoH, 1997) and *Saving Lives: Our Healthier Nation* (DoH, 1999) introduced primary care groups and trusts to work with local authorities to develop more integrated services; health improvement programmes to establish local strategies for implementing national targets for health and healthcare; and NICE, an independent organization providing guidance on effective prevention and treatment interventions.

Health action zones were established to reduce health inequalities and promote better access to services in areas of poor health and high levels of deprivation. Further innovations included NHS Direct for healthcare advice and information by phone (and later by internet) and NHS walk-in centres for quick access without appointment for the assessment and treatment of minor injuries or advice and information.

National service frameworks (NSFs) set out the principles and standards of provision for a range of conditions (coronary heart disease, diabetes, renal) and groups (mental health, older people) developed with the assistance of health professionals, service users and carers, managers and agencies or organizations.

The NHS Plan (DoH, 2000) set out the government's vision of a health service designed around the patient. In particular, it:

1. Restated the principle of free care at the point of delivery and established nursing care as free to all in residential and nursing homes.
2. Set targets for new hospital schemes, extra beds, and more frontline staff (nurses, consultants, GPs) by 2010.
3. Restated a commitment to reduce major causes of mortality and morbidity, and set further targets to reduce health inequalities.
4. Gave PCTs responsibility to commission care services and allowed those trusts that performed well more financial freedom.
5. Sought clarity around new roles and responsibilities among the health professions and promoted collaboration and interprofessional working.
6. Called for greater patient or user involvement on committees, trusts and boards to help develop services.
7. Offered private sector management teams the opportunity to take over failing hospitals.

The following legislation has been enacted:

● The NHS Reform and Healthcare Professions Act 2002 brought in structural and organizational changes through reform of the distribution of functions between strategic health authorities and PCTs; reform of structures for patient and public involvement in the NHS; and reform of the regulation of the healthcare professions.

- The Health and Social Care (Community Health and Standards) Act 2003 allowed NHS trusts and non-NHS bodies to apply for independent foundation trust status. In response to concerns regarding the inaccessibility of dental services, the Act allows PCTs to commission NHS dental treatment by paying dentists for the number of patients they see. Foundation status makes trusts accountable to a board of employers, staff and local residents and gives trusts more financial and organizational freedom. Foundation hospital trusts operate in England as independent not-for-profit hospitals.

- The NHS Redress Act 2006 reforms how lower value clinical negligence cases can provide appropriate redress or compensation without the need to go to court.
- The Health Act 2006 allows for the prohibition of smoking in certain premises and locations, and for the amendment of the minimum age of persons to whom tobacco may be sold. It also covers the prevention and control of healthcare infections and how NHS organizations ensure that patients are cared for in a clean environment with a low risk of infection from MRSA or *Clostridium difficile*.

The 'third way' as a mixture of the welfare system and the market approach is apparent in the policies outlined above. There remains a strong emphasis on ensuring value for money or 'best value', with the Healthcare Commission responsible for reviewing and rating performance. New Labour is committed to continuing PFI, having announced a new wave of hospital building at a cost of £1.5 billion (DoH, 2007). PCTs and foundation hospital trusts should mean that decisions on health services are made locally with user involvement. Consumerism is evident in the legislation tackling redress in cases of clinical negligence. State intervention is permissible, to regulate both the professions and individual behaviour, for example the smoking ban.

Current health issues on the social policy agenda

Funding of health and social care

The question of how healthcare should be funded and how comprehensive services should be continues to be a problem for policy-makers. Public expectations of health services continue to rise as medicine develops new techniques and treatments to which the public demands fair and equitable access.

Example 7.3

FAIR AND EQUITABLE ACCESS TO TREATMENT: THE CASE OF HERCEPTIN

Herceptin is a drug that is effective in the treatment of early-stage breast cancer. In February 2006, a Swindon woman took her local PCT to the High Court following its refusal to give her the drug. The PCT argued that it would only fund the drug for patients in 'exceptional circumstances' and the drug was not licensed for treatment of early-stage breast cancer. A year's treatment with the drug is estimated to cost £20,000. The High Court upheld the PCT's refusal to fund Hercpetin but this ruling was overturned in

April 2006 by the Court of Appeal in a judgement that said it was irrational to treat one patient but not another. In June 2006, NICE issued guidance to health services in England and Wales that the drug had

received its European licence and should be available on the NHS. Women in Northern Ireland had had access to the drug since November 2005.

Source: BBC News 2006a

CONNECTIONS

Chapter 10 examines the rational basis for resource allocation within the NHS.

Rationing is not simply a consequence of the health service reforms of the 1990s, but is also a consequence of professional judgement. GPs decide which patients to refer to specialist services, based on their own ideas, beliefs and interpretation of need. Research on access to renal dialysis and other kidney treatments, for example, has shown that older people are systematically discriminated against through decisions not to refer them for specialist treatment (Allsop, 1995; New and Mays, 1997).

The needs of older people and others with chronic disorders have raised questions on what constitutes healthcare. In particular, problems remain concerning the boundary between health and social care. This is particularly acute for service providers and, more importantly, service users because healthcare is free at the point of delivery while social care is subject to charges. This issue impedes the development of integrated care.

The increase in the number of older people being supported by a diminishing working population is seen as putting a strain on available welfare resources. The high social value placed on independence places older people in a position of relative powerlessness and low social status whereby they become characterized as a burden. Despite this stereotyping, ageing is not a uniformly experienced phenomenon due to varying factors such as health, access to physical and emotional support, class, gender and race (Giddens, 2006). While retirement is likely to lead to a loss of income, living standards and status, there is a view of older people as gaining greater political influence ('the grey vote') as they experience more independence in this 'third age', free from the responsibilities of employment and parenthood.

The government's White Paper *Security in Retirement* (DWP, 2006) proposed that the state pension age would rise to 68 for men and women by 2044; that state pensions would be made more generous in the next Parliament and tied in future to earnings rather than prices; and that from 2012 people would be automatically enrolled on a low-cost national savings scheme to help save towards their future pension.

The provision of healthcare for older people demonstrates the difficulty of determining what a health issue is. The relationship between social factors and health is shown particularly clearly in old age. Medical advances and an improvement in the standard of living have led to increased longevity in general, but social inequality tends to become more pronounced in old age.

The acute model of healthcare dominant in the NHS can be seen as problematic for older people. The acute model's focus on curing and restoring people to full function does not take account of the high incidence of chronic illness in old age. Chronic disorders receive less attention in policy and resource terms, although the introduction of NSFs for some chronic conditions suggests this imbalance is being addressed.

A goal of *Saving Lives: Our Healthier Nation* (DoH, 1999) was to increase the length of people's lives and the number of years that people spend free from illness. Longevity continues to be a policy goal but this may be seen as problematic, as nearly half of all NHS expenditure goes on people aged 65 and over. Higher levels of need and demand for healthcare in old age have been presented as an economic problem. Williams (1997) argued that age should be a criterion for rationing decisions and that older people should not assume a right to healthcare equal to that of younger people. The charity Age Concern responded that to identify a class of people with less entitlement to services would be grossly inequitable.

When policies for community care were developed in the late 1980s, older people were regarded as a priority for attention. There was widespread agreement that an alternative to institutionalized regimes in geriatric hospital wards and residential care homes was needed (Means and Smith, 1998). Enabling older people to live in their own homes through reorganized services had, and still has, widespread appeal.

Community care is organized through a system of professional practice known as 'care management'. The care manager (from the purchasing local authority) establishes what an individual's needs are and then develops a 'package of care' that suits them, which is then purchased from a range of providers. Care management should ensure that the older person's needs are met in an integrated way, the individual having some say in how services are delivered, and the mixed economy of care offering a degree of choice over provision. The reality has been more problematic. The 1990 NHS and Community Care Act maintained the organizational and financial separation between health and social care services, which has militated against integrated service provision.

There are important differences in older people's entitlement to services, with healthcare being free and social care being means-tested. An example of this is that one old person may be bathed for free by a district nurse, whereas another may have to pay social services for a care assistant to bathe them. This has had implications for older people's access to services where some have been moved from one service to the other as each attempts to cut costs.

The Royal Commission on the Long-term Care of the Elderly (1999) argued for a collectivist approach in which the cost of care in old age should be spread across the generations. It argued that personal care (including bathing, hygiene and toileting) should be included as healthcare and provided free, whereas housing and ordinary food costs should be means-tested. A minority group argued against this approach, stressing individual responsibility and self-reliance and maintaining that targeted services were more appropriate, given limited resources. The disagreement is over how the costs of care should be met and by whom. The response to the Royal Commission from policy-makers has been varied.

In Scotland, free personal and nursing care for those aged over 65 living in their own homes was introduced in 2002. Not all members of the Scottish Parliament agreed with this new policy, arguing that it subsidizes the better off (Christie, 2002). People in care homes receive varying levels of payments depending on need that substantially reduce their costs. In effect, this creates a two-tier system of care for older people within the UK. It results in older people in Scotland being better off than those in the rest of the UK, where entitlement to personal care continues to be means-tested.

Consumerism and empowerment

There is an ongoing debate about whether policy should take a consumerist or empowerment approach to the provision of welfare. Consumerism may be characterized by customer, choice, complaint and compensation. It can be seen in policies such as direct payments and in proposals such as a 'patient's passport', where patients would receive funding to enable them to move around different providers – NHS, not-for-profit, private and voluntary. Such a scheme is regarded as a means of privatizing the NHS as it allows people to spend public money in the private sector. An empowerment approach is apparent in policies encouraging service user involvement and control over services. Empowerment can be collectivist through the promotion of support systems, networks and self-help groups.

Need and risk

A different way of framing and developing policy would be to use the concept of welfare risk rather than welfare need. This would require policy-makers to define those at risk or regarded as vulnerable, such as children and older people, and then devising protection policies. The concept can be extended into areas of health risk such as smoking, high cholesterol, obesity and heart disease.

The historical outline in this section has shown how ideas and values concerning the role and the relative responsibilities of the state, individuals, families and the private and voluntary sectors have been developed to deal with social problems. Policy-making and implementation are part of a political process that is influenced by pragmatism and expediency as well as ideology. The next section turns to the policy process and presents perspectives and frameworks for analysis to help the reader develop a critical view of proposed and actual social policies.

Theoretical and methodological approaches

The development of the discipline

The discipline of social policy is inextricably linked with the processes of policy-making and practice in welfare provision. At the beginning of the twentieth century, there was an upsurge of interest in the education and training of occupational groups in public sector welfare services. Because there were no texts written at the time, academic courses relied on casework records, including those of the Charity Organization Society, as sources of data. Other sources included government statistics, census data and official reports.

Empirical research data, such as those produced by Booth (1902) and Rowntree (1901), were important to the development of the academic study of welfare. However, the intention was that the data they produced should not simply be available for study but also be a means of stimulating government action to address social problems. This conceptual linkage in social policy between academic work and action by the state was influential in the development of welfare state policies in the Fabian Society and the Labour Party in the early twentieth century.

The idea of the welfare state had an increasingly broad appeal. By the time the Beveridge Report was published in 1942, all political parties were interested in developing welfare along broadly similar lines. The period of intense political activity as the welfare state was established after the Second World War was reflected in academic circles. During the postwar years, the discipline of social administration flourished in British universities as the public sector expanded and more professional education was required. The broad consensus over the role of the state in developing welfare services was evident in the style and content of the discipline. It was generally concerned with the design and development of effective services, largely informed by professional ideas relating to the best ways of meeting human need.

Titmuss (1974) developed a model for classifying welfare systems according to their ideological basis. He distinguished between residual and institutional models of welfare. *Residual systems* offer welfare as a last resort, or safety net, to those in danger of becoming destitute. The principle of individual responsibility is encouraged, and welfare targeted at those in greatest need. Recipients may be means tested to prove themselves poor through no fault of their own. In residual systems, welfare is often experienced as stigmatizing to recipients.

In contrast, *institutional systems* favour universal benefits, collectively financed through taxation. These are less likely to be experienced as stigmatizing because they benefit a wide cross-section of society and are intended to reduce inequality.

? Institutional welfare has characterized Britain in the postwar years. How has it been challenged?

Research in the 1960s led to the 'rediscovery' of poverty as researchers exposed ongoing problems that had not been adequately addressed by the welfare state (Abel-Smith and Townsend, 1965). Concern about homelessness, depicted in the 1966 film *Cathy Come Home*, prompted the formation of the voluntary organization Shelter. During the 1960s, there was a growing realization that the welfare state was not necessarily benevolent and included some highly questionable practices. The concept of institutionalization – the loss of personal identity that occurs when people are subjected to institutional regimes – was developed (Goffman, 1961). In addition, evidence of the abuse of patients and residents in institutions was publicized (Robb, 1967). This raised more fundamental questions concerning the role of the welfare state as an instrument of social control, engaged in oppressive acts against vulnerable people.

It was at this time that the discipline became known as social policy rather than social administration, indicating a shift in perspective from a study of how to deliver welfare to a critical analysis of welfare policies and the role of the state. These critiques can be divided into cultural, materialist, feminist, postmodern and comparative.

Cultural critiques of welfare

Cultural critiques have challenged the way in which welfare services are designed and provided and the assumptions that are made about the needs and expectations of, for example, women, black and minority ethnic groups, and disabled and older people. The uniformity of services and lack of understanding of the differences between service users have been criticized. For example, many people whose first language is not English require support with gaining access to health services. Since equality of access is a fundamental principle of the NHS, it could be argued that such support should be provided as a right.

CONNECTIONS

Chapter 6 explores the significance of cultural identity and beliefs to health.

The NHS Plan (DoH, 2000) called for wider availability of interpreting and advocacy services; however, the provision of these services remains patchy. The NHS Direct website offers information in a dozen languages including Arabic, Polish, Somali and Urdu, alongside a tele-interpreting service by phone and online. An estimate that the NHS spends £55 million on translation services has led to the suggestion that GPs should encourage users to learn English (Adams, 2007).

Materialist critiques of welfare

Materialist critiques focus on the needs and demands of working-class people for more welfare in the context of diminishing resources, and commentators in the 1980s pointed to an emerging crisis of welfare as supply failed to meet demand (Hayek, 1983; Taylor-Gooby, 1985). The 'New Right' Conservative government in the 1980s also identified welfare as placing an unmanageable burden on the economic system. Its response, however, was that there was too much welfare and it needed to be privatized.

These perspectives have been influential in the shift in health policy from a postwar consensual model to a more market-oriented conflictual model. Key debates in social policy concern how much difference social policies can make and whether egalitarian social policies can compensate for unequal societies (Tawney, 1964; Blakemore, 2003).

Chapter 4 examines health inequalities in greater detail.

Feminist critiques of welfare

Feminist critiques have questioned assumptions about women's dependent status, caring roles and their opportunities for paid work, and the failure to take gender roles into account when analysing welfare (Finch and Groves, 1980). Women's daily work to ensure the health and safety of family members is not regarded as productive activity in the same way as paid healthcare is, even though there is evidence that formal healthcare systems have always depended on informal family care to enable them to function. When the NHS was established, assumptions were made about mothers being available to provide care as and when professionals required them to. The schedules of child health clinics made no concession for mothers in paid employment. In the 1950s, assumptions about women's dependency on their husbands was so strong that women in teaching and nursing were expected to leave their jobs when they married. Women were classified according to their husbands' occupation in census returns and other social research.

The traditional division between caring work in the public and private spheres is artificial, and a 'reconception of caring' is required to take account of women's caring work (Graham, 1983). Since the implementation of the NHS and Community Care Act in 1990, a great deal of research has been conducted into the effects of caring on carers' physical and mental health, finances, employment opportunities and participation in social life. One study (SPRU, 2004) concluded that carers often have additional healthcare needs as a result of their caring responsibilities. They are more likely than non-carers to report emotional and mental health problems including anxiety and depression. Feminists have identified how assumptions relating to women's caring roles continue to be made in both policy and practice (see, for example, Pascall, 1997).

Critiques of feminist perspectives have also emerged that take inequality between women into account in their analysis of women's position in the welfare systems. Disabled women have pointed out that the depiction of women carers as exploited victims is not only deeply offensive to disabled people, but also presents a distorted picture of the relationships between disabled and non-disabled people. The contribution of disabled people to family life also needs to be recognized (Morris, 1992). Black women have argued that feminists have neglected to take account of their experiences. Racist and discriminatory values have meant that black women have been expected to take on low-grade, menial work. In the NHS, for example, black nurses have been routinely offered jobs below their level of qualifications and skills.

Postmodernist critiques of welfare

Postmodernism questions a range of assumptions underpinning the provision of welfare services, for example whether all groups in society attach the same meaning and value to welfare services. Postmodernism also contributes to theoretical and methodological analyses in social policy. For example, post-modern analyses challenge the traditional divisions of welfare into categories of service users. Within mental health, the needs and demands of patients from different ethnic groups vary significantly, yet these variations are often neglected as services are organized along rigid lines. Postmodernism questions whether particular needs can be met within universalist models of welfare (Thompson and Hoggett, 1996; Williams, 1992).

Postmodernism has itself been critiqued. Taylor-Gooby (1994) argues that postmodern analyses overemphasize the importance of changes to economic and social systems, and suggests that some aspects of modern life, for example levels of insecurity, poverty and exploitation, demonstrate continuity rather than change and are reminiscent of pre-welfare state conditions.

Postmodernism is useful in questioning whether universalistic policies are appropriate in a fragmented world. A postmodern approach to policy-making can be seen in New Labour's willingness to change policy directions, often in the face of media responses, without adequate public consultation, piloting and evaluation of options (Blakemore, 2003).

Comparative critiques of welfare

As the discipline of social policy has developed, ideas about how welfare can be organized in order to gain maximum benefit from state, private, occupational, voluntary and informal sectors have benefited from comparative perspectives. Comparative models of welfare follow Titmuss's (1974) classification of residual and institutional models of welfare (see above).

Analysing the relationship between state welfare and the market is important in tackling some questions posed at the beginning of this chapter:

- Who benefits from social policies?

- Whose values do social policies reflect?

- What is the relationship between social policies and broader social inequalities?

A simple comparison of spending on welfare does not answer these questions. In the USA in 2004, for example, healthcare absorbed 15.3% of gross domestic product (GDP) compared with 10.9% for Germany and 8.3% for the UK; yet state welfare is residual and minimal in the USA but well developed in the UK. However, by looking at sources of funding, one sees different values at play. In the UK, 86% of health spending was funded by public sources in 2004, while in the USA the figure was 45%, reflecting a greater reliance on private healthcare there (OECD, 2006).

Esping-Anderson (1990) has developed a classification of three welfare 'regimes' that attempts to take into account issues of citizen rights and inequalities:

1. Emphasis on the government's role in providing comprehensive welfare services funded through taxation, so a high level of employment is necessary. Social equality an important aim. Examples are Sweden and Denmark.

2. Government involvement in the organization of welfare through both private and state insurance schemes and through the voluntary sector. Tends to be conservative in approach to family values. Examples are Germany and France.

3. State welfare provided at a minimal level, targeted at the poorest. The voluntary and informal sectors are expected to play a major role, and the private markets are relatively unregulated. Also known as 'residual' or 'laissez-faire' welfare states. Examples are the USA and Spain.

Two dimensions of comparison are of particular importance:

- the extent to which the state enables individuals to enjoy an acceptable standard of living independently of the labour market ('decommodification')

- the extent to which the state promotes equality and social integration through welfare.

Classifications such as Esping-Anderson's are useful in helping us to identify similarities and differences between countries. However, it only identifies three regimes within Western developed democracies. The regimes focus on income maintenance and the labour market, while the focus on formal welfare provision neglects the contribution of the informal sector and the family in producing welfare (Daly, 1994). Daly argues that the family is the most significant provider of welfare in all welfare states.

The classifications need updating and expanding to recognize other welfare state regimes in, for example, Eastern Europe. The collapse of the Soviet bloc and the re-emergence of independent nation states in Eastern Europe have seen a transition in welfare provision, from the Soviet state-managed, secure economy with guaranteed employment and service provision to more liberal, democratic, market-oriented but insecure systems that do not guarantee employment or rights to services (Deacon, 2000).

? **What other factors would need to be taken into account if comparisons were to include developing countries?**

Gough (2004) expands Esping-Anderson's classifications to include developing countries. In distinguishing between welfare regimes, he notes different patterns of colonization and decolonization. For example, 'insecurity' welfare regimes of sub-Saharan Africa are characterized by late decolonization and independence. In these countries, the main livelihood comes from agriculture, families and clans take care of welfare needs, and key roles are played by political or military elites and by external agencies such as the United Nations or the World Bank. The 'productivist' welfare regimes of East Asia such as Taiwan and Malaysia have different patterns of colonization. These are dynamic emerging capitalist economies where the aim is high economic growth, with social policy regarded as social investment and where the state acts as regulator rather than provider of welfare. The 'conservative-informal' welfare regimes of South America experienced early decolonization and independence. Their economies were principally driven by exports that led to wealth and the development of a capitalist class and urban workers. While those in the formal employment sector benefited from the emergence of social insurance and protection schemes, those in the informal economy remained unprotected and unregulated.

The United Nations Development Programme provides useful data for comparisons between countries and produces an annual Human Development Report. Its 'human development index' (HDI) is calculated from data on the per capita GDP, life expectancy and adult literacy in any country. It is used to indicate whether a country is developed, developing or underdeveloped. Giving a world overview, the *Human Development Report 2006* (UNDP, 2006) noted stagnation in the world HDI as the continued improvement of developed countries was offset by the general decline of the developing world, especially countries in sub-Saharan Africa and South Asia. It is necessary to take account of a range of social as well as economic factors because there is a clear difference between countries in how resources are used for welfare.

Deacon (1997) refers to the levels of global inequity and the way in which the welfare of people in some developing countries is adversely affected by dependency on the West and mounting debts. In addition, continued and widening economic inequity, food deprivation, enforced migration and exposure to organized crime need to be taken into account.

Comparative social policy contributes to our understanding of both how and why welfare is organized in a particular way. In Ireland, for example, there is a long tradition of Church involvement in healthcare. In Sweden, women's participation in paid employment has been higher than that in many other European countries, and this affects how the informal sphere operates. Comparative approaches demonstrate how concepts such as needs, rights, equity, autonomy and responsibility are expressed through policies in different ways in different contexts.

Methodologies of social policy in understanding health

A range of methodologies, empirical and non-empirical, qualitative and quantitative, can be identified in social policy. For example, the works of social researchers, such as Townsend's (1979) surveys of poverty, have contributed significantly to theory development. Townsend's research led to the development of the concept of 'relative deprivation', which describes the standard of living of any individual or group in comparison with the vast majority of the population. He argued that **policies** to tackle poverty needed to take into account social and cultural factors as well as individual human needs.

Example 7.4

USING TEXTUAL ANALYSIS TO UNDERSTAND POLICY

'Policy is both text and action, words and deeds' (Ball, 1994). Scott (2000, p. 18) observes that 'policy texts are characterized as official texts which operate to influence public perception of a policy agenda'. He notes how words are used and positioned to sound authoritative and to present a case for policy change as though there is no challenge or room for debate. A close reading of policy texts is a useful way to begin policy analysis.

A starting point is a content analysis through a systematic reading of a policy document. A quantitative approach involves counting the number of times key words or ideas are used. A qualitative approach or narrative analysis considers the meanings, contexts, subjects and descriptions of the policy, for example who is the policy talking about and what is intended for them. A comparison between policy texts is a useful means of spotting similarities and contradictions.

A reading of The NHS Plan (2000) might note how the use of words, such as 'modern', 'reform' and the much-repeated phrase 'for the first time', indicates the message being presented. The context is set by phrases such as 'the NHS failing to deliver', 'a 1940s system operating in a 21st century world', 'a lack of national standards' and 'old-fashioned demarcations between staff' to justify reform and modernization. Further narrative analysis would pick up who the reforms are aimed at – patients and staff; when, where and how the reforms will happen; and the setting of targets to know if and when they are achieved – such as 7,000 extra hospital beds and 20,000 extra nurses. A close reading can lead on to other questions such as what values underpin the text.

Data from qualitative research, such as that published by the Joseph Rowntree Foundation and others, have been crucial in, for example, encouraging the voices of service users to be included in social policy theorizing. Williams et al. (1999) argue that there is a need to understand the relationship between the personal history and experiences of people who use welfare services and the material and social world. The idea of welfare users as passive recipients or victims of the system has been profoundly challenged by a range of organizations, such as disabled people's and women's groups. Research that enables the voice of the service user to emerge presents a particular problem to policy-makers and service providers, as the demand to be more sensitive to service users' own constructions of their needs sits uncomfortably with demands to provide more efficient and cost-effective services.

Policy analysis

Social policy analysis concerns not only welfare systems but also individual policy development. Policy analysis is a core activity of research and theory-building. Policies may be analysed on the basis of whether they achieve their objectives. Le Grand et al. (1998), for example, examined the evidence on whether the radical ideas behind the NHS reforms and creation of the internal market achieved what was intended. They concluded that there were fewer changes to the functioning of the NHS than might have been expected. More recently, writers have been evaluating New Labour's welfare reforms in health (Paton, 2002) and social care (Baldwin, 2002).

However, policy analysis goes deeper than simple evaluations of policies against their stated aims and objectives. Policy analysis can be divided into the analysis *for* policy and the analysis *of* policy (Hill, 2005):

- analysis *for* policy contributes to solving social problems through a focus on evaluating the impact of policy, gathering data and information to assist policy-makers, and advocacy to present policy options or choices.

- analysis *of* policy is an academic activity concerned with advancing understanding and knowledge through studies of policy content, outputs and process such as decision-making.

Although this distinction is useful, there is a relationship between the two types as each influences the other: the development of knowledge has implications for policy-making, and policy-making is the subject of academic analysis.

Hudson and Lowe (2004) introduce a framework for policy analysis that considers policy at a macro-, meso- and micro-level. A macro-level analysis considers concepts such as globalization, the political economy, and changes in the world of work, technology and governance. For example, the impact of globalization and technology in connecting people around the world has economic and social implications. Multinational corporations are able to shift production to countries where labour costs are cheap. Easier intercontinental travel raises concerns about health and the spread of infections such as SARS.

A meso-level analysis looks at structures of power, policy networks, institutions and policy transfer. For example, the differential power exerted by the state and various policy stakeholders such as political elites, organizations, pressure groups and service users in introducing, shaping or undermining social policies. Policy transfer is about the exchange or sharing of policy ideas, as seen where elements of US 'workfare' are apparent in New Labour's New Deal policies that put paid employment to the fore rather than the right to welfare.

A micro-level analysis focuses on decision-making and makers, implementation and delivery, and evaluation and evidence. Decision-making is limited by the choices available in the chaotic real world of policies developing incrementally and building on what has gone before, rather than being a rational choice that starts with a blank sheet of paper. Individuals and charismatic leaders have an impact, such as Aneurin Bevan, the minster of health, in establishing the NHS, and the frontline workers or 'street-level bureaucrats' (Lipsky, 1979) who implement and deliver social policies. The latter's role may be crucial in promoting, interpreting, hindering or delaying a policy.

The policy process

Social policies can be understood as dynamic processes influenced by a range of groups and individuals that have a stake in the process. Understanding the policy process enables us to understand relationships of power between the people involved and, beneath the surface, the relationship between policies and social divisions and inequalities. Ham and Hill (1993, p. 12) maintain that a policy is a 'web of decisions rather than one decision', also arguing that non-decision-making is as important as decision-making to the policy analyst.

A traditional approach to the policy process as a system is shown by Hogwood and Gunn's (1984, p. 24) model that lists the stages in a policy cycle: deciding to decide; deciding how to decide; issue definition; forecasting; setting objectives and priorities; options analysis; policy implementation, monitoring and control; evaluation and review; policy maintenance, succession and termination. This is useful but policy development is rarely neat and tidy, moving in an orderly linear fashion from one completed stage to the next. Indeed, policy initiation 'may start anywhere in the system' (Hill, 2005, p. 21).

Figure 7.2 shows different elements of the policy process and how they affect each other. The relationship between policy-making and output, for example, may be examined to assess the efficiency of implementation systems. On the other hand, understanding the way in which issues get on the policy agenda in the first place can shed light on outcomes. There are several elements to the process.

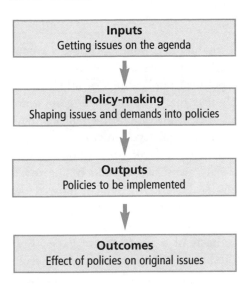

Figure 7.2 The policy process

Inputs

The way in which issues emerge as problems requiring government action reflects particular social and cultural values. Human needs and suffering do not always attract attention, and even where there is an awareness of a problem, this does not always translate into political action. Social phenomena may be perceived as problems by some but not others. Lone parenthood, for example, is consistently characterized as a social problem, but this characterization is open to dispute.

Policy inputs may come from within governments as well as from external interest groups. For example, in 1988, following a funding crisis in the NHS, the prime minister's review was established. Unusually for a review of the health service, this group did not include any medical professionals but was limited to a small group of Cabinet ministers, chaired by Prime Minister Margaret Thatcher. This review needs to be understood in the light of the political importance of the NHS and the need for the government to take decisive action.

Getting an issue onto the agenda requires effective organization and access to sources of power and influence. The ability of any group to lobby effectively is crucially important. Some groups are more privileged than others in having access to formal or informal networks of power. Professional and commercial groups, for example, have enjoyed greater influence over health policy than health service users (Allsop, 1995). However, where lay or user groups have organized effectively around particular issues, such as the need for better services for people with HIV, they have been successful.

Policy-making

The process of formulating issues or demands into policy proposals comes next in the policy process. Policy-makers have to consider how any issue fits in with their overall agenda, what the political implications of adopting an issue as policy might be, and how likely it is that proposals will gain wider support and pass through the legislative process. Consultation enables policy-makers to test and listen to opinion. At a national level, this may be in the form of Green Papers, such as *Independence, Wellbeing and Choice* (DoH, 2005a) seeking views on how adult social care services could be improved and *Your Health, Your Care, Your Say* (DoH, 2005b), which allowed the public to speak directly to ministers, health professionals and each other about how improvements could be made in local services.

These two consultations formed the basis of a single White Paper, *Our Health, Our Care, Our Say* (DoH, 2006a), which is a firm proposal from government for legislation. Following this, a government bill is introduced to Parliament, to be followed by a long process of reading, debate and amendment within the House of Commons, the House of Lords and parliamentary committees.

Example 7.5

POLICY-MAKING: THE EXAMPLE OF A SMOKING BAN IN WORKPLACES AND PUBLIC PLACES

In July 2006 a bill to ban smoking in virtually all workplaces in England was approved by Parliament and came into effect on 1 July 2007. This follows on from smoking bans introduced in Scotland (from March 2006) and in Wales and Northern Ireland (from April 2007).

The call for a ban was based on scientific evidence that exposure to other people's smoke is dangerous to health. Reports such as that from the government's Scientific Committee on Tobacco and Health (SCOTH, 2004) and studies such as Jamrozik's (2005) have raised public awareness of the risks of passive smoking. The pressure group Action on Smoking and Health (ASH) commissioned a MORI poll in 2004 that showed overwhelming public support for new legislation to end smoking in the workplace. A government report on public health (Wanless, 2004) considered the evidence of smoking bans implemented in other countries such as Ireland. In November 2004, the government responded with the White Paper *Choosing Health: Making Healthier Choices*

Easier (DoH, 2004) that included proposals to end smoking in the majority of workplaces and public places except for private clubs and pubs not serving food.

Ultimately, the smoking ban went further than the government intended. Concern in the Cabinet that many Labour MPs would not support the exemptions of clubs and pubs led to the decision to allow a free vote, where MPs make up their own minds rather than follow the party line. This resulted in a total ban in all enclosed areas. The legislation introduces fines of £50 for individuals caught smoking in a banned area and up to £2,500 for those in charge of premises failing to stop people smoking in a restricted area.

While welcomed by anti-smoking groups like ASH, trade unions concerned for the health and safety of their members, and the Health Secretary Patricia Hewitt, as a change that would 'save thousands of people's lives', others regard it as an infringement of civil liberties. Organizations such as the Tobacco Manufacturers Association believe that people should continue to have the opportunity to make informed choices about whether to smoke or not. Smoking support groups funded by the tobacco industry, such as FOREST (Freedom of the Right to Enjoy Smoking Tobacco), argue that people will continue to smoke and may do so more at home around children. Legal challenges are expected from large hotel and pub groups.

Sources: DoH, 2004; ASH, 2006; BBC News, 2006b

Outputs

If a bill goes through all the stages mentioned above, it becomes an Act of Parliament that requires implementation through central or local government or other agencies. At this stage, there is scope for further modification. Local conditions and priorities differ, and this will influence the implementation process. For example, the relationship between the overall strategic aims of the Department of Health and health authorities is not straightforward. The government may give guidance on putting policies into operation, but how this is interpreted at the local level varies. The relationship between central government and local authorities is an important focus for analysis in social policy.

Pressure to change implementation procedures also often emerges. The Carers' National Association, for example, conducted research on the implementation of the 1995 Carers (Recognition and Services) Act, which revealed a gap between policy and practice in general and variations between local authorities in how they implemented the policy. In addition, legislation may meet some but not all the demands of interest groups: the Disability Discrimination Act 1995 met some of the demands of disabled people's groups for action to promote equality of opportunity but stopped short of establishing a commission for disability equality along the lines of the Commission for Racial Equality.

Outcomes

What difference does a policy make to people's lives? Given the scope for modification and change at all stages of the process, it is not surprising that policy outcomes can be quite different from what was envisaged by stakeholders at the beginning. This often means that the process of campaigning and lobbying begins again as further reforms and changes are demanded. Policies also often have unforeseen consequences that may stimulate pressure for further policy action.

At this stage, the experiences of patients and service users also need to be taken into account. Policies to improve efficiency in the NHS have, for example, led to problems over the discharge from hospital of frail and chronically sick people, who may be regarded as 'bed-blockers'. How do individual patients experience problems over hospital discharge? How does it feel to be a 'bed-blocker'? In what way can such feelings and experiences be articulated and heard by policy-makers and service providers?

The policy process is therefore not neat and linear but continuous and complex, influenced by the context in which it occurs. This involves social policy analysts in identifying the links between policy processes and broader economic, political and social systems, as well as taking into account the experiences of service users.

CASE STUDY Obesity

This case study takes up themes identified in the chapter including the application of frameworks for policy analysis and answers key questions:

- How is obesity as a health issue defined?
- Who should address obesity and how?
- Whose views and values are reflected in policy decisions?

Defining a health issue

Obesity is seen as an important risk factor for chronic diseases, mental ill health and a poorer quality of life. A UK government report (NAO, 2001) recommended that the NHS should use demographic evidence to ensure a consistent approach to obesity management. NICE (2006) has produced a review of interventions that effectively tackle obesity.

Responding to the issue

In May 2004, the health secretary announced that the government was concerned about the serious health impact of obesity and that this would be addressed in the White Paper on public health to be published later that year.

The White Paper *Choosing Health* (DoH, 2004) set out three core principles of its 'new public health' approach:

- *Informed choice:* where the public make decisions about health choices based on credible and trustworthy information.
- *Personalization:* recognition that support in making and sticking with healthy

choices must fit with the reality of individual lives.
- *Working together:* progress on healthier choices depends on effective partnerships between local government, the NHS, businesses, the voluntary sector, communities, the media, and others.

In 2004, a target on tackling obesity was laid down for the first time. Under a public service agreement (PSA) setting out key improvements the public can expect from government, the target was to halt the year-on-year rise in obesity among children under eleven by 2010. This was a target shared by the Department of Health, the Department of Culture, Media and Sport (DCMS) and the Department for Education and Skills (DfES). It is illustrative of New Labour's 'third way' approach of target-setting and joined-up thinking and action between departments.

In February 2006, the departments gave a policy response update on progress (DoH, 2006b). The public health minister (DoH) spoke of changing attitudes through the '5 A Day' campaign and school fruit scheme. The schools minister (DfES) referred to a transformation in the health content of school meals, with £220 million made available to improve lunches. The sport minister (DCMS) announced investment of over £1.5 billion in school sport to encourage more physical activity.

Views and values in decision-making

Who determines what is a health problem and defines the associated issues? For whom is it a problem or issue – the state, the individual, organizations, professionals? The historical context shows where UK policy on obesity was initiated and how it developed. By applying Hudson and Lowe's (2004) framework for analysis at a macro-level, one could see UK policy on obesity as emerging from the global context set out by the WHO (1998). Considering the political economy, questions emerge on the aims and purpose of the policies such as the need for an effective, efficient and healthy workforce.

The 'new' public health approach of the government was evident in the establishment of the School Food Trust in 2005, with £15 million funding from the DfES to promote the education and health of children by improving the quality of food in schools. This was addressing the core principles by providing information and guidelines through 'food education', supporting healthier choices and working together with schools and the food industry. However, some feel these areas should be left to the free choice of the individual, families, organizations or local authorities.

The dilemma for government and the values encompassed in its approach to health policy are apparent in Prime Minister Blair's response on BBC *Breakfast* to a question about health inequalities. Blair sees the role of government is to raise awareness of the importance of healthy lifestyle but argues that the difficulty 'is trying to balance not becoming a nanny state and telling everyone what to do, with trying to educate people that there are real choices which you make' (Weaver et al., 2006).

Media stories can help to initiate or maintain a policy drive; one, with the headline 'Britons most obese in Europe' (Weaver et al., 2006), for example, quoted a report showing that 23% of adults in the UK are obese compared to countries such as France and Italy where the rate is below

10%. In addition, public response to media stories can impact on policy.

The television series *Jamie's School Dinners* (Channel 4, 2005), which revealed poor quality and low investment in school meals, produced a widespread audience reaction in support of celebrity chef Jamie Oliver's campaign to improve school dinners. This impacted directly on the catering companies supplying schools, with a drop in the numbers of parents opting for school dinners and thus a drop in sales of their products, which were seen as being unhealthy. The government responded with a pledge to invest £220 million over three years to improve standards and to set minimum recommendations for spending on ingredients.

Future policy directions and debates

While this case study has mainly considered obesity policy in England, a visit to the websites for the Scottish Parliament, the National Public Health Service for Wales and the Health Promotion Agency for the Northern Ireland Executive presents a range of approaches and priorities in tackling obesity. For example, the Scottish Parliament is considering introducing universal free school meals partly in response to NHS statistics that put the number of obese children in Scotland as double the UK average.

In terms of welfare needs and risks, this case study raises the question of where responsibility lies for tackling obesity. The WHO labels obesity as a problem and this view is endorsed by the UK government, health organizations and health workers. Policy responses are initiated, with targets set, then implemented and evaluated. Cautionary tales appear in the media and medical reports or journals to demonstrate that obesity remains an ongoing problem for those who do not accept the responsibilities for their own or their children's health.

A mother was called to a child protection conference with the local social services and health experts to discuss whether her eight-year-old son weighing 14 stone should be taken into care (BBC News, 2007). The parent argues about choice, saying 'When (he) won't eat anything else, I've got to give him the food he likes.' The local PCT talks of working with the family over a period of time and seeing the 'child's interests as paramount'. Who should determine the interests of a child aged eight? Aged 14?

A report from the Medical Research Council's human nutrition research centre links bad parenting to obesity in children, according to the *Guardian* (Boseley, 2007). Researchers interviewed midwives, obstetricians and other professionals from maternity units in the northeast of England and published findings that obese mothers-to-be need significantly more NHS care than pregnant women of a healthy weight (Heslehurst et al., 2007).

Those wanting to make healthier choices may be rewarded and supported with NHS health trainers, advice and support. NICE offers guidance on the prevention, management and treatment of obesity. It presents support tools for NHS staff in assessing the risk of obesity in patients and works with the independent sector to develop alternative approaches in behaviour change. Where behaviour change is not possible, then there is the medical solution. In December 2006, NICE recommended guidelines about the use of anti-obesity drugs and stomach-stapling surgery (bariatrics) to tackle obesity.

This case study has illustrated how obesity becomes defined as a health issue requiring a policy response. Government response to the issue is based on evidence and values, and media coverage is a powerful tool in framing issues for public consumption. What emerges is not consistent or consensual, but a mixture of policies informed by popular beliefs and values as well as scientific evidence and evidence about cost-effectiveness. The policy agenda is never static, but constantly shifting and evolving.

Summary

- The discipline of social policy enables us to understand how ideas about people's health and wellbeing are put into practice through welfare systems. Social policy also enables us to recognize that interventions are not always beneficial and policies may not, in practice, enhance health and wellbeing. Critical approaches in social policy probe deeper to analyse the complex nature of welfare systems

- An analysis of the policy process provides further illumination of the relationship between policies and the economic, political and social contexts in which they are developed

- Social policy includes fundamental philosophical questions about the ways in which a society secures the health and wellbeing of its most vulnerable members, such as older people

- Social policy continues to experience a tension between the need to analyse and critique welfare policies and the need to provide information that can be used to develop policies. Social policy is, simultaneously, about values, principles and pragmatism

- The importance of social policy to health studies is that it enables us to see how ideas about people's health and wellbeing are shaped into policies and practices, and how this is a dynamic process that is continually being analysed and changed

Questions for further discussion

1. Over the next two or three days, study reports or articles on health issues in one of the broadsheet newspapers. Think about the following:

    - Who is raising the issue and whom do they represent?
    - Is the issue on the policy agenda locally, nationally or internationally?
    - Where is pressure being directed?
    - What values are being expressed through this issue?

2. 'On the principle of the equal moral worth of all people, healthcare should not be rationed.' Discuss this proposition, with particular reference to old age.

3. Visit the Department of Health website at www.dh.gov.uk. Click on 'health topics' and follow the link to the topic of your choice such as communicable diseases, HIV, obesity or older people's services. Track how the policies associated with your topic are being implemented and consider their likely impact on the lives of schoolchildren, people of working age and retired people.

Further reading

There are several useful introductory texts on social policy. These will enable you to follow up general points related to the discipline.

Baggott, R. (2004) *Health and Health Care in Britain* (3rd edn) Basingstoke: Palgrave Macmillan.
A concise and detailed introduction to all aspects of health care in Britain that takes account of many recent changes in the NHS and health policy.

Blakemore, K. and Griggs, E. (2007) *Social Policy: An Introduction* (3rd edn). Buckingham: Open University Press.
This is a readable text looking at the general themes of welfare and at particular areas. Chapter 9, on health policy and health professions, will enable you to explore this issue in greater depth.

Buse, K., Mays, N. and Walt, G. (2005) *Making Health Policy*. Maidenhead: Open University Press.
Helps to gain an understanding of policy process and offers international perspectives.

Busfield, J. (2000) *Health and Health Care in Modern Britain*. Oxford: Oxford University Press.
Aimed at those studying the sociology of health and healthcare. Examines key issues affecting healthcare in contemporary Britain.

Dean, H. (2006) *Social Policy*. Cambridge: Polity Press.
Explores the foundations of social policy, the issues it addresses and the economic, political and sociological dimensions.

Drake, R. (2001) *The Principles of Social Policy*. Basingstoke: Palgrave – now Palgrave Macmillan.
Introduces concepts and key issues in social policy and how policies are shaped by political values and beliefs.

Orme, J., Powell, J., Taylor, P. and Grey, M. (2007) *Public Health for the 21st Century: New Perspectives on Policy, Participation and Practice* (2nd edn). Maidenhead: Open University Press.
Offers an overview of the public health field, analysis of contemporary practice and policy changes, and exploration of debates around the meaning of public health.

The following are some useful websites:

- hdr.undp.org/ for access to the United Nations Development Programme's annual Human Development Reports.
- www.dh.gov.uk to visit the Department of Health website to explore current and recent activities by central government in health.
- www.kingsfund.org.uk The King's Fund publishes a range of reports, papers and guides on policy and practice in health and social care.
- www.northernireland.gov.uk Select Department of Health, Social Services and Public Safety to access information on policies, services and news on health and social care services in Northern Ireland.
- www.nphs.wales.nhs.uk The National Public Health Service for Wales delivers a full range of public health services and provides resources, information and advice to the Welsh Assembly, trusts and other NHS health bodies.

References

Abel-Smith, B. and Townsend, P. (1965) *The Poor and the Poorest*. London: G. Bell.

Acheson, D. (1998) *Independent Inquiry into Inequalities in Health: A Report*. London: Stationery Office.

Adams, K. (2007) 'Should the NHS curb spending on translation services?' *British Medical Journal* **334**: 398.

Allsop, J. (1995) *Health Policy and the NHS: Towards 2000*. London: Longman.

ASH (Action on Smoking and Health) (2006) Factsheet no. 14: Smoking in Workplaces and Public Places, www.ash.org.uk/html/factsheets/html/fact14.html, accessed 09/03/2007.

Baggott, R. (2004) *Health and Healthcare in Britain* (3rd edn). Basingstoke: Palgrave Macmillan.

Baldwin, M. (2002) New Labour and social change: continuity or change?, in M. Powell (ed.) *Evaluating New Labour's Welfare Reforms*. Bristol: Policy Press.

Ball, S. (1994) *Education Reform: A Critical and Post-Structuralist Approach*. Buckingham: Open University Press.

BBC News (2006a) Woman wins Herceptin court fight, news.bbc.co.uk/go/pr/fr/-/1/hi/health/4902150.stm and NHS drug watchdog backs Herceptin, news.bbc.co.uk/go/pr/fr/-/1/hi/health/ 5058952.stm, accessed 28/02/2007.

BBC News (2006b) Campaigners welcome smoking ban, news.bbc.co.uk/1/hi/uk_politics/4714992.stm, accessed 15/02/2007.

BBC News (2007) Care hearing due for obese child, news.bbc.co.uk/1/hi/health/6396457.stm, accessed 09/03/2007.

Beveridge, W. (1942) *Social Insurance and Allied Services* (The Beveridge Report). London: HMSO.

Blakemore, K. (2003) *Social Policy: An Introduction* (2nd edn). Buckingham: Open University Press.

Booth, C. (1902) *Life and Labour of the People of London*. London: Macmillan – now Palgrave Macmillan.

Boseley, S. (2007) Parents are focus of new childhood anti-obesity education campaign, *Guardian*, 15 March.

Christie, B. (2002) 'United Kingdom divided as Scotland introduces free personal care for elderly people'. *British Medical Journal* **324**: 1542.

Daly, M. (1994) Comparing welfare states: towards a gender friendly approach, in D. Sainsbury (ed.) *Gendering Welfare States*. London: Sage, pp. 101–17.

Davey Smith, G., Dorling, D. and Shaw, M. (2001) *Poverty, Inequality and Health in Britain: A Reader*. Bristol: Policy Press.

Davey Smith, G., Dorling, D., Mitchell, R. and Shaw, M. (2002) 'Health inequalities in Britain: continuing increases up to the end of the 20th century'. *Journal of Epidemiology and Community Health* **56**: 434–5.

Deacon, B., with Hulse, M. and Stubbs, P. (1997) *Global Social Policy: International Organisations and the Future of Welfare*. London: Sage.

Deacon, B. (2000) 'Eastern European welfare states: the impact of the politics of globalization'. *Journal of European Social Policy* **10**(2): 146–61.

DHSS (Department of Health and Social Security) (1983) *NHS Management Inquiry*. London: HMSO.

DoH (Department of Health) (1987) *Promoting Better Health*, White Paper on primary care. London: Stationery Office.

DoH (Department of Health) (1991) *Patient's Charter*. London: Stationery Office.

DoH (Department of Health) (1992) *The Health of the Nation: A Strategy for Health in England*. London: Stationery Office.

DoH (Department of Health) (1997) *The New NHS: Modern, Dependable*. London: Stationery Office.

DoH (Department of Health) (1998) *Our Healthier Nation*. London: Stationery Office.

DoH (Department of Health) (1999) *Saving Lives: Our Healthier Nation.* London: Stationery Office.

DoH (Department of Health) (2000) *The NHS Plan: A Plan for Investment, A Plan for Reform.* London: Stationery Office.

DoH (Department of Health) (2004) *Choosing Health: Making Healthy Choices Easier.* London: Stationery Office.

DoH (Department of Health) (2005a) *Independence, Wellbeing and Choice,* Green Paper. London: Stationery Office.

DoH (Department of Health) (2005b) *Your Health, Your Care, Your Say*, Green Paper. London: Stationery Office.

DoH (Department of Health) (2006a) *Our Health, Our Care, Our Say*, White Paper. London: Stationery Office.

DoH (Department of Health) (2006b) Government response to report on tackling childhood obesity. Press release 2006/0077. London: DoH.

DoH (Department of Health) (2007) Mapping the success of NHS building schemes since 1997. Press release 2007/0043. London: DoH.

Doyal, L. and Gough, I. (1991) *A Theory of Human Needs.* Basingstoke: Macmillan – now Palgrave Macmillan.

DWP (Department of Work and Pensions) (2006) *Security in Retirement: Towards a New Pensions System*, White Paper. London: Stationery Office.

Esping-Anderson, G. (1990) *The Three Worlds of Welfare Capitalism.* Cambridge: Polity Press.

Finch, J. and Groves, D. (1980) 'Community care and the family: a case for equal opportunities'. *Journal of Social Policy* 9(4): 487–511.

Giddens, A. (1998) *The Third Way: The Renewal of Social Democracy.* Cambridge: Polity Press.

Giddens, A. (2006) *Sociology* (5th edn). Cambridge: Polity Press.

Goffman, E. (1961) *Asylums: Essays on the Social Situation of Mental Patients and other Inmates.* Harmondsworth: Penguin.

Gough, I. (2004) Welfare regimes in development contexts: a global and regional analysis, in I. Gough and G. Wood, with A. Barrientos, P. Bevan, P. Davis and G. Room, *Insecurity and Welfare Regimes in Asia, Africa and Latin America: Social Policy in Development Contexts.* Cambridge: Cambridge University Press.

Graham, H. (1983) Caring: a labour of love, in J. Finch and D. Groves (eds) *A Labour of Love: Women, Work and Caring.* London: Routledge & Kegan Paul, pp. 13–30.

Ham, C. and Hill, M. (1993) *The Policy Process in the Modern Capitalist State.* Hemel Hempstead: Harvester Wheatsheaf.

Hayek, F.A. (1983) *Knowledge, Evolution and Society.* London: Adam Smith Institute.

Heslehurst, N., Lang, R., Rankin, J. et al. (2007) 'Obesity in pregnancy: a study in the impact of maternal obesity on NHS maternal services'. *BJOG: An International Journal of Obstetrics and Gynaecology* **114**(3): 334-342.

Hill, M. (2005) *The Public Policy Process* (4th edn). Harrow: Pearson.

Hogwood, B. and Gunn, L. (1984) *Policy Analysis for the Real World.* Oxford: Oxford University Press.

Hudson, J. and Lowe, S. (2004) *Understanding the Policy Process.* Bristol: Policy Press.

Jamrozik, K. (2005) 'Estimate of deaths attributable to passive smoking among UK adults: database analysis'. *British Medical Journal* **330**: 812.

Le Grand, J. and Bartlett, W. (1993) *Quasi-markets and Social Policy.* Basingstoke: Macmillan – now Palgrave Macmillan.

Le Grand, J., Mays, N. and Mulligan, J. (1998) *Learning from the NHS Internal Market: A Review of the Evidence.* London: King's Fund.

Lipsky, M. (1979) *Street Level Bureaucracy.* New York: Russell Sage.

Malin, N., Wilmot, S. and Manthorpe, J. (2002) *Key Concepts and Debates in Health and Social Policy.* Buckingham: Open University Press.

Marshall, T.H. (1950) *Citizenship and Social Class and other Essays.* Cambridge: Cambridge University Press.

Means, R. and Smith, R. (1998) *From Poor Law to Community Care: The Development of Welfare Services for Elderly People 1939–1971.* Bristol: Policy Press.

Miller, C. (2004) *Producing Welfare: A Modern Agenda.* Basingstoke: Palgrave Macmillan.

Morris, J. (1992) '"Us" and "them"? Feminist research, community care and disability'. *Critical Social Policy* **33**(Winter): 22–39.

NAO (National Audit Office) (2001) *Tackling Obesity in England: Report by the Comptroller and Auditor General.* London: Stationery Office.

New, B. and Mays, N. (1997) Age, renal replacement therapy and rationing, in *Healthcare UK 1996/7: The King's Fund Annual Review of Health Policy.* London: King's Fund, pp. 205–23.

NICE (National Institute for Health and Clinical Excellence) (2006) 'Obesity: guidance on the prevention, identification, assessment and management of overweight and obesity in adults and children', clinical guideline 43, www.nice.org.uk.

OECD (Organisation for Economic Co-operation and Development) (2006) *OECD Health Data 2006: How Does the United Kingdom Compare,* www.oecd.org/dataoecd/29/53/36959993.pdf.

Pascall, G. (1997) *Social Policy: A New Feminist Analysis.* London: Routledge.

Paton, C. (2002) Cheques and checks: New Labour's record on the NHS, in M. Powell (ed.) *Evaluating New Labour's Welfare Reforms.* Bristol: Policy Press.

Powell, M. (2000) 'New Labour and the third way in the British welfare state: a new and distinctive approach?' *Critical Social Policy* **20**(1): 29–60.

Robb, B. (1967) *Sans Everything: A Case to Answer*. London: Nelson.

Rowntree, B.S. (1901) *Poverty: A Study of Town Life*. London: Macmillan – now Palgrave Macmillan.

Royal Commission on Long-term Care of the Elderly (1999) *With Respect to Old Age: Long-term Care – Rights and Responsibilities*. London: Stationery Office.

SCOTH (Scientific Committee on Tobacco and Health) (2004) *Update of Evidence of Health Effects Secondhand Smoke*. London: SCOTH.

Scott, D. (2000) *Reading Educational Research and Policy*. London: Routledge Falmer.

SPRU (Social Policy Research Unit) (2004) *Hearts and Minds: the Health Effects of Caring*. London: Carers UK.

Tawney, R.H. (1964) *Equality* (4th edn). London: George Allen & Unwin.

Taylor-Gooby, P. (1985) *Public Opinion, Ideology and State Welfare*. London: Routledge & Keegan Paul.

Taylor-Gooby, P. (1994) 'Post-modernism: a great leap backwards?' *Journal of Social Policy* 23(3): 385–404.

Thompson, S. and Hoggett, P. (1996) 'Universalism, selectivism and particularism: towards a postmodern social policy'. *Critical Social Policy* 16(1): 21–43.

Titmuss, R.M. (1974) *Social Policy: An Introduction*. London: Allen & Unwin.

Townsend, P. (1979) *Poverty in the United Kingdom*. Harmondsworth: Penguin.

Townsend, P. and Davidson, N. (eds) (1982) *Inequalities in Health the Black Report*. Harmondsworth: Penguin.

UNDP (United Nations Development Project) (2006) *Human Development Report 2006*. New York: Oxford University Press.

Wanless, D. (2004) *Securing Good Health for the Whole Population, the Wanless Report*. London: HM Treasury.

Weaver, M. and agencies (2006) 'Britons most obese in Europe', Guardian Unlimited 10/10/06, www.society.guardian.co.uk/print/0,,329597469-105965,00.html.

WHO (World Health Organization) (1998) *Obesity: Preventing and Managing the Global Epidemic: Report of WHO Consultation on Obesity*. Geneva: WHO.

Williams, A. (1997) 'Rationing healthcare by age: the case for'. *British Medical Journal* 314: 820–2.

Williams, F. (1992) 'Somewhere over the rainbow: universality and diversity in social policy'. *Social Policy Review* 4: 200–19.

Williams, F., Popay, J. and Oakley, A. (1999) *Welfare Research: A Critical Review*. London: UCL Press.

Politics and health

Outline of chapter

This chapter will enable readers to:

- Compare competing definitions of politics and variants of political science

LEARNING OUTCOMES

- Understand the political nature of health

- Examine the influence of politics and political ideology on health

- Assess the emerging contribution of politics to health studies

Overview

The discipline of politics examines the debates, ideas and institutions that surround community organization and collective decision-making about resources. In this chapter, the contribution of politics to health studies is examined. The first part of the chapter considers how politics is defined and how this underpins the various strands of political science. It also examines some of the key concepts of political study: power, ideology, democracy, government and the state. It also explores what contribution politics has made and can make to health studies. The second part considers some of the theoretical and methodological approaches within politics. It looks at political ideologies, how they offer competing definitions of politics, varied views of the social and political world, and divergent views on health and health improvement. A case study explores how recent changes in many contemporary societies, associated in particular with neoliberal economic policies, have led to a greater emphasis on freedom through choice. Individuals are called upon to take a greater role in self-care and risk management in relation to their bodies. At the same time, the development of large multinational companies has given rise to a system of production whereby their size and dominance have provided them with an ability to structure the food market.

Introduction

In broad terms, politics is about **community** organization, how people choose to live together, and collective decision-making about resources or, as Laswell (1936) has claimed, 'who gets what, when, how'. A variety of competing definitions have been utilized over time and by different political ideologies, and it has been suggested that the definition of politics is itself a political act (Leftwich, 1984). Following Heywood (2000), a broad fourfold classification is possible:

- *Politics as government:* the word 'politics' is derived from *polis*, the Greek for city-state. Traditionally, politics has been associated with the art of government and the activities of the state and its academic study focuses on the personnel and machinery of government, excluding the many arenas in which political activities take place in civil society.

- *Politics as public life:* politics is primarily concerned with the conduct and management of community affairs through the institutions of the state (for example the courts, police, the NHS), excluding the political activity of families, personal relationships and so on.

- *Politics as conflict resolution:* politics is concerned with the expression and resolution of conflicts through compromise, conciliation, negotiation and other strategies. Politics is thus seen as a process privileging debate and discussion.

● *Politics as power*: politics is the process through which the production, distribution and use of scarce resources is determined in all areas of social existence – including personal relationships.

This classification shows a large variation in the conceptualization of politics; for example, the first concept is very narrow and the last is very broad. The first concept, which is the most prevalent definition within mainstream political discourse in the UK, places restrictive boundaries around what politics is – the activities of governments, elites and state agencies – and therefore also restricts who is political and who can engage in politics (that is, the members of governments, state agencies and other elite organizations). It is a 'top-down' approach that essentially separates politics from the community. This should be contrasted with the last definition, which offers a more encompassing view of politics: politics, effectively, is everything. While politics may be seen as concerned with compromise and conciliatory activity, for many it is the exercise of power and how legitimacy for the exercise of that power is achieved. Authority is one means alongside wealth, strength or violence. Politics is thus a term that can be used to describe any 'power-structured relationship or arrangement whereby one group of persons is controlled by another' (Millett, 1969). This is a 'bottom-up' approach, which suggests that any and every issue is political and, likewise, anyone and everyone can engage in a political act.

THINKING ABOUT

Why are there calls to take the politics out of health?

These competing definitions of politics have also permeated the contemporary discipline of political science (the study of politics), where the different academic approaches similarly operate divergent conceptualizations about what should be studied (Stoker, 2002).

The contribution of political science to health studies

The concepts and methods of political science have a clear potential to contribute to the study of health. However, to date (aside from specific discussions about healthcare), health has not been widely considered as a political entity within academic debates or, more importantly, broader societal ones. In this section, we examine some of the reasons behind this, and then discuss more recent arguments which suggest that health is political and, therefore, that political science has much to offer our understanding of health.

The political and the non-political

The marginalization of the politics of health is unlikely to have a simple solution because the treatment of health as apolitical (that is, not political) is almost certainly the result of a complex interaction of a number of different factors.

Health equals healthcare

Health is often reduced and misrepresented as healthcare (or in the UK, as the National Health Service). Consequently, the *politics of health* becomes significantly misconstructed as the *politics of healthcare* (see, for example, Freeman, 2000), and, more specifically, as the politics of the NHS. For example, the majority of popular political discussions about health concern issues such as NHS funding and organization, NHS service delivery and efficiency, or the demographic pressures on the future provision of healthcare. The same applies in most other 'developed' countries.

Chapter 9 and Chapter 7 both study health as ways in which care is organized and delivered.

The limited, one-dimensional nature of this political discourse surrounding health can be traced back to two ideological issues: the definition of health and the definition of politics (Carpenter, 1980). The definition of health that has conventionally been operationalized under Western capitalism has two interrelated aspects to it: health is considered as the absence of disease (a biomedical definition) and as a commodity (an economic definition). Both these definitions focus on individuals, as opposed to society: health is seen as a product of individual factors such as genetic heritage or lifestyle choices, and as a commodity that individuals can access either via the market or, in the UK's case, the health system (Scott-Samuel, 1979).

Health in this sense is an individualized commodity that is produced and delivered by the market or the health service. Inequalities in the distribution of health are therefore either a result of the failings of individuals through, for example, their lifestyle choices, or the way in which healthcare products are produced, distributed and delivered.

CONNECTIONS

Chapter 10 claims that health is produced and that the study of economics enables a society to decide how much and to whom scarce resources should be allocated in relation to healthcare. It discusses the advantages and limitations of using the market to allocate resources such as healthcare.

It is important to note that this limiting, one-dimensional view of health is common across the political spectrum, with left-wing versus right-wing health debates usually focusing on the role of the NHS. This 'NHS illusion' has resulted in the naive perspective among health activists that societal ill health can be cured by better NHS services (Carpenter, 1980).

To what extent do you agree with David Hunter (2003, p. 111) that: 'All available evidence suggests that the NHS, essentially a "sickness" service, will never take the wider public health seriously.'

Health and concepts of politics

Earlier we outlined four broad definitions of politics and suggested that the first one, politics as the art of government and the activities of the state, was the most prevalent within current political discourse. The **hegemony** of this conceptualization of politics influences which aspects of health are considered to be political. Healthcare, especially in countries like the UK where the state's role is significant, is an immediate subject for political discussion as it involves differences over funding and delivery. While such differences may be partly resolved through negotiation and conciliation, there has been recourse to the economic marketplace and rational decision-making. The establishment of the NHS as a service free at the point of delivery might have been expected to be a fair and acceptable mechanism for delivering healthcare. Yet the allocation of treatment and care has come to be determined by market mechanisms and this has caused dissatisfaction and conflict.

Chapter 7 discusses the historical and social context for the establishment of the welfare state in the UK.

Calls to replace politics with managerialism especially in relation to healthcare emerged in the 1970s. Using available information to conduct detailed option appraisals might be expected to be a rational form of decision-making. Instead, this process also caused dissatisfaction – professional judgement was thought to be sacrificed to managerial expertise and the interests of the community were thought to play too little a role.

CONNECTIONS
CONNECTIONS

Chapter 9 discusses the factors influencing the structure of the NHS and what has driven its various reorganizations.

Health and political science

To date, health has not been seriously studied within political science – nor for that matter has politics within health. This has compounded its exclusion from the political realm. Health, to a political scientist (in common with more widely held views), often means only one thing: healthcare and, usually, the NHS. Some political scientists will argue that they do study health as a political entity but what is usually under analysis is the politics of healthcare.

Understanding why this has happened requires us to consider the various schools of thought within political science and their corresponding definitions of the political, as discussed in the introduction. These schools of thought have not been equally successful in political science and the discipline is dominated, especially in the USA, by the behaviouralist, institutionalist, and rational choice strands. To adherents of these schools, politics – and therefore political science – is concerned with the processes, conditions and institutions of mainstream politics and government. As the politics of healthcare revolves around the politics of institutions, systems, funding and elite interactions, it fits the priorities of these mainstream schools of political science. Health, in its broader sense, therefore tends to be thought of as apolitical and of academic concern only to disciplines such as sociology, public health or medicine.

CONNECTIONS ....

Chapter 5 examines two strands of concerns about health: inequalities and the ways in which groups and societies perceive and experience health.

The political nature of health

The hopes, aspirations and expectations of the advances in scientific and medical knowledge in improving human health and wellbeing, forecast at the beginning of the twentieth century, have not been realized (Townsend and Davidson, 1992; Whitehead, 1992; Acheson, 1998). As one of the reasons for establishing the NHS in 1948 had been to reduce inequalities in health, it came as a surprise to many in the 1970s when a growing body of evidence began to emerge which suggested that the provision of access to free healthcare had done little to reduce the contrasting health experiences of different groups in Britain. In 1977, David Ennals, the then secretary of state for health and social security, established a working group to investigate the reasons behind these increasing health inequalities, resulting in the now famous Black Report (Black et al., 1980), which emphasized the importance of material and structural factors in explaining variations in health status by social class. To many, this was a chance to put health, not just healthcare, on the political agenda. However, as the newly elected Conservative government dismissed the recommendations of this report virtually wholeheartedly (see Berridge and Blume, 2003), the 1980s saw a continued policy focus on *healthcare* rather than health. Where public health was discussed at all, the focus was on improving overall population health (rather than reducing health inequalities), largely through attempts to get individuals to change their lifestyle behaviours (for example DoH, 1992). By the mid-1990s, however, a backlash against individualistic, lifestyle behavioural approaches to health was clearly evident. Not only did a growing body of post-Black

Report research provide further evidence of the importance of social and economic factors in the distribution of health experiences (for example Fox et al., 1985; Dahlgren and Whitehead, 1991), but Crawford's (1977) claim that the heavy policy emphasis on lifestyle behaviours constituted nothing less than 'victim-blaming' had become widespread in academic discussions (for example Labonte, 1986). By this stage, there was a consensus among many of the people involved in public health research and activity that health was very much a political issue.

CONNECTIONS

The way in which inequalities in health became an issue on the political agenda is discussed in Chapter 5 and Chapter 7.

However, this consensus did not automatically result in political scientists taking an interest in health and it is not until relatively recently that a body of work has emerged which overtly argues that health is itself a political issue (see, for example, Navarro, 2004; Borrell et al., 2007), and should therefore be examined using political science perspectives (Bambra et al., 2005, 2007); by, for example, examining why and how policy decisions about health are made and identifying the role that political ideologies play in these decisions (Smith, 2007).

CONNECTIONS

Chapter 7 shows how the welfare state reflects the degree to which societies take care of their citizens. The welfare state and labour market policies have an effect on income and social inequalities in the population.

Bambra et al. (2005) have argued that 'health, like almost all other aspects of human life, is political in numerous ways'. They identify four key aspects of the political nature of health:

- unequal distribution
- health determinants
- organization
- citizenship.

Ultimately, health is political because power is exercised over it. The health of a population is not entirely under the control of an individual citizen but is under the control of the wider political relations of society. Changing society is only achievable through politics and political struggle.

Unequal distribution

Evidence that 'the most powerful determinants of health in modern populations are to be found in social, economic, and cultural circumstances' (Blane et al., 1996) comes from a wide range of sources and is also, to some extent, acknowledged by government (Townsend and Davidson, 1992; Acheson, 1998; DoH, 1998; SEU, 1998). Yet differences in health experiences between areas and social groups (socioeconomic, ethnic and gender) remain. How these inequalities in health are approached by society is highly political and ideological: are health inequalities to be accepted as 'natural' and inevitable results of individual differences both in respect of genetics and the silent hand of the economic market, or are they abhorrences that need to be tackled by a modern state and a humane society? Underpinning these different approaches to health inequalities are not only divergent views of what is scientifically or economically possible, but also differing political and ideological opinions of what is desirable.

Health determinants

While genetic research is helping us to better understand why some people are predisposed to experience certain diseases, and other causes of ill health are becoming better understood, it is evident that environmental triggers are, in most cases, even more important and that the major determinants of health or ill health are inextricably linked to the social environment (Dahlgren and Whitehead, 1991; Acheson, 1998; Wilkinson and Marmot, 2006; www.euro.who.int/document/e81384.pdf). In this way, factors such as housing, income, employment – indeed many of the issues that dominate political life – are all important determinants of health and wellbeing. The importance of these factors, which are beyond the realm of the health sector, also help to demonstrate why non-healthcare policies are of such importance to health (Townsend and Davidson, 1992; Acheson, 1998; Whitehead et al., 2000; Wanless, 2004).

CONNECTIONS

Chapter 5 gives a detailed description of the social determinants of health.

Organization

Health is political because any purposeful activity to enhance health needs 'the organised efforts of society' (Secretary of State for Social Services, 1988) or the engagement of 'the social machinery' (Winslow, 1920): both of these require political involvement and political actions. Population health can only be improved through the *organized* activities of communities and societies. In most countries, the organization of society is the role of the state and its agencies. The state, under any of the four definitions of politics outlined earlier, is a (and more usually, *the*) subject of politics. Furthermore, it is not only who or what has the power to organize society, but also how that organizational power is processed and operated that makes it political.

Health and citizenship

Health is political because the right to 'a standard of living adequate for health and well-being' (UN, 1948) is, or should be, an aspect of citizenship and human rights. According to the *Universal Declaration of Human Rights* (UN, 1948):

> Everyone has the right to a standard of living adequate for the health and well-being of himself and of his family, including food, clothing, housing and medical care and necessary social services, and the right to security in the event of unemployment, sickness, disability, widowhood, old age or other lack of livelihood in circumstances beyond his control.

Citizenship is 'a status bestowed on those who are full members of a community. All who possess the status are equal with respect to the rights and duties with which the status is endowed' (Marshall, 1963). Following Marshall, it is possible to identify three types of citizenship rights: civil, political and social. While the right to health includes the right to healthcare, it goes beyond healthcare to encompass the underlying determinants of health, such as safe drinking water, adequate sanitation and access to health-related information and a standard of living adequate for health and wellbeing.

Example 8.1

HEALTH AND HUMAN RIGHTS

An outstanding feature of the 1996 South African Constitution is the inclusion of a Bill of Rights, in which section 27 states that (Republic of South Africa, 1996):

  (1) Everyone has the right to have access to:
    (a) healthcare services, including reproductive healthcare;
    (b) sufficient food and water; and
    (c) social security, including, if they are unable to support themselves and their dependants, appropriate social assistance.

  (2) The state must take reasonable legislative and other measures, within its available resources, to achieve the progressive realization of each of these rights.
  (3) No one may be refused emergency medical treatment.

The South African courts, particularly the Constitutional Court, have often been called upon to interpret and give effect to some of these rights in relation to those living with HIV/AIDS and confidentiality, HIV testing, and access to medication.

In the UK, the welfare state ensured that certain health services and a certain standard of living became a right of citizenship. However, the extent to which health is a right of citizenship is a continued and constant source of political struggle in other parts of the world. For example, 45 million US citizens currently lack access to healthcare and even in the UK's NHS, access to healthcare is rationed through high charges for drug prescriptions, dentistry and optometry services (Bambra et al., 2007).

Thus, to maintain that politics and health can remain separate is incoherent, because many of the determinants of health are themselves politically determined, the technical agenda of medicine is set by political forces, and the provision of healthcare involves the distribution of a scarce commodity.

Example 8.2

POLITICS IN MEDICAL PUBLICATIONS

Rightly, many medical journals have never subscribed to this distinction between political and technical, trying instead to widen their readership's perspective on health. The *BMJ*'s stated aim is to publish 'papers commenting on the clinical, scientific, social, political, and economic factors affecting health'. Similarly, the *Journal of the American Medical Association* recognizes a 'responsibility to improve the total human condition' and to 'inform readers about non-clinical aspects of medicine and public health, including the political ... '. Thomas Wakley, MP and 'medico-political polemicist', founded the *Lancet* with the aim of introducing a 'radical slant' to the 'corrupt medical establishment'.

This approach does present some difficulties. One problem is that political bias may creep into a profession that requires objectivity. Maintaining high standards of evidence can guard against such subjectivity. Yet the current evidence is that many high-impact general medical journals ignore major medico-political issues altogether. Since September 2001, neither the *New England Journal of Medicine* nor the *Annals of Internal Medicine* has published any article containing the text word 'Afghanistan' or 'Iraq'. The suppression of important health issues is even more worrying than the threat of subjective bias, which can be countered.

Source: Barr et al., 2004, pp. 61–2

Theoretical and methodological approaches

The nature of politics as an academic discipline is much debated, some seeing it as branch of philosophy or history and others as a science. Aristotle (384–322 BC), the Greek philosopher, claimed politics was the 'master science', in that all we do in life, in society, in arts and in science is influenced by politics. His classification of the constitutions of the Greek city-states was both systematic and rigorous. Many social scientists have since tried to build a body of political **theory** using 'scientific' methods of **empirical** observation. Karl Marx, for example, sought to uncover scientific laws driving historical development. However, in the latter half of the twentieth century, the main academic strand of political science was behaviourism, reflecting a view that only that which could be observed and quantified should be studied, leading to a focus on voting behaviour and electoral systems. The modern discipline of politics combines many approaches and focuses:

- Political theory examines theories of institutions, forms of government and systems of representation

- Political philosophy looks for answers to more philosophical questions concerning freedom, justice, equality and rights

- Comparative government tries to generalize about political power and systems from the analysis of groups of countries, international relations being the study of how countries relate through war and diplomacy

- Political ideology is concerned with ideas about the ways states should be organized.

In addition, politics includes many subdisciplines examining the role of the state in the economic system (political economy); the formation of political attitudes; the exercise of power in society; and the policy-making processes of government.

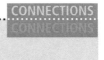

Chapter 2 provides a summary of a Marxist approach to the study of history. Chapter 7 describes a systems model of the political process.

The politics of health can be analysed from each of these perspectives. Signal (1998), for example, argues for a political analysis of health promotion and employs different forms of analysis. In common with a consensus view of politics as reconciling competing interests, Signal discusses pluralist interest group theory, or pluralism, which holds that public policy is developed according to the interests of a range of groups who compete with each other in order to influence the policy process. Like tobacco and alcohol companies, food companies exert enormous influence on public policy, lobbying officials, coopting experts and expanding sales by marketing to children, members of minority groups and people in developing countries. Their corporate social responsibility is increasingly called into question (Lang et al., 2006).

CONNECTIONS

The making of food and health policy is discussed in the case study in Chapter 7.

In this section, we focus on political ideologies and how these have informed health policy and approaches to health in the UK. Ideology is a system of interrelated ideas and concepts that reflect and promote the political, economic and cultural values and interests of a particular societal group (Bambra et al., 2007). Ideologies, like societal groups, are therefore often conflicting and the dominance of one particular ideology within a society to a large extent reflects the power of the group it represents. Ideology can be used to manipulate the interests of the many in favour of the power and privileges of the few (Ledwith, 2001). So, for example, liberal democratic ideology, with its emphasis on the individual, the market and the neutral state, can be seen as a reflection of the power of business interests within capitalist society (Bambra et al., 2005). A hegemonic (that is, universally prevailing) ideology is usually one that has successfully incorporated and cemented a number of different elements from other competing ideologies and thereby fuses the interests of diverse societal groups and classes

(Gramsci, 1971). There is emerging evidence that ideology plays a key role in determining mortality and population health (Navarro, 2004).

 What are the key characteristics of dominant ideologies?

Conservatism

The literal interpretation of Conservatism is to 'conserve', that is, to maintain what has been tried and tested, rather than to seek radical change. As Eccleshall (1994, p. 63) puts it:

> Whereas other ideologies stand *for* something – a more even distribution of resources, for example, or an extension of civil liberties – conservatism *warns* against dismantling established institutions.

Part of maintaining the traditional order of things includes a belief that human talent varies naturally and, consequently, that attempts to 'level' things out (in the way many socialists advocate) are artificial and destined to fail. The existence of a social hierarchy is not only viewed as inevitable but also desirable as it is thought to promote innovation and success, and allows the majority to benefit from the leadership of particularly talented individuals. Rich people tend to be thought of as creators of prosperity rather than plunderers of the poor (a view that contrasts with socialist and Communist ideas about wealth). Hence, Conservatism differs from many other political ideologies in its vindication of inequality (Eccleshall, 1994).

Conservative preferences for maintaining tradition are associated with preserving the dominance of particular groups (for example wealthy, white men) or a religion (for example Christianity) or culture (for example 'Britishness'). Taken to an extreme, these preferences may be linked to xenophobia, nationalism and racism. More often, these preferences are associated with a morality emphasizing the importance of self-discipline, decency, the 'nuclear family unit' and a respect for the rule of law.

As well as a tendency towards tradition, other features of Conservatism include a view of society as a collection of self-interested individuals, a belief underlying Margaret Thatcher's infamous claim made in the 1980s that 'there's no such thing as society'. Of particular importance to health, Conservatives tend to see the role of the state as minimal, with a preference for limited (if any) welfare provision. While some Conservatives favour a society in which the privileged classes provide basic welfare (for example housing) to the 'deserving poor', there is agreement that too much provision by the state removes incentives from the poor to improve themselves, creating a dependency culture and a permanent underclass of what Thatcher called 'moral cripples'. The only exception to Conservative preferences for minimal government intervention in society tends to be around law and order, where significant state intervention is often viewed as essential to maintain the smooth running of society.

Despite the association between Conservatism and tradition, some strands of Conservatism have involved advocating for radical change. For example, although the 'New Right' movement of the 1980s (strongly associated with Thatcherism in the UK, and Reaganism in the USA) employed a traditionally Conservative moral rhetoric, the drive towards the free market and competitive individualism (see Friedman and Friedman, 1980) took its inspiration from liberal thinking (Dearlove and Saunders, 1991). Such ideas, when applied to health and healthcare, resulted in the widespread restructuring and privatization of the welfare state in the 1980s.

Understanding Conservative and New Right ideologies can help us to understand why Thatcher's government made the decision to reject the recommendations put forward in the Black Report (1980), which claimed that health inequalities were largely a result of material inequalities in wealth. The New Right Conservatism of 1980s British governments involved a commitment to reducing tax (and therefore public expenditure), so it was unlikely that a party elected on this basis would agree to policy recommendations which depended on increased public expenditure. Traditional Conservative acceptance of societal inequalities also played a role; quite simply, Thatcher's Conservatives did not view health inequalities as a policy problem, but rather as a 'natural' feature of society (see Berridge, 2002). As the New Right ideological hold over the Conservative Party lessened under John Major in the early 1990s, it became more legitimate to discuss the issue of health differences in policy circles but only by employing the less emotive term, 'health variations'. In 1997, the new Labour government (traditionally associated with more egalitarian values) made it clear that it considered health inequalities to be a significant policy problem and, for the first time in over a decade, explicit political commitments were made to reducing 'health inequalities' (for example Department of Health, 1997). However, in keeping with the 'third way', these commitments were accompanied by a promise not to increase public spending for at least two years.

From the early 1990s onwards, the popularity of New Right ideas among Conservatives declined. For example, the Scottish Conservative Party manifesto on health in 2007 (Scottish Conservatives, 2007) states:

Our families pay tax, and are entitled to expect high quality healthcare services in return. Too often, though, they don't receive it. Families need to know that they have acute services like A&E and maternity facilities close to their homes, a choice over where they receive elective treatment, access to a dentist, and improved mental health facilities.

? What political concepts and values are implicit in this statement?

Liberalism (and neoliberalism)

At its heart, liberalism is essentially an economic approach but, like all economic doctrines, it has far-reaching political and social repercussions. With its focus on freedom and choice, liberalism emphasizes the importance of individual rights over those of social groups. Classical liberals believe a free market guarantees social justice, allowing all those with talent and a willingness to work to succeed. The flip side of this presumption is that poor social circumstances are explained by liberals in rather social Darwinian terms, as a result of individual weakness and/or laziness (Heywood, 1992). This genre of liberalism was popular in the eighteenth and nineteenth centuries, when its proponents advocated minimal state intervention in the economy and the importance of the 'invisible hand of the market' and free trade. Popular discontent with the social consequences of this approach (including extensive material deprivation such as that of the Great Depression in the 1930s) resulted in the emergence of strong political opposition (from Communism, socialism and social democracy) and put pressure on liberals to adapt. Out of this situation, 'modern liberalism' emerged, which conceded that state intervention to reduce the excesses of market economics and mitigate its negative effects was desirable. In postwar Britain, this resulted in the emergence of Keynesian welfare capitalism.

The crisis of welfare in the late 1970s led to the re-emergence of classical liberal ideas, especially in relation to economics, exemplified by the approaches of the Thatcher and Reagan governments. This form of liberal thinking, which resurrected market economics, is known as **neoliberalism** (neo meaning new). Under the neoliberal governance of Thatcher in Britain, state intervention was scaled back and public expenditure cut, the economy was deregulated and state-owned companies were privatized. Once again, the primacy of the individual came to the fore (with a corresponding rise in the emphasis placed on traditional morality and responsibility). Politically, neoliberalism is associated with the USA in particular but economic **globalization** means it has increasingly become perceived as hegemonic (that is, globally dominant) to the extent that some commentators argue there is now no alternative (Fukuyama, 1989).

Neoliberalism has been criticized for its negative impact on health by a range of commentators. David Coburn (2000), for example, claims that neoliberal policies damage health in the following three ways:

- Neoliberal economic policies result in increased inequalities in wealth, which many health researchers believe are directly related to health inequalities (for example Wilkinson, 2005)

- The liberal emphasis on individuals corrodes social cohesion, which is also thought to be important for health (Wilkinson, 2005)

● Neoliberal attacks on the welfare state reduce the 'safety net' available to people living on low incomes, exacerbating poverty in some groups and making access to health-related services (such as dentistry) more difficult.

Other critiques of neoliberal policy in relation to health focus on the individualistic nature of the ideology. Authors such as Rose Galvin (2002) claim that neoliberal governments have deliberately emphasized the importance of avoiding 'risky behaviours' in such a way that individuals are positioned as responsible for their own health status. This, Galvin (2002, p. 119) argues, leads to assertions about individual culpability for those living with chronic diseases, 'for if we can choose to be healthy by acting in accordance with the lessons given us by epidemiology and behavioural research, then surely we are culpable if we do become ill'. In achieving public consensus that risky behaviours (such as excessive consumption of alcohol, lack of exercise and poor diet) cause chronic disease, governments are able to shift responsibility for health improvement away from themselves and onto individuals, thereby allowing the kind of minimal state intervention advocated by liberalism.

In a critique of the 2001 Commission on Macroeconomics and Health Report (Sachs Report), Katz (2004) compares a neoliberal approach to health with a social justice perspective (Table 8.1).

Table 8.1 Neoliberal and social justice approaches to health

Neoliberal approach to health	Social justice/human rights approach to health
Underlying assumptions	**Alternative assumptions**
Economic growth, within a globalized 'free' market, is the aim	Fair distribution and sustainable use of resources is the aim
Health is what you get from a health service	Health is what you get from meeting basic needs
International aid, with conditionalities to enforce certain policies, is the only way to finance health	Sovereign and solvent states must provide for their people's basic needs without outside interference
Democracy is alive and well in the developed world and is the model for the developing world	Democracy is in crisis everywhere; self-determination of nation states and a rules-based system of international governance are required
Key features	**Key features**
Addresses symptoms, short term	Addresses root causes, long term
Promotes 'magic medical bullets'	Promotes the meeting of basic needs
Promotes interventions delivered through health services	Promotes public works to free people from miserable living conditions
Identifies charity and international aid as the only sources of funds for health	Identifies redistribution and economic justice as sources of funds for health
Maintains the status quo of extreme concentrations of wealth and power	Demands a fair and rational international economic order
Focuses on individual behaviour and tends to blame victims	Focuses on structural poverty and violence and tends to blame 'the system'

Source: Adapted from Katz, 2004, p, 756

Socialism and social democracy

According to Heywood (1992), socialism is the broadest of political ideologies containing a variety of perspectives from revolutionary Communists to reformist social democrats. The meaning of socialism is therefore not fixed and it differs by place and time. Originally socialism was associated with the Marxist/Communist tradition, and used to describe material equality (common ownership of the productive wealth and a classless society) in contrast to the purely political equality (right to vote and be represented) of capitalism (Heywood, 1992). The Social Democratic Parties (SDP) of Western Europe were originally based within the Marxist tradition but by the early twentieth century a split occurred: the Communist Parties continued to advocate revolution and the overhaul of capitalism, while the SDP supported the reform of capitalism and proposed a parliamentary road to socialism. The SDP were therefore no longer committed to the abolition of capitalism but to reforming it on moral grounds (in the UK particularly, social democratic ideology was strongly influenced by the utopian socialism of Morris and Owen). In the immediate postwar period, this entailed using increased state intervention (such as public ownership of key parts of the economy and the establishment of the welfare state) to mitigate the effects of capitalism and thereby achieve needs-based social justice (Heywood, 1992). However, there is little agreement among social democrats about how much state intervention is required in the economy and this has been notable in policy differences between countries (compare, for example, the UK and Sweden). The most recent evolution of social democracy – the 'third way' (associated with Blairism in the UK) (Giddens, 2002) – has seen the abandonment of previous commitments to public ownership and a dilution in views of the extent to which capitalism is seen to require reform (Giddens, 1998). This, alongside the collapse of actually existing socialism in the Eastern bloc, has led to speculation as to whether socialism is dead.

Example 8.3

SOCIALIST APPROACHES TO IMPROVING THE HEALTH OF POPULATIONS

A recent comparison of the level of population health among 29 developed countries over the period 1945–80 (Navarro and Shi, 2001) demonstrates that population health fared best in countries that had social democratic governments in rule for most of this period. In this period, these countries (Sweden, Finland, Norway, Denmark and Austria) all had extensive welfare states, funded by relatively high taxation that allowed higher expenditure on social security (for example health, education and family support services) than in countries under other types of governance. This suggests that socialist values of equality, redistribution of wealth and a strong welfare state are beneficial for health, which makes sense in light of recent and growing consensus around the importance of social determinants of health. Evidence from regions of India (Kerala) and northeast Italy, where significant improvements in population health outcomes (reduced health inequalities and associated population health improvement) have also occurred under socialist governance (Navarro and Shi, 2001), adds support to those who argue that socialist programmes are most compatible with healthy populations. Even Cuba, which is governed by a non-elected socialist government, demonstrates impressive health outcomes, with life expectancy rates that are on a par with developed countries that spend twenty times as much on health (Veeken, 1995).

? What might account for the purported better health outcomes in social democratic/socialist countries?

Whether the key to these health improvements lies in a more egalitarian society, as Wilkinson (2005) would suggest, or in better government responses to material deprivation, as Lynch et al. (2000) might argue, is debatable. Whatever the cause of reduced health inequalities and improved population health in these countries might be, the dominance of governments of a socialist persuasion demonstrates the importance of political ideology for health.

Nationalism (and Fascism)

Unlike other political ideologies discussed in this section, nationalism does not describe an interrelated set of values and is probably better thought of as a belief, rather than an ideology (Heywood, 1992). This belief, that all nations should be self-governing, spread from the French Revolution of 1789, so that countries previously thought of as 'realms' or 'kingdoms' began to be thought of as 'nation states', and their inhabitants as 'citizens' rather than 'subjects'. As an idea, nationalism straddles the political spectrum; at various times and places, nationalism has been associated with both democratic and authoritarian governments, and with left-wing and right-wing political movements. For example, ideas about nationalism have been employed to promote the importance of social cohesion, order and stability by right-wing parties in Britain and France, while they have also been adopted by left-wing (Marxist) movements advocating 'national liberation' in countries like China and Vietnam. This is partly because the concept of a 'nation' is difficult to pin down, sometimes being used interchangeably with 'state', 'country' and even 'race' (Heywood, 1992).

Nationalism is an embedded feature of most modern societies (Billig, 1995), as demonstrated in the pervasiveness of flags, national anthems, public ceremonies, and national currencies and languages. However, important debates about nationalism remain. On the one hand, some commentators suggest that the growing importance of regional and global institutions (such as the European Union and United Nations) mean that nationalism is becoming irrelevant. On the other, the recent devolution of power to countries such as Wales and Scotland and the persistence of some separatist movements (for example the pressure for Basque independence in Spain) suggest nationalism is alive and well.

An extreme interpretation of some of the ideas involved in nationalism forms the basis of Fascism, which focuses on establishing the dominance of a particular community or social group (often referred to as the 'dominant race'). Under Fascism, subservience to the glory of a particular 'nation' or 'race' is demanded and, consequently, individual liberties are eliminated. Fascism is therefore both extremely elitist and patriarchal – the dominance of one group over others is seen as desirable and inequality between this group and others is actively promoted. Aside from this central belief, many of the ideas involved in Fascism are vague and inconsistent; it is more identifiable with particular movements and individuals, such as the Fascist dictatorships of Hitler (Germany, 1933–40), Mussolini (Italy, 1922–43) and Franco (Spain, 1938–75), than with any systematic ideology.

It could be argued that some level of shared national identity is likely to be beneficial for health, on the basis that it is seen to promote social cohesion – a feature that authors such as Richard Wilkinson (2005) argue is closely linked to health. However, as nationalist ideas have been employed by such a wide variety of political movements, it is difficult to draw any clear conclusions about nationalism's implications for health. Navarro and Shi's (2001) comparison of 29 countries found that the poorest health outcomes of all the countries they looked at were in Spain, Greece and Portugal, all of which had undergone significant periods of Fascist rule in the period of study. This suggests, at the very least, that extreme incarnations of nationalism are likely to be health-damaging. The authors claim that the causes of poor health outcomes in these ex-Fascist countries are likely to result from a combination of regressive fiscal policies (that is, policies that tend to favour the wealthy, without benefiting the poor), underdeveloped welfare states, and the general repressive nature of such regimes.

Feminism

There are a number of different feminisms, such as liberal, socialist or radical, and each has a different approach to politics. This reflects the fact that **feminism** is an evolving social movement. However, what unifies each approach is the idea that gender inequalities are unjust and need to be tackled.

Chapter 5 discusses explanations for gender inequalities in health.

Central to this focus is the belief that 'the personal is political'. Previously, the private domestic and family sphere and relations between men and women were considered as 'non-political'. Feminism brought these issues into the public sphere, therefore politicizing them and getting them on the political agenda (Chapman, 1995).

The origins of feminism date back to the French Revolution in the late eighteenth century and Mary Wollstonecraft's tract on the rights of woman. In the context of the nineteenth and early twentieth century, women (particularly those in wealthier countries with emerging democracies) argued for the same legal, political and economic rights that men had begun to obtain. In the UK, women gained the same voting rights as men in 1928, the Equal Pay Act was passed in 1970 and the Sex Discrimination Act in 1975.

This equal rights approach of liberal feminists – to gain access to the public sphere on the same terms as men by overcoming discrimination – was challenged in the 1960s and 70s by both socialist and radical feminists. Socialist feminists argued that women would only gain full equality with men under socialism and that the oppression of women was a vital element of the capitalist system – in this context, the legal equal rights gained during the twentieth century could only have a limited impact on the systemic power inequality between the sexes. Only the removal of the private sphere altogether (by the collectivization of domestic work and childcare) would ensure equality (Chapman, 1995).

Radical feminists shifted attention further, to the nature of domestic relations between men and women, and other more cultural aspects of male domination and oppression. They highlighted the 'oppressive dualism of gender' and argued that we live in a patriarchal society in which women are systematically dominated by men in all areas of life (Randall, 1987). The goal was no longer to be 'just like men', but to challenge societal assumptions about masculinity and femininity, arguing that they were social constructs rather than fixed natural phenomena. They also drew attention to the limits that unequal and restricting traditional gender roles placed on women (and also men). This meant that women's individual experiences of oppression were collectivized and considered as a consequence of their political relationship of subordination and oppression by men and therefore something that could be changed – primarily by women's political empowerment and liberation from gender socialization.

While it is quite widely accepted that patriarchy has negative health consequences for women (for example Doyal, 1995), more recent research suggests male dominance in society also has important negative health effects for men (Stanistreet et al., 2005). By comparing data from 51 countries, Stanistreet et al. demonstrate that societies with higher rates of female homicide (female murder victims) also have higher rates of male mortality. They claim that female homicide rates can be viewed as an indicator of the extent to which a society is patriarchal, on the basis that most female homicides are carried out by men, and therefore suggest that patriarchy reduces male life expectancy.

Example 8.4

PATRIARCHY AND HEALTH

Patriarchy, defined by Chapman (1995) as 'the systematic domination of women by men and domination of men by other men', is a complex phenomenon and so it is difficult to measure and research is conflicting: is patriarchy damaging to male health and the source of their higher mortality or is it, by bestowing power and privilege, the source of better health? Data from societies where relationships between men and women have been more equal over a long time period (for example Israeli kibbutz) demonstrate increased male life expectancy, resulting in smaller differences in life expectancy between men and women (Leviatan and Cohen, 1985). On the other hand, an international study by Stanistreet et al. (2007) found that in societies in which women are still unequal but beginning to gain equality in areas such as employment, increased economic activity by women correlated with increased mortality from injury and poisoning among men *but not* women. Stanistreet et al. (2005, pp. 873–6) concluded that some men may initially respond to improvements in gender equality by engaging in risky or self-destructive behaviours:

It may be that, as women increasingly occupy traditionally masculine roles, thus challenging the stereotypes of hegemonic masculinities, some men engage in compensatory risky behaviours as a means of asserting what appears to be a diminishing masculine identity.

Environmentalism

Many, if not all, of the political ideologies discussed so far have tended to perceive nature as nothing more than a resource for human beings to exploit. However, since the 1960s, when Rachel Carson published *The Silent Spring* (1962), there has been an increasing awareness of a growing ecological crisis. As both the number of human beings, and the demand for higher standards of living increase, a growing number of people are predicting that a global catastrophe (for example through climate change) will soon challenge the way we live. As with all the other ideologies discussed, the term 'environmentalism' is often applied to a broad range of ideas and theories, from those which fundamentally question conventional assumptions about nature to far less radical responses to specific environmental issues. Generally, environmentalists claim that, by conceiving of nature as an ever plentiful resource, humans have placed not only their own future in jeopardy, but that of the whole global ecosystem. To avoid disaster, environmentalists advocate that all policies should be judged by their sustainability (that is, the extent to which a particular policy can be maintained without damaging the fragile ecosystem).

This ideological perspective criticizes a basic assumption of the other ideas discussed in this section, namely the central position of human beings. This sets environmentalists apart from the usual Left–Right political spectrum. Since the 1980s, 'Green' parties have emerged in most industrialized countries, including the UK, with the aim of moving environmental concerns up the political agenda. Pressure groups such as Greenpeace and Friends of the Earth have also helped to increase awareness of environmental concerns such as acid rain and nuclear waste. Currently, most major political parties in Britain claim to be concerned with the environment, but their various responses tend to suggest environmental concerns can be accommodated without the need for radical change. In contrast, an increasing number of scientists and environmentalists believe that the damage to the ecosystem caused by humans is now so great that significant climate and environmental change is inevitable. If this is the case, all humans can hope to achieve, even through radical change, is damage limitation (for example Lovelock, 2006). Despite increasingly pessimistic predictions by these groups, the more radical branches of environmentalism are unlikely to be taken seriously by mainstream politics as they suggest there are limits on human, material ambitions – a suggestion which challenges the core of many influential ideologies.

An awareness of links between the environment and human health are not new; many of the nineteenth-century achievements in improving public health were a result of changes to the environmental conditions in which people lived (for example around sanitation and air pollution). Following the success of environmental activists in promoting the political nature of their cause, from the 1960s onwards, clear links between the public health and environmental movements began to develop. In 1990, Maurice King wrote a now-famous commentary in the medical journal, the *Lancet*, in which he argued that an ecological approach to public health was essential in order to avoid the likelihood of humans being caught in a 'demographic trap'. Increasingly, it became clear that public health could not afford to focus solely on human health, for without a sustainable, healthy environment in which to live, human health would inevitably decline. By the mid-1990s, the term 'ecological public health' was being used as a means of highlighting the dependence of public health on the survival of the ecosystem (Nutbeam, 1998). Since then, it has become increasingly accepted by mainstream public health activists that the two issues ought to be viewed as a shared agenda. In 2006, the UK Public Health Association and the Faculty of Public Health published a joint manifesto, *The Convergence of Health and Sustainable Development*, which aimed to establish a network incorporating both environmental and public health activists. The manifesto, signed by a wide range of public health practitioners and advocates, makes links between environmental degradation and health inequalities and commits signatories to, for example, 'undertaking carbon audits and ecological footprint analyses' and bringing together social, environmental and economic policies 'to achieve synergy'.

CASE STUDY The politics of 'fat'

Tackling obesity involves tough political choices. Food choices are seen as personal choices, and this notion is deliberately pursued in advertising and has also become part of political rhetoric. The notion of choice now dominates discourse around health and social care, education and lifestyles (DoH, 2004). This prominence of individual choice is itself part of political discourse, premised on neoliberal concepts of individualism. Yet the choices people make which lead them to be overweight or obese are not free ones at all. Patterns of food consumption are strongly linked to socioeconomic status, as well as displaying national trends. The link between obesity and poverty in the UK has a political dimension and is in part fuelled by the political lobbying and influence of processed and fast-food companies. The term 'obesogenic' is now used to describe a toxic environment that encourages obesity. This case study on obesity explores, in turn, the UK regulatory bodies' decisions regarding food price, availability, marketing and advertising; the influence of the food industries' lobbying; and the broader political context of globalization and how this affects food choices and obesity.

The exponential increase in media coverage and the inherently individual blaming tone adopted in relation to obesity seem to have the elements of what social scientists call a 'moral panic'. Moral panics are typical during times of rapid social change and involve projecting increased anxiety onto vulnerable or marginalized groups. As Guthman and Dupais (2005) note, such unprecedented media attention on obesity and health has resulted in a situation whereby obesity is more than simply a threat to individual and public health. Obesity reportedly raises airline costs (through increased fuel costs), affects worker productivity through ill health and disability, and is even a security threat, as fitness levels among armed and civilian or public security personnel fall due to overweight. Thus obesity per se is far bigger than fat. It is a moral, social and political issue.

Food choices are determined by multiple factors, many of them subject to legal regulations and controls. These factors include price, availability, promotion, marketing and advertising. Price and availability are key determinants of food choices, and the growth of cheap and readily available fast food has been linked to the rising levels of obesity (French et al., 2000; Prentice and Jebb, 2003). Within free-market economies, price levels are set by the producers and there is no regulation by government. The only way in which governments can intervene is to tax products that are deemed to be unhealthy or unsafe – the route used in the case of tobacco and alcohol. In the UK, there have been calls for unhealthy 'junk' food to be taxed (Marshall, 2000), but these have not yet materialized. According to members of the British Medical Association, taxing unhealthy food is much more complicated than taxing single commodities such as tobacco; what is the definition of 'healthy' or 'unhealthy' food? To what extent is this concept socially (and therefore morally) constructed? Moreover, it will be those people in the lower socioeconomic groups and with the least purchasing power who will suffer financially if taxes are successfully introduced and also, therefore, ultimately, in terms of health. In the US by contrast, New York Assembly member Felix Ortiz proposed a 'fat tax' on foods and entertainments such as video games that contribute to a sedentary lifestyle. Most liberal governments balk at such proposals, which they see as interfering with individual liberties. As J.S. Mill observed in the classic treatise 'On Liberty', the harm principle holds that each individual has the right to act as he wants, so long as these actions do not harm others. If the action is self-regarding, that is, if it only directly affects the person undertaking the action, then society has no right to intervene. The only example of large-scale direct intervention by a UK government into people's diets and food intake came from wartime rationing, when food shortages and government priorities allowed for a suspension of normal market economic activity.

The underlying political principle can be seen to be liberalism, with freedom of economic activity and choice as the goal. The government has acted in a limited number of areas – food labelling, advertising to children and school meals. The Food Labelling Regulations, introduced in 1996, require food manufacturers to list the ingredients and processes used in their food products, as well as other details such as geographical origin (www.food.gov.uk). Falsely describing, advertising or presenting food is an offence. There are additional regulatory frameworks such as the Food Safety Act 1990, which sets out the composition of various food items such as bread, meat products and spreadable fats, and the European Marketing Standards set nutritional standards for products such as organic food and olive oil. Since 2005, it has been mandatory for the labelling of prepacked food sold in the UK or the rest of the EU to state whether it includes a number of items linked to allergic reactions, for example nuts. The principles underlying these regulations appear to be the necessity of facilitating an informed choice, and the need to ensure food safety, that is, avoiding unintended exposure to allergens. Here, then, legislation, government policy, serves to regulate and control, arguably for the benefit of the majority.

Marketing and advertising are also thought to affect people's food choices. Research has shown that television advertising has a modest direct effect on children's food choices (Hastings et al., 2003; Paliwoda and Crawford, 2003). Given this knowledge, whether or not to regulate television advertising and promotion therefore becomes a salient political issue. This long-running debate has been framed in terms of protecting children from undue pressures to eat unhealthily versus the freedom of legal commercial enterprises to advertise and market their products. Ofcom, the regulatory body for the communication industries in the UK, has announced a television ban on fast foods before, during and after programmes aimed at children. The ban on programmes aimed at 4–9-year-olds was implemented in 2007 and will be extended to programmes aimed at 10–15-year-olds by 2009 (www.ofcom.org.uk).

CONNECTIONS

The ethical issues and principles of harm and freedom raised by a ban on advertising are discussed in Chapter 11.

Advertising in the media is the end product of the food industries' marketing activities, which also encompass sponsorship of public events, political lobbying and funding of research. Nestle (2002) has documented her first-hand experience as a nutritionist confronting the food industry regarding healthy eating messages. Given the fact that almost twice as much food as is required is produced annually in the USA, the priority of the food industry is to get people to buy more of its products, regardless of any health messages. Nestle (2002) illustrates how food companies use the political system, marketing strategies and nutrition experts to encourage people to buy their products, regardless of their impact on health. Paradoxically, Campos et al. (2006) argue that overweight and obesity are not significant public health problems, but that they have been represented as such due to the influence of the pharmaceutical and weight loss industries. These industries obviously stand to gain financially if obesity increases and becomes seen as a medical issue. Here again, the influence of private industries is the dominant factor; it is just their business and hence their interests in terms of lifestyle that varies. According to Guthman and Dupais (2005), many of the world's leading authorities on obesity, who operationalize criteria and definitions of obesity, happen to be funded by the pharmaceutical and weight loss industries, as have certain members of the International Obesity Task Force (responsible for WHO reports). Indeed, the pharmaceutical, weight loss and food industries all have a vested interest in maintaining what is currently a narrow public health focus on the obesity issue and amounting to moral panic.

Once again, the political priorities of free-market economies and free individual choices appear to be the dominant principle and philosophy. Even when confronted with such a significant and avoidable public health issue as obesity, governments are loath to regulate and legislate to improve nutrition and diets. In order for such regulations to be implemented, there needs to be evidence of health risks, significant positive media coverage and indications of public support.

The attention given to rising trends in obesity reflects the neoliberal agenda of global public health in its insistence on analysing health issues in terms of individual behaviour, exaggerating the extent to which people control their lives. How the processes driving the integration of global food markets – specifically trade, foreign investment and the growth of transnational food companies – affect health have been relatively ignored. With globalization comes:

1. Highly processed, energy-dense food from multinational companies that cheapens calories

2. Growth opportunities for the food industry to market foods and beverages with the highest profit margins in developing countries
3. Less physical labour needed to raise and secure food
4. The rise of service-based economies and technological advances that further erode physical activity (Brownell and Yach, 2006).

Transitions in diet that took more than five decades in Japan have occurred in less than two in China (Chopra and Darnton-Hill, 2004). For example, in only four years between 1989 and 1993, the share of rich urban Chinese households consuming a low-fat diet (less than 10% of calories from fat) fell from 7% to less than 1%.

While this case study has focused on the problem of obesity and overeating in all countries, it is ironic that, alongside this burgeoning problem, the converse is also happening. Millions of people lack food security, meaning that they are without access to sufficient safe and nutritious food to enable an active and healthy life. In 2003, The UN Food and Agriculture Organization (FAO) reported that around 852 million people are chronically hungry due to extreme poverty, while up to 2 billion people intermittently lack food security due to varying degrees of poverty. Building sustainable and secure food supplies to feed the world's population remains a global political and economic priority.

Summary

- There are a number of different definitions of politics. These underpin different approaches to political science and competing political ideologies. Politics focuses on the debates, ideas and institutions that

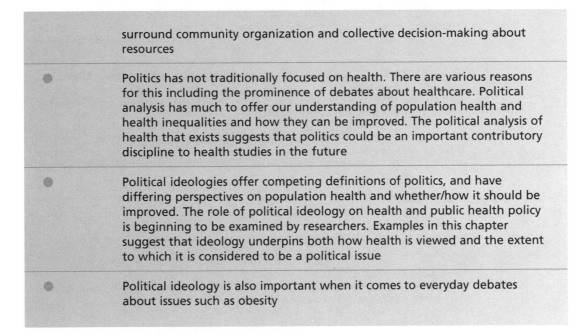

surround community organization and collective decision-making about resources

● Politics has not traditionally focused on health. There are various reasons for this including the prominence of debates about healthcare. Political analysis has much to offer our understanding of population health and health inequalities and how they can be improved. The political analysis of health that exists suggests that politics could be an important contributory discipline to health studies in the future

● Political ideologies offer competing definitions of politics, and have differing perspectives on population health and whether/how it should be improved. The role of political ideology on health and public health policy is beginning to be examined by researchers. Examples in this chapter suggest that ideology underpins both how health is viewed and the extent to which it is considered to be a political issue

● Political ideology is also important when it comes to everyday debates about issues such as obesity

Questions for further discussion

1. Over the next few days examine media reports about health:
   ● What issues are up for discussion?
   ● Do they relate to health or healthcare?
   ● What ideological values underpin the issue, how it is presented and the solutions that are proposed?
   ● Which political interests are being promoted?

2. 'As anyone who has lived among villagers or slum-dwellers knows only too well, the health of the people is influenced far more by politics and power groups and by the distribution of land and wealth than it is by the prevention and treatment of disease' (Werner, 1981). Discuss this proposition with particular reference to obesity.

3. 'Health is far too important to be decided by politicians.' Why do people say this? How realistic is the suggestion?

4. The mix of voluntary codes and self-regulation, together with some regulatory codes used to tackle obesity, is typical of a neoliberal approach to politics and food. How would an environmentalist, or a socialist, approach differ?

Further reading

There are several introductory books on politics and political ideologies. These will enable you to follow up general points related to the discipline.

Heywood, A. (2000) *Key Concepts in Politics*. Basingstoke: Macmillan – now Palgrave Macmillan.
This provides an accessible and readable guide to political concepts and how they are used as tools for analysis.

Heywood A. (2003) *Political Ideologies: An Introduction*. Basingstoke: Palgrave Macmillan.
This is the essential textbook for any student wishing to understand contemporary ideological discourse, including 'new' ideologies such as feminism and environmentalism, and covers the impact of developments such as globalization.

Jones, B., Kavanagh, D., Moran, M. and Norton, P. (2006) *Politics UK*. London: Longman.
This provides a general introduction to the British political and electoral system and examines the influence of various institutions such as the judiciary, local government and the media.

Marsh, D. and Stoker, G. (eds) (2002) *Theory and Methods in Political Science*. Basingstoke: Palgrave Macmillan.
A discussion of different methodologies used in political science.

In addition, these accessible journal papers discuss the role of politics in the study of health:

Bambra, C., Fox, D. and Scott-Samuel, A. (2005) 'Towards a politics of health'. *Health Promotion International* **20**: 187–93.
Bambra, C., Fox, D. and Scott-Samuel, A. (2007) 'A politics of health glossary'. *Journal of Epidemiology and Community Health* **61**: 571–4.

Acknowledgements

This chapter draws on two Bambra et al. articles (2005, 2007). We would therefore like to acknowledge the co-authors Debbie Fox and Alex Scott-Samuel, as well as other members of the Politics of Health Group, www.pohg.org.uk/.

References

Acheson, D. (1998) *Independent Inquiry into Inequalities in Health: Report*. London: Stationery Office.

Bambra, C., Fox, D. and Scott-Samuel, A. (2005) 'Towards a politics of health'. *Health Promotion International* **20**: 187–93.

Bambra, C., Fox, D. and Scott-Samuel, A. (2007) 'A politics of health glossary'. *Journal of Epidemiology and Community Health* **61**: 571–4.

Barr, D., Fenton, L. and Edwards, D. (2004) 'Politics and health'. *Quarterly Journal of Medicine* **97**: 61–2.

Berridge, V. (2002) 'Witness seminar: the Black Report and the health divide'. *Contemporary British History* **16**(3): 131–72.

Berridge, V. and Blume, S. (2003) *Poor Health: Social Inequality before and after the Black Report*. London: Frank Cass.

Black, D., Morris, J. N., Smith, C., and Townsend, P. (1980) *Inequalities in Health: Report of a Research Working Group*. London: DHSS.

Blane, D., Brunner, E., and Wilkinson, R. (eds) (1996) *Health and Social Organization: Towards a Health Policy for the Twenty-first Century*. London: Routledge.

Borrell, C., Espelt, A., Rodríguez-Sanz, M. and Navarro, V. (2007) 'Politics and health'. *Journal of Epidemiology and Community Health* **61**: 658–9.

Brownell, K.D. and Yach, D. (2006) 'Lessons from a small country about the global obesity crisis'. *Globalization and Health* **2**: 11.

Campos, P., Saguy, A., Ernsberger, P. et al. (2006) 'The epidemiology of overweight and obesity: pharmaceutical crisis or moral panic?' *International Journal of Epidemiology* **35**(1): 55–60.

Carpenter, M. (1980) 'Left orthodoxy and the politics of health'. *Capital and Class* **11** (Summer): 73–98.

Carson, R. (1962 [2000]) *Silent Spring*. London: Penguin.

Chapman, J. (1995) The feminist perspective, in D. Marsh and G. Stoker (eds) *Theory and Methods in Political Science*. Basingstoke: Macmillan – now Palgrave Macmillan.

Chopra, M. and Darnton-Hill, I. (2004) 'Tobacco and obesity epidemics: not so different after all?' *British Medical Journal* **328**: 1558–60.

Coburn, D. (2000) 'Income inequality, social cohesion and the health status of populations: the role of neoliberalism'. *Social Science and Medicine* **51**: 135–46.

Crawford, R. (1977) 'You are dangerous to your health: the ideology and politics of victim blaming'. *International Journal of Health Services: Planning, Administration, Evaluation* **7**(4): 663–80.

Dahlgren, G. and Whitehead, M. (1991) 'What can be done about inequalities in health?' *Lancet* **338**: 1059–63.

Dearlove, J. and Saunders, P. (1991) *Introduction to British Politics* (2nd edn). Polity Press: Cambridge.

DoH (Department of Health) (1992) *The Health of the Nation: A Strategy for Health in England*. London: HMSO.

DoH (Department of Health) (1997) *Public Health Strategy Launched to Tackle the Root Causes of Ill-health*, press release. London: DoH.

DoH (Department of Health) (1998) *Saving Lives: Our Healthier Nation*. London: HMSO.

DoH (Department of Health) (2004) *Choosing Health: Making Healthy Choices Easier*. London: DoH

Doyal, L. (1995) *What Makes Women Sick? Gender and the Political Economic of Health*. New Brunswick: Rutgers University Press.

Eccleshall, R. (1994) Conservatism, in R. Eccleshall, V. Geoghegan, R. Jay et al. (eds) *Political Ideologies: An Introduction*. London: Taylor & Francis.

Fox, A.J., Goldblatt, P.O. and Jones, D.R. (1985) 'Social class mortality differentials: artefact, selection or life circumstances?' *Journal of Epidemiology and Community Health* **39**(1): 1–8.

Freeman, R. (2000) *The Politics of Health in Europe*. Manchester: University of Manchester Press.

French, S.A., Harnack, L. and Jeffery, R.W. (2000) 'Fast food restaurant use among women in the Pound of Prevention study: dietary, behavioural and demographic correlates'. *International Journal of Obesity* **24**(10): 1353–9.

Friedman, M. and Friedman, R. (1980) *Free to Choose*. London: Martin Secker & Warburg.

Fukuyama, F. (1989) 'The end of history?' *The National Interest* **16**: 3–18.

Galvin, R. (2002) Disturbing notions of chronic illness and individual responsibility: towards a genealogy of morals. *Health: An Interdisciplinary Journal for the Social Study of Health, Illness and Medicine* **6**(2): 107–37.

Gard, M. and Wright, J. (2005) *The Obesity Epidemic: Science, Morality and Ideology*. London: Routledge.

Giddens, A. (1998) *The Third Way: The Renewal of Social Democracy*. Cambridge: Polity Press.

Giddens, A. (2002) *Where Now for New Labour?* Cambridge: Polity Press.

Gramsci, A. (1971) *Prison Notebooks*. New York: International Publishers.

Guthman, J. and Dupais, M. (2005) 'Embodying neoliberalism: economy, culture, and the politics of fat'. *Environment and Planning D: Society and Space* **24**: 427–48.

Hastings, G., Stead, M., McDermott, L. et al. (2003) *Review of Research on the Effects of Food Promotion to Children*. Report commissioned by the Food Standards Agency, http://www.foodstandards.gov.uk/multimedia/pdfs/promofoodchildrenexec.pdf.

Heywood, A. (2000) *Key Concepts in Politics*. Basingstoke: Macmillan – now Palgrave Macmillan.

Hunter, D.J. (2003) *Public Health Policy*. Cambridge: Blackwell.

Katz, A. (2004) 'The Sachs Report: investing in health for economic development or increasing the size of the crumbs from the rich man's table, Part 1'. *International Journal of Health Services* **34**(3): 751–73.

King, M. (1990) 'Health is a sustainable state'. *Lancet* **336**(8716): 664–7.

Labonte, R. (1986) 'Social inequality and healthy public policy'. *Health Promotion International* **1**(3): 341–51.

Lang, T., Rayner, G. and Kaelin, E. (2006) *The Food Industry, Diet, Physical Activity and Health: A Review of Reported Commitments and Practice of 25 of the World's Largest Food Companies*. London: Centre for Food Policy, City University.

Laswell, H.D. (1936) *Politics: Who Gets What, When, and How*. New York: Peter Smith.

Ledwith, M. (2001) 'Community work as critical pedagogy: re-envisioning Freire and Gramsci'. *Community Development Journal* **36**: 171–82

Leftwich, A. (1984) *What is Politics? The Activity and its Study*. Oxford: Blackwell.

Leviatan, U. and Cohen, J. (1985) 'Gender differences in life expectancy among kibbutz members'. *Social Science and Medicine* **2**: 545–51.

Lovelock, J. (2006) *The Revenge of Gaia: Why the Earth is Fighting Back – and How We Can Still Save Humanity*. London: Allen Lane.

Lynch, J.W., Davey Smith, G., Kaplan, G.A. and House, J.S. (2000) 'Income inequality and mortality: importance to health of individual income, psychosocial environment, or material conditions?' *British Medical Journal* **320**: 1200–4.

Marshall, T.H. (1963) *Sociology at the Crossroads*. London: Hutchinson.

Marshall, T. (2000) 'Exploring a fiscal food policy: The case of diet and ischaemic heart disease'. *British Medical Journal* **320**: 301.

Millett, K. (1969) *Sexual Politics*. London: Virago.

Navarro, V. (ed.) (2004) *The Political and Social Contexts of Health*. New York: Baywood.

Navarro, V. and Shi, L. (2001) 'The political context of social inequalities and health'. *Politics of Policy* **31**(1): 1–21.

Nestle, M. (2002) *Food Politics: How the Food Industry Influences Nutrition and Health*. Berkeley, CA: University of California Press.

Nutbeam, D. (1998) 'Health promotion glossary'. *Health Promotion International* **13**(4): 349–64.

Paliwoda, S. and Crawford, I. (2003) *An Analysis of the Hastings Review*. Commissioned by the Food Advertising Unit for the Advertising Association, www.adassoc.org.uk/hastings_review_analysis_dec03.pdf, www.ofcom.org.uk, accessed 24/8/07.

Prentice, A.M. and Jebb, S.A. (2003) 'Fast foods, energy density and obesity: a possible mechanistic link'. *Obesity Reviews* **4**(4): 187–94.

Randall, V. (1987) *Women and Politics*. Basingstoke: Macmillan – now Palgrave Macmillan.

Republic of South Africa (1996) *Constitution of the Republic of South Act 108 of 1996*, www.info.gov.za/documents/constitution/1996/ a108-96.pdf.

Scott-Samuel, A. (1979) 'The politics of health'. *Community Medicine* **1**: 123–6.

Scottish Conservatives (2007) *Standing Up for Families* manifesto, www.scottishconservatives.com.

Secretary of State for Social Services (1988) *Public Health in England: The Report of the Committee of Inquiry into the Future Development of the Public Health Function*, Cm 289. London: HMSO.

SEU (Social Exclusion Unit) (1998) *Bringing Britain Together: A National Strategy for Neighbourhood Renewal*. London: HMSO.

Signal, L. (1998) 'The politics of health promotion: insights from political theory'. *Health Promotion International* **13**(3): 257–64.

Smith, K.E. (2007) 'Health inequalities in Scotland and England: the contrasting journeys of ideas from research into policy'. *Social Science and Medicine* **64**(7): 1438–49.

Stanistreet, D., Bambra, C. and Scott-Samuel, A. (2005) 'Is patriarchy the source of men's higher mortality?' *Journal of Epidemiology and Community Health* **59**: 873–6.

Stanistreet, D., Swami, V., Pope, D. et al. (2007) 'Women's empowerment and violent death among women and men in Europe: An ecological study'. *Journal of Men's Health and Gender* **4**: 257–65.

Stoker, G. (2002) Introduction, in G. Stoker and D. Marsh (eds) *Theories and Methods in Political Science*. Basingstoke: Palgrave Macmillan.

Townsend, P. and Davidson, N. (1992) The Black Report, in P. Townsend and N. Davidson (eds) *Inequalities in Health*. London: Penguin.

UK Public Health Association (2006) *The Convergence of Health and Sustainable Development*, www.ukpha.org.uk/media/Word_Documents/sdmanifestoagreed.doc, accessed 7/2/07.

UN (United Nations) (1948) *Universal Declaration of Human Rights*. General Assembly Resolution 217A(III), UN Doc A/810 at 71. New York: UN.

Veeken, H. (1995) 'Cuba: plenty of care, few condoms, no corruption'. *British Medical Journal* **311**(7010): 935–7.

Wanless, D. (2004) *Securing Good Health for the Whole Population*. London: HM Treasury.

Whitehead, M. (1992) The health divide, in P. Townsend and N. Davidson (eds) *Inequalities in Health*. London: Penguin.

Whitehead, M., Diderichsen, F. and Burstrom, B. (2000) Researching the impact of public policy on inequalities in health, in H. Graham (ed.) *Understanding Health Inequalities*. Buckingham: Open University Press.

Wilkinson, R. (2005) *The Impact of Inequality: How to Make Sick Societies Healthier*. New York: The New Press.

Wilkinson, R. and Marmot, M. (eds) (2006) *Social Determinants of Health* (2nd edn). Oxford: Oxford University Press.

Winslow, C. (1920) 'The untilled fields of public health'. *New Scientist* **51**(1306): 923–33.

Organization and management and health

This chapter will enable readers to:

LEARNING OUTCOMES

- Gain a sound understanding of modern management theories and be able to relate them to examples of practical situations and issues, particularly in relation to healthcare

- Better understand the nature and operation of health services and how they can be managed

- Understand the influences on large, complex organizations and the skills and abilities needed by practitioners

Overview

Management, the professional administration of business concerns, public undertakings and organizations in general – as well as its many shortcomings – is a topical subject, particularly in relation to the health services. This chapter will explore why this topic should form part of the health studies curriculum for students, regardless of their professional background or personal inclination to be involved in management. The chapter outlines some of the major theoretical concepts relating to organization and management studies, and applies these to the NHS in the UK. The NHS is a unique organization with a huge and diverse remit and workforce. Its scale of operations makes the NHS a major British organization, and within its area of operations, many different organizational and management styles have been tried and tested. The first part of the chapter focuses on theories relating to organizations and how they operate within a broad political and policy context. The second part of the chapter discusses different management theories and models and their relevance to the NHS, and discusses contemporary issues such as what best motivates workers, and how leaders can enthuse their staff. The chapter concludes with a case study on the development of a local obesity strategy.

Introduction

We all relate to organizations of various kinds – the local authority, the GP practice, local retailers, online stores, schools and colleges – and we are all affected by the way they are managed, the way they interact with us and deliver (or not) the goods and services we need. The more we are aware of the way these organizations operate, how they are structured and managed, the more successful we are likely to be in our dealings with them.

Organizations vary enormously in their size and complexity: the UK NHS is one of the largest and, arguably, most complex organizations in the industrialized world, with responsibility for prevention, curing and caring and a huge workforce. Applying theories that examine organizations, their culture, workforce and leadership to the NHS is therefore a good test of their adequacy and usefulness.

Management is the act – or art – of managing resources, whether they are human, technological or financial. It is about conducting business, from initiating and developing ideas for new or improved products to leading, supervising and delivering the result. It is concerned with the arrangements for carrying out organizational processes and executing work (Mullins, 2005) and depends on the skill, competence, knowledge, dedication, vision and integrity of those who manage – managers' skills are closely connected to the success, or otherwise, of the organization's work.

About 100 years ago, Henri Fayol, one of the founding fathers of management theory, described the central tasks of management (Pugh and Hickson, 1996) as:

- planning
- organizing the structure
- organizing human resources (people)
- coordinating or harmonizing the various functions
- controlling the operation and outcome of the organization.

Most healthcare systems have, at various times, problems with one, more or all these tasks. The pace of change in the UK NHS has accelerated in the past 20 years, with frequent changes of structure, efforts to 'grow' new sorts of practitioner from the traditional nurse and doctor roles and variable success with staying within budget and treating people safely and effectively.

Before 1948, healthcare was paid for by individuals or charities. This gave way to a nationalized system – the NHS, which is free at the point of delivery – in 1948. There were periodic efforts during the 1950s and 60s to adjust the new system so that it provided care in the most economic way, but the 1970s brought the first focused effort on effective and rational management of healthcare in the wake of the oil crisis, recession and the squeeze on all services funded from taxation. The past 40 years have seen many more efforts to achieve equitable access to effective healthcare – healthcare that improves people's lives at a price that the economy can bear – by changing the way healthcare is organized and managed.

The contribution of management to health studies

The structure of organizations

First of all, what is an organization? Various answers have been advanced, but it comes down to there being a set of rules, or social arrangements, for achieving agreed goals. In the NHS, such goals include the prevention of illness, caring for and/or healing the sick and advancing our knowledge of health and illness. Organizations are necessary because individuals are unable to accomplish the same outcomes as effectively, if at all, as an organized group (Mullins, 2005). Some organizations require extensive premises from which to deliver services such as hospitals or local authority 'one-stop shops', while others are focused around community-based activities and have more modest accommodation requirements. Obviously the building, whatever the size, is not the organization and neither are the individuals that comprise the staff. The organization refers to the way those individuals are organized to work together.

Two essential management attributes mark out successful organizations: good management and sound organizational structure. Good management enables the organization to adjust and respond to the pressures placed upon it. It could be argued that the largest public sector health service organization in the world was slow to wake up to these essentials. Regional strategic planning was not formally introduced into the NHS until about 1970 and the concept of management, as differentiated from **administration**, came largely as a result of the Griffiths Report of 1983 (DHSS, 1983). It was only after this report was adopted by government in 1984 that, for example, fully developed personnel departments became the norm, and this was in an organization of well over one million workers.

What do we mean by organizational structure? Essentially, we mean a set of roles and recognized relationships between them, usually interdependent, where each role depends on others to achieve the organizational purpose.

THINKING ABOUT

How would you go about finding out how an organization such as a university or your workplace is structured?

An organization's structure not only gives it an identity but also a framework for the allocation of responsibility and authority, which shows:

● the division of work

● lines of accountability

● spans of control and command

● levels of remuneration.

Since its inception, the NHS has been organized in some form of hierarchy with local organizations (for the most part) providing services within a largely centralized policy framework. Currently, the NHS comprises some 152 organizations known as **primary care** trusts (PCTs), which commission community-based and hospital services from, largely, 270 NHS provider organizations – acute trusts, mental health trusts and NHS foundation trusts (Figure 9.1).

Currently, the main policy document guiding the development of the NHS in England is *The NHS Plan*, published in July 2000 (www.library.nhs.uk/healthmanagement/). This document details a 10-year investment and reform plan for the NHS, which includes plans to increase workforce numbers, reduce waiting lists and improve IT systems. The principle underpinning this form of organization is that high-quality care (and better health in general) will result from clear specifications for service devised by people who understand local needs (PCTs), and providers that compete with each other to deliver those services. Thus public funds are distributed on the basis of services delivered.

The structure of the NHS as an organization has grown in size and complexity in response to changes in the requirements demanded of it. Larger organizations need rules and regulations to hold them together and, among other things, to prevent loss of budgetary control. While there are large organizations bound by relatively few such rules, public services in the UK have tended to develop a greater degree of bureaucracy in their structure and control. These types of organization have hierarchies, rules, regulations and job descriptions that delimit responsibility and ensure both order and rigidity. Handy (1993) sees the function of these organizations as to impose order and control on a turbulent world.

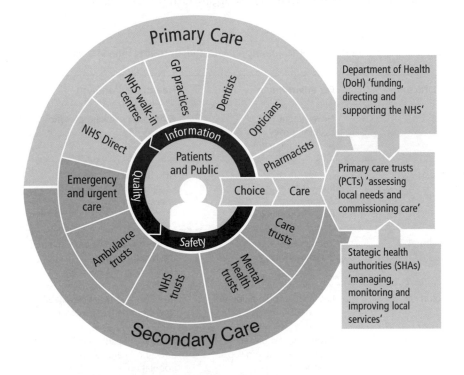

Figure 9.1 Structure of the NHS in England

THINKING ABOUT

Consider an organization you are familiar with. How many people report to each manager (their span of control)? How many layers or levels of management are there? Is the organization's hierarchy tall or flat? How much autonomy does each worker have? Is authority centralized or decentralized? Does the organization employ functional experts for some tasks (for example a finance department)?

Changing healthcare organizations

The provision of health services in the UK is the second highest item of Treasury expenditure after social services and reflects the high priority afforded to it by the voting public. As such, it demands serious attention in the shape of good management. Moreover, health services compete for resources with other major government responsibilities, such as social care, education, defence and local authority funding.

All organizations operate in an environment, usually regarded as everything that lies outside organizational boundaries. The NHS is constantly subject to change as the policy context changes, as well as the resources and materials received. It can be helpful to classify the environmental factors that may influence (and be influenced by) an organization (Table 9.1).

Table 9.1 PESTEL analysis: some examples of environmental pressures

PESTEL factor	Far environment	Health environment
Political	Government policy Taxation policy Acts of Parliament	Policies on smoking cessation and obesity
Economic	Money supply Interest rates Employment Financial wellbeing	NHS budget Local health service priorities Prices of drugs
Sociocultural	Demographics Social mobility	Prevailing patterns of ill health: the health burden Health-related behaviour
Technological	Research and development New discoveries	New drugs and their availability New treatments and procedures
Environmental	Environmental protection laws, for example disposal of asbestos	Healthy/unhealthy environment affecting health of the population
Legal	Laws	Employment laws, for example working hours directive

CONNECTIONS

Some of these issues are discussed in other chapters: Chapter 4 examines the socioeconomic patterns of health and ill health; Chapter 10 looks at issues of rationing and public spending; and Chapter 11 looks at the legal context for health service delivery.

The PESTEL (or PEST) analysis is used to assess the external influences that might influence, or be influenced by, an organization; political, economic, sociocultural, technical developments, environmental or legal. Moreover, we may conveniently divide organizational environments into 'near' and 'far' environments: the 'near' consisting of those factors that impinge on each organization directly; and the 'far' consisting of broader changes at national or international level that impact on the organization.

The 'far' environmental factors include the overall economic performance of the country, the labour supply and the costs of other government commitments such as defence and education. There may be political pressure to match government spending on healthcare with those of comparable EU countries, such as France and Germany.

? How does increasing globalization affect the internal and external environments of organizations?

Instability in the environment may give rise to various degrees of turbulence for organizations. An important part of good management is being vigilant to forthcoming changes and taking action in time to anticipate as well as respond to them. Ansoff and McDonnell (1990) suggest a five-point scale on which to consider environmental turbulence, from a stage in which the organization can easily respond to the situation in which an environmental event occurs, as in 1948, to major changes that are introduced so quickly that the organization is overwhelmed. Table 9.2 shows how the environment for health and social care has increased in turbulence since the beginnings of the NHS in 1948 to the present day, 2007.

Chapter 7 describes the development of the welfare state and some of the political drivers influencing change.

? Practitioners in the NHS may point to numerous reorganizations in the past decade including the establishment of foundation hospitals, proposals for 'poly clinics', changing roles towards more generic workers as well as many changes in structure. What accounts for this level of turbulence?

Organizational culture

All organizations will be influenced by their:

- history
- primary function
- goals and objectives
- size
- location
- management and staff
- external environment.

Table 9.2 Environmental turbulence

Date	History	Level of turbulence	Events
1948	Start of the NHS	**1** Environmental turbulence is calm. The future is expected to be the same as the past. Change is slower than the organization's ability to respond	Pre-existing health facilities were nationalized, but not rationalized. Funding levels remained unaltered and followed historic patterns. Healthcare provision was essentially low tech. Health services were now free at the point of use, including prescriptions. Demand for health services rose steeply. Unanticipated costs rose but general inflation was low at around 2.5%. The NHS was run by administrators and doctors
1960s	Several attempts made to rationalize the NHS. Only minor changes were made	**2** Environmental turbulence more complex but calm. The future deemed to be forecastable by extrapolation	The rise in technical development. Big increases in NHS clinical support staff. The heart-lung machine and kidney dialysis now widespread and experiments with transplantation. Variety and costs of available drugs increase. NHS funding increased, but spending deficits were made up by the Treasury by a system of secondary estimates. Inflation mostly low
1970s	First major reorganization of the NHS to change the national structure. A top-down bureaucratic imposition to achieve uniformity of structure and grading (1974)	**3** The organization's ability to respond to turbulence becomes more complex yet the future can still be predicted with some degree of confidence	Continued rise in technical development and application and in the numbers of clinical support staff. NHS planning system introduced. First attempt to rationalize funding to local areas. Steep rise in inflation. The IMF loan conditions ended the secondary estimates scheme and imposed cash limits. The rise of the NHS manager and managerial function of senior clinical staff and clinical support staff. Reforms opposed by many clinicians
1980s	Second reorganization of the NHS rescinding some of the 1974 reforms. The *NHS Management Inquiry* introduced general managers who were in charge of clinical staff. Further reforms introduced in 1989 to differentiate providers from purchasers or commissioners of healthcare	**4** Future less predictable, with introduction of global and sociopolitical change	These reforms were introduced in the context of other reforms of the Thatcher Conservative government, with the attempt to make the public services function similar to those of the private sector. Many non-NHS managers introduced to the NHS for the first time. Many funding cutbacks and bed numbers' reduction. The introduction of the private finance initiative. Further cost escalation. Inflation high
1990s	Full implementation of the 1989 reforms and many other changes introduced by central government. GP fundholding. Further reform under the new Labour government	**4/5** Turbulence increased, with unexpected events occurring more quickly than the organization can respond	Strict imposition of cash limits led some local health authorities to selectively cut services. Postcode provision arose and became a political issue. Regional health authorities abolished, with functions shared between regional offices and expanded health authorities. Several 'scandals' given very high profile (paediatric cardiac surgery, mistaken cancer test results) with consequences for the healthcare safety agenda. NHS trusts and GP fundholding introduced. Fundholding subsequently abolished. Local primary care groups established. Clinical governance and modernization agenda established
2000s	Further changes to NHS structure imposed by government. Significant additional funds applied to the NHS, which serve mostly to fill long-standing deficits. Trend to establish 'independent' organizations to oversee NHS practice, in the form of regulators (Healthcare Commission and Commission for Social Care Inspection) and 'guiders' – National Institute of Health and Clinical Excellence, National Patient Safety Agency	**5** Turbulence as above	The *NHS Plan* published, which promotes patient and public involvement in decisions about healthcare, reintroduction of market-like principles to NHS through payment by results and practice-based commissioning. Primary care groups become primary care trusts. Abolition of Community Health Council, establishment of the Commission for Patient and Public Involvement in Health – and then its abolition in favour of locally based organizations. Health authorities combine into strategic health authorities, and then reduce in number from 28 to 10. Greater client focus illustrated through Choose and Book, sharing doctor's letters with patients and decreased time to treat initiatives. Direct payment for social care services takes hold

The NHS, together with social care, is the largest organizational enterprise in the UK and consists of many different types of smaller component organizations each having to work together. They, in turn, are made up of smaller organizational departments and units, which must also work together if people are to have coherent services. It is at the interface of these organizational boundaries that problems and inefficiencies often occur. For example, an older person finds that they are not able to cope at home following treatment in hospital and may need residential care in the longer term. The consultant makes a referral to social care services when the patient has completed their treatment. The adult social services department of the local authority gives the referral a low priority because the case is complex, there are more urgent cases pressing and the patient is 'safe in hospital'. The consultant believes that institutionalization and the possibility of a hospital-acquired infection mean that the patient is not at all safe and makes his views plain. The local authority feels as if the NHS is trying to shift responsibility, and costs, to social services, and that seamless care is being compromised.

Part of this clash is due to the **organizational culture** in which professionals such as doctors work. Organizational culture includes everything from the visible structures and processes to more deeply held values that underpin observed behaviour. Practitioners understand what is meant by the culture of the organization – it is the 'way things are done around here' (Deal and Kennedy, 1982, p. 4). Handy (1995, p. 182) has developed a useful typology of organizational cultures based on four Greek gods (Table 9.3).

Handy declares that no organization consists of a single culture but within the smaller unit there will be a more or less consensual culture about, for example, the degree of individual autonomy. When a change in values is required, resistance to that change is very likely.

The NHS became the social equivalent of mass production; largely state directed and managed, built on a paternalistic relationship between state donor and individual recipient. Patient expectations were a low or non-existent priority. The Act of 1946 had, however, encapsulated doctors' clinical freedom in their right to prescribe and refer, that is, to spend the NHS budget, in the interest of their patients, as they saw necessary. The size and complexity of the NHS has led to an extensive bureaucratic structure, which includes relevant Acts of Parliament, the decisions of trust boards, standing financial instructions, health and safety regulations, codes of practice and human resource policies.

Top-down initiatives designed to promote changes in clinical activity – such as the national service frameworks – introduce monitoring systems that are viewed as signs of a lack of trust, thus eroding commitment to the NHS itself and often resulting in resistance to change. One response by government is to look beyond the NHS to the private sector, which is seen as being more flexible and less resistant to 'modernization'.

Table 9.3 Analysis of organizational culture

Nomenclature	Description	Health services
Person culture: Dionysus	Professionals who thrive on autonomy and personal decision-making. Their organizations exist to serve their needs and are flexible	GPs and other doctors and practitioners who have developed a degree of clinical autonomy
Role culture: Apollo	An organization based on rules and rule-following with defined and limited degrees of enterprise and discretion. Staff and job functions are clearly defined	NHS attempts to define roles, for example Knowledge and Skills Framework, Agenda for Change
Club or power culture: Zeus	An organization based on a single autocratic person who makes all the rules (which may be varied at any time) and who is intolerant of disloyalty	Most frequently found in some hospital consultants running clinical 'firms' or departments
Task culture: Athena	A team whose members acquire recognition through expertise and skill rather than grade. Tend to focus exclusively on the task in hand and favour collective decision-making	Research departments, A&E departments and other specialist units where there are few status differences among staff. However, being essentially fluid, they are often managed by Zeus people

Source: Based on Handy, 1995, p. 182

The NHS includes many different work cultures at different organizational levels that regularly test the decision-making structures of the NHS. There have been other, more recent tests:

- outsourcing or contracting out services

- developing partnerships with other organizations that have an interest in, or influence over, people's health

- the move to engage patients and the public in decisions about their own healthcare and health services in general.

Outsourcing is having an external vendor provide services that were previously provided in-house. Many trusts have taken decisions to outsource cleaning, catering, portering, laundry and security services. It could be argued that the use of agency nurses and other professionals also constitutes a form of outsourcing.

Outsourced workers are not NHS employees and are managed by the company providing them. Their loyalty is to their employer rather than to the organization in which they are deployed, and teamworking among them is dependent on the calibre of leadership available in the outsourced, as well as the 'host', company. This can present a further challenge to the main organization that has to 'manage' these workers through non-NHS-employed managers and by written contracts covering their precise duties.

Delivering services through **partnerships** between health, social care and other organizations has developed from an operational necessity (coordinating the work of health and social care professionals around the care of individual clients and patients) to a strategic goal for the organizations involved. Early experience of this way of working took the form of joint planning activities among health and local authorities providing services to the same communities. The professional, political and practical benefits of closer working led to pooled budgets, joint service management arrangements, and on to the more formal exercise of partner bodies' responsibilities and new organizational forms, for example local strategic partnerships and local drug action teams, which include health services, local authorities, education and police services and voluntary organizations. Voluntary sector organizations, including charities, are now actively engaged in providing both mainstream and specialist services, commissioned by PCTs with public funds. Independent, for-profit organizations commissioned in the same way also increase plurality in service provision. Forming effective partnerships between these agencies is not easy. Differences in approach, belief, priorities and governance mean that the partners have to be committed to each other at all organizational levels and concentrate effort on making their partnership work for the people they serve.

Perhaps the most recent source of cultural tension in health services has emerged from the policy to engage patients and the public in decisions about healthcare and health services. The policy has twin goals: make people take more responsibility for their own wellbeing by helping them to engage actively in decisions about their own healthcare; and make health services more relevant to people who need them by involving patients and the public in designing and monitoring services.

? What cultural challenges to the NHS are posed by the new initiatives for patient and public involvement?

Managing healthcare services

Health and social services were for many years 'administered' rather than managed, that is, centrally devised policies were carried out and administrators were publicly accountable for doing this (Stewart, 1989). The search for a more rational and effective way to deliver health services saw service planning emerge as a serious discipline and 1976 saw the first thoroughgoing reorganization of the NHS based on the principle of consensus management and a new population-based system of funding for health services. Following the Griffiths Report in 1983, in 1984 general managers were appointed to health services at many levels and they were then expected to 'manage' the various semi-autonomous professional disciplines and services that constitute the NHS. Consensus management, the principle that all management decisions should be implemented only after an agreement between all the stakeholders, was at an end. The 20 years that followed saw several structural changes, not least that which created the now familiar 'super disciplines' of commissioning, as distinct from providing, services. But the development underpinning and common to all the structural changes has been to do with leadership in organizations, by which is meant the work to create the conditions in which individuals and teams can do their best work. Thus, the most difficult challenge that large organizations like the health service face is how to use their scale and strength effectively while remaining sufficiently flexible to adapt to new circumstances. As Moss Kanter (1989) put it in her guide to successful change management: How do you teach the giant to dance?

Teamwork

The organization of health services has tended to devolve into smaller and more compact groupings, for example clinical care groups, divisions, disease-specific teams, for example cancer networks and infection control teams. Teamwork is a significant factor in healthcare delivery and **team-building** an essential aspect of organizational development. Two important things flow from this; first, smaller units are often more flexible and, second, this approach requires many more 'leaders', or workers with leadership skills, at every level of the health services.

The words 'group' and 'team' are often used interchangeably. A group can be described as any collection of people defined by a common purpose: located together, classified together or sharing beliefs. In an organizational context, however, a team may be defined as a group of workers selected by an organization for a defined purpose. Teams exist in many different forms, as can be seen in Table 9.4.

Table 9.4 A team classification

Types of team	Examples
Groups reporting to the same supervisor	Departmental teams, management teams
Groups of people with common aims	Research teams
Temporary groups for specific tasks	Project teams introducing new buildings, new services or the reconfiguration of services
Groups of people with interdependencies	Community nursing teams, hospital at home schemes; such teams may cross organizational boundaries
Groups of people with no formal links but who cannot accomplish tasks as individuals	Some project teams and some teams of experts involved in problem-solving

Difficulties may arise, however, when team members are drawn from quite disparate disciplines, as when addressing health promotion issues, for example. Teams might include schoolteachers, local authority staff, psychologists, nutritionists, health promotion workers, trade union representatives, shopkeepers and parents.

 ## What is needed to turn such a group into a team?

Team membership is different from being an employee in a large organization. Large organizations ascribe roles or job functions to each position in the hierarchy and the role is performed irrespective of who the role occupant happens to be. It is easy to feel like a cog in a wheel and then the role can become mechanistic and impersonal. This can result in a weakened sense of personal responsibility for work performance and a subsequent loss of personal satisfaction from employment.

Teams are more flexible and provide support to all team members to achieve agreed goals and outcomes. Team leaders need to lessen the rigidity with which each team member regards their role, without the accusation of exploitation. Tuckman (1965) observed that teams go through observable stages of development, which he called the forming, storming, norming and performing stages:

- The *forming* stage: interactions are polite and guarded.

- The *storming* stage: interactions are made to test fundamental differences between group members. Different members may be professionally committed to their own ways of doing things. Various conflicts are likely to emerge, and even the leadership may be challenged.

- The *norming* stage: norming involves getting organized, confronting and resolving issues, focusing on the task ahead instead of the group and generally establishing systems and procedures. Kakabadse et al. (1988) believe that the duration of this phase depends on the skills and abilities of the leader.

- The *performing* stage: this is dependent upon the group members' willingness to resolve their differences, and again the leader can facilitate this. When this occurs, group members become more supportive and communicative, rely on each other more readily and combine in joint problem-solving rather than mutual blaming when problems are encountered.

These stages are, however, by no means progressive. External and internal changes can cause the team to revert to earlier phases, particularly if team membership or the leader is changed. Although it is assumed that any team will progress through all four stages, this is not always so. Changes in team composition or strong professional or political agendas may inhibit team development and thus effectiveness. The *Journal of Interprofessional Care* regularly publishes papers on interprofessional teams such as community mental health teams, Sure Start teams and others where professionals are clear about their own individual roles but perceive that their roles are not recognized or understood by other members of the team.

The greater the decision-making responsibility, the higher the standard of training and competence that is required if increased throughput is to be accompanied by an increased quality of service. There is a constant evolution in both structure and relationships, and professional and service developments, largely as a consequence of the environmental pressures of three main factors: available finance, available technology and the health needs–demand equation – all of which are fundamentally political issues.

Leadership

 Are all managers leaders?

If we agree with Mullins that leadership is 'essentially … a relationship through which one person influences the behaviour or actions of other people' (Mullins, 2005, p. 253), then we are faced with the problem of differentiating leadership from management. But why bother, surely both are required, and at every level of the organization? While management may be regarded as having responsibility for organizational structure, strategy and systems – the hard Ss as Watson (1983) identified them, leaders tend to work with people – staff, skills, style (culture) and shared goals – the so-called soft Ss.

If the leader's prime function is to inculcate followership, what power does he or she have?

The ability to punish and reward, or 'resource power', will not necessarily produce willing followers. 'Referent power', where would-be followers admire the leader's characteristics and wish to copy them for themselves (French and Raven, 1968), is more effective. In the professional world of health services, referent power is greatly enhanced by expertise or 'expert power'. The requirement for a leader to be a charismatic superman was one of the mythologies debunked in a survey of 2,000 NHS managers (Alimo-Metcalfe and Alban-Metcalfe, 2000). The most important characteristic emerged as concern for others, followed by the ability to communicate and inspire. As health and social care delivery has grown more complex, the requirements of leaders have had to change. The director, general manager or chief executive must lead clinical, professional and support staff and cannot rely on shared professional experience and qualifications for credibility and authority. The requirements to listen, take advice, explain, convince and, wherever possible, secure agreement are common to all situations. Inevitably, some decisions will trigger opposition among one or more of the interested staff groups and securing support, or acquiescence, will demand an approach that is flexible and appropriate to the situation. Neither a purely task nor a people orientation alone is adequate to resolve the leadership complexities presented in the modern NHS.

THINKING
ABOUT

Think of people you know whom you perceive to be leaders. What personal qualities do they possess? Are they able to command respect from a wide range of different people? Why do you trust them? Why do you, or would you, follow them?

Rosemary Stewart (1989) has set out some leadership characteristics that enable leaders and/or managers to gain a degree of respect in any organization. To these we have added some more of our own.

Leaders require:

Vision: to imagine what might be better and communicate that to everyone

Values: a demonstrable commitment to the work, service and to people

Valour: courage to take risks, to make difficult decisions, to hold firm in periods of turbulence

Virtue: integrity and constancy in dealing with individuals; keeping one's word. This means not making promises that one cannot keep or one is unlikely to be able to keep

Vigour: to pursue goals, to support individuals and groups, energize by example

Vigilance: to watch over the organization by constantly scanning the horizon and assessing the effects of the changing environment

Visibility: to be seen, to be known and to be approachable by workers at all levels.

One might also add 'vicarious liability', that is, taking responsibility when things go wrong and not shifting the blame onto others.

Managing change

Effecting change within any organization has been likened to managing a contest between opposing and resisting forces – the so-called force field approach (Lewin, 1951). David Gleicher et al. (1987) have proposed an approach known as the change equation:

$$D \times V \times F > R$$

- 'D' stands for the *dissatisfaction* with the present situation: where employees are comfortable in an inefficient situation, education is required to demonstrate current disadvantages

- 'V' represents a shared *vision* of a better future or way of working: this can raise morale and increase motivation and thus commitment for the change

- 'F' is an acceptable *first step*: a way of initiating the change that is least threatening to all

- 'R' is *resistance* to change: the cost to the individual or group of making the change.

Good communication is a vital underpinning of this equation. Leadership which attends to all four components of this equation is most likely to bring about the desired change. Where successful, the system will suffer minimal disruption and is likely to self-heal any damage that occurs.

This common-sense formula is often forgotten in many organizations where change is announced from the top and implemented with minimal, if any, consultation. Even when the situation is urgent (for example the changes in practice concerning the retention of human organs and tissue demanded by the government and public), attention to the change equation can facilitate positive development. Using von Bertalanffy's (1951) biological model, we can draw an analogy between messages conveyed by nerves in a biological organism and the role of communications in organizations. Neither entity can operate successfully without them.

Theoretical and methodological perspectives

? How can theory help us to understand organizations and people at work, and manage them effectively?

Theories about the way people and organizations behave have developed over more than 100 years and reflect changing social attitudes and ideas about manufacture and service. They offer descriptions and analyses of the way employees and organizations behave in different sets of circumstances, which can help people to understand what they observe around them when they are at work. There is no one 'right' theory of organization or behaviour: some were products of their age, all have both proponents and critics. Attention to theory can, however, help students, practitioners and managers understand, and therefore influence, the people and organizations around them.

For example, it is obvious that not all organizations are alike and it often seems that the similarities between organizations as entities are outweighed by their considerable differences. General practices and hospitals both employ clinical and support staff and deliver healthcare but are profoundly dissimilar in scale and culture. Such disparities generate distinctive variations in structure and rules, ways of working and even value systems, which affect efficiency and people's experience of their work. There is no one 'right' way to manage organizations: much depends on a combination of factors which may include the organization's history, size and function.

The purpose of this part of the chapter is to sketch out the types of management and organization theory that have developed in recent times, and to indicate where each might be of value to people concerned with healthcare organizations.

Scientific management

The progenitors of modern management theory were F.W. Taylor (1856–1915) in the USA and Henri Fayol (1841–1925) in France. Taylor (2003), whose operational sphere was a steelworks, prescribed precise methods and practices for his manual workers and rewarded them with pay commensurate with their compliance and output. He discounted the ability of his workers and their managers to both identify and use the most efficient methods of work for any particular task. Today, his 'scientific management' has its counterpart in many clinical procedures such as the avoidance of contamination in barrier nursing. These (prescribed) procedures are now carried out without additional monetary reward but as part of accepted professional practice. Moreover, improvement in such practices can come from the results of research, often conducted by health professionals themselves. While the rather remote and directive nature of Taylor's approach is deemed no longer appropriate, the essential methodology is still reflected in professional practice informed by scientific evidence.

Fayol (1949), also an engineer, wrote about the formal structure of organizations, with the emphasis on planning, technical requirements and the principles of management, with the concomitant assumptions of logical and rational behaviour. His five elements of management – to forecast and plan, organize, command, coordinate and control – clearly stem from an era when autocracy was the predominant and accepted approach to management. Fayol, like his contemporary Max Weber, developed a model of the organization as a well-designed and well-run machine, which would always respond to the levers of control, provided they were correctly applied, and this represented 'good management'.

? Would the levers of scientific management help today's managers?

The initial but transient enthusiasm for Taylor's ideas occurred at the time when America was attempting to re-establish its industrial base and output following the Civil War. Pure Taylorism foundered because of its rigidity and a flawed assumption of workers' rationality. However, his ideas have endured for over 100 years in efficiency surveys, work study and method study, which survive in various forms, either in their own right (for example clinical pathway reviews) or in combination with other review methods (for example business process re-engineering).

Bureaucracy and organizations

The notion of an organization based on rules is popularly attributed to Weber (1964), who used the term **bureaucracy** to label the phenomenon and regarded the term as one synonymous with efficiency (rather than the mildly abusive connotation of today). Although he did not define the term, he described the characteristics of a bureaucracy as having a hierarchy of authority, a system of rules and thus impersonality (each individual had to follow the rules rather than personal preferences) and many specialized roles. One can readily recognize some of these characteristics in the larger parts of the health services and indeed size appears to be positively correlated with bureaucratic characteristics, which Handy (1995) has named the role culture.

There have been many criticisms of bureaucracy as an organizational form, not least in its potential to stifle initiative (which Weber regarded as a positive function) and restrict personal growth and development. In a bureaucracy, people are rewarded for following rules rather than attaining goals and so the rules and associated processes can become ends in themselves. In fact, the rules can and do become the goals in some instances. The nature of health and social care, however, both demands a clear framework in which practitioners work (licensing, regulation, accreditation), and requires those same professionals to exercise clinical discretion. An accommodation is required between, for example, a list of drugs and procedures that may be prescribed under NHS arrangements and the need to provide patients with the best care available. Rules generally allow organizations to exercise control at long range, whereas at close range, there is usually someone who has been vested with sufficient discretion to give or amend a ruling.

? To what extent is the NHS a bureaucratic organization?

The human relations approach

The mid-1920s saw the next major development in management theory – the human relations approach, frequently associated with Elton Mayo, who, at the time, was a researcher at the Graduate Business School at Harvard University. The significant work discussed here was undertaken by his two colleagues, Roethlisberger and Dixon (1943).

Unlike scientific management, which regarded workers as robotic servants, the human relations school discovered that workers responded to their working conditions, to leadership, group dynamics, managerial behaviour and, above all, to recognition. Where Taylorism had dehumanized workers, the human relations approach sought to humanize work organizations, sometimes to the detriment of economic efficiency.

The 'discovery' of this seemingly obvious phenomenon occurred during the famous Hawthorne experiments conducted from the mid-1920s in the Western Electric Company in America.

Example 9.1

THE HAWTHORNE EXPERIMENTS

The Hawthorne experiments consisted of several phases. In the first phase, six women were segregated in a 'test' room and told to work normally on their assembly of relay switch gear. Over a period of two years, the physical conditions, lighting, ventilation and temperature control were changed, as were their pay arrangements, incentives, benefits, work breaks and so forth. However adverse their conditions became, their productivity rose with each change of the conditions – even when all privileges were temporarily removed.

These workers were made aware that they were taking part in an experiment. Although the methodology employed was flawed, the explanation for this unanticipated finding was that the recognition afforded to the workers was the source of their motivation. This phenomenon became known as the Hawthorne effect.

For a thorough analysis of all the Hawthorne experiments, see Rose, 1978, Chapter 11.

Although of enormous significance, these experiments were poorly conducted, badly flawed and subject to much criticism. The major lesson they offer, however, is the importance of managerial behaviour and of the informal organizations that arise among workers trying to do good work – something that Weberian bureaucracy ignores and, indeed, seeks to suppress. Mullins (2005) believes these experiments, with all their faults, were the first approach to organization and management that had an appreciation of industrial sociology.

We can see that whereas Taylor sought to design systems of work without regard to the needs of people, the human relations approach took an opposite direction, placing the needs of people above the requirements of the organization. Both are now regarded as inadequate management models. Attaining a workable balance between these two requirements appears to be a major and necessary skill of the manager and much later research on shift working, for example, demonstrated and highlighted this fact.

Behavioural theory

Research in the 1940s in the University of Michigan and in the 1950s in Ohio State University investigated management and leadership styles. Managers were categorized as 'job centred' or 'employee centred', which were broadly aligned to the Taylorist and the human relations approaches respectively. Many thought that these orientations were personality traits and reflected the way leaders regarded their subordinates and the assumptions they made about the subordinates' attitude to work. This was developed into a popular theory by Douglas McGregor (1987), which described theory X and theory Y leaders. Theory X leaders believed their subordinates disliked work and responsibility and would avoid it if they could. These leaders would therefore become highly directional towards their staff, emphasizing task accomplishment above all else. Theory Y leaders held the opposite view and thus took an approach that gave greater weight to engaging with employees and their needs and preferences at work.

It was clear that neither extreme was necessarily helpful and that leader behaviour, if it were to be effective, had to be flexible and appropriate for the different situations that leaders encountered. Indeed, the Ohio studies were able to demonstrate that these two characteristics were independent variables and the most effective leaders, rather than having a fixed leadership 'style', selected the most appropriate behaviour for each situation.

Situation theory

Situation theory grew from the recognition that no one management or leadership style could serve all situations and that flexibility was required. Tannenbaum and Schmidt (1973) described a matrix which identified several factors that might influence the leadership approach in a given situation:

- factors in the manager, for example his or her experience, confidence, expertise

- factors in their subordinates, for example maturity and training, willingness and ability to take decisions

- factors in the situation, for example degree of urgency, nature of the task to be undertaken.

In highly complex organizations such as the NHS, the decision of direction (that is, 'what is to be done') is taken at the top of the hierarchy and imposed on the organization beneath. How that direction is to be achieved is frequently left to local leaders, and it is here that situation theory can have its most frequent application.

Contingency theory

Contingency theory provides a further development of situation theory. Extensive research by Fred Fiedler (1967) of the University of Washington led him to postulate that the amount of *influence* a leader possesses should determine leadership approach. Where this influence was relatively moderate, for example where technical expertise was similar to or less developed than that of subordinates, the preferred approach needed to be employee centred.

Where influence was either weak or strong, a task orientation could be adopted. Fiedler's theory has been contested as far too simplistic an approach and contradicted by evidence from other sources. Nevertheless, it is interesting to note that in the complex world of health and social care, leaders may have only moderate influence in what are highly technical situations. The title, salary and budget that may go with a leadership position do not necessarily bring legitimate and ultimate authority. The goals of health and social care organizations are more often achieved collaboratively, contingent on situational factors.

Does a lack of specialist expertise limit a person's ability to manage?

Motivation theories

League tables, reports of regulators and individuals' experiences tell us that health and social care institutions do not all perform to the same standard. Why is this? Many types of factors may be at work (see the PESTEL analysis above), and the issues are complex, but staff motivation, and therefore individual performance, is a significant factor in organizational performance. Motivation is a complex concept, but put simply it refers to 'the will to work', particularly when unsupervised. Quality, persistence, endurance, energy, patience and many other attributes are involved.

The motivation to work, and its link with job satisfaction, is clearly a large and important aspect of management theory. Motivation theories may be divided into two groups: content and process theories.

Content theories

Content theories postulate that all humans are driven by a similar set of needs. Good organization and management ensure that these needs are satisfied at work and can increase the motivation of workers. But to what extent is this really true? The most familiar content theorist is Abraham Maslow (1943), who suggested that there is a hierarchy of people's needs: they will first be motivated to satisfy essential physiological needs and then move on to psychological needs, via security, social and self-esteem needs. When one need is satisfied, the next higher level need becomes the motivation for action on their part.

THINKING
ABOUT

Think about the last job you enjoyed. What was the basis for your satisfaction – pay, status, autonomy, or its purpose and significance?

The salience of each need varies with the individual. Some workers value job security far more than a risky challenge. Traditionally, public sector workers have been thought to fall into this category, while others, such as entrepreneurs, are thought to do their best work in conditions of high risk. However, risk is understood differently by different people. The dot com entrepreneur might regard the public sector worker's daily contact with clients and patients as extremely risky, while the public sector worker might value the autonomy of the self-employed entrepreneur. Moreover, it is by no means certain that an individual will seek to satisfy all such needs in a work context. Hobbies, sports, social interests and competitions may provide the opportunity for self-actualization, which Maslow describes as the highest need of all. For self-actualizing to occur at work, appropriately challenging jobs must be available during times of full employment, together with the recognition that accompanies excellent performance. Maslow's hierarchy was not developed in a management but in a clinical context and has been applied by enthusiastic management theorists (Fincham and Rhodes, 1999): it has not, however, enjoyed much empirical support.

Clayton Alderfer (1972) grouped individuals' basic needs into:

- existence, for example job security, pay

- relatedness, for example social interaction

- growth, for example professional development.

These are not necessarily hierarchical needs; rather a continuum along which one might travel in either direction depending on circumstance and stage of career development. This theory might explain the importance of training and career development and the benefits they might bring in both the retention and motivation of health service workers. However, Alderfer also believed that workers who could not satisfy their growth needs would settle for taking larger 'helpings' of existence and relatedness satisfaction. The worker's effort–reward 'psychological' contract with the employer would favour the worker rather than the organization, for example workers would satisfy more of their social needs at work, perhaps at the expense of effic-iency. This might present a particular challenge for managers.

Frederick Herzberg (1966) thought that not all needs were motivating because his definition of motivation included the additional effort and energy contributed by the worker, beyond the minimum normally required by the organization. Supervision, salary, the work environment, company policy and even relationships with colleagues, however satisfying, would not generate the additional input that met his definition. Although important, he called these the *hygiene* factors because they related to the context in which work is performed. His *motivators* related to work content, for example achievement, recognition for achievement, responsibility, interesting/meaningful work and an opportunity for career development and advancement. This theory appeals to health and social care workers because of the high number of professionals employed, where there is considerable scope for exercising professional judgement and where recognition can come from several sources, for example patients, their relatives, colleagues and managers. However, Herzberg's methodology has been criticized, as have the conclusions he has drawn from his oft-repeated research projects. Not all people are the same and ultimately his theory is limited by the same constraints that bind all the content theorists, namely, the impossibility of devising a universal formula to motivate all staff.

Process theories

Process theories are based more on the precise value of the reward to the individual in exchange for particular behaviour. Adam's equity theory (1965), for example, considers the output required for the input given; is it worth it – what's in it for me? This is linked with social comparison: what is the effort–reward contract for other similar workers, or workers in my social comparison group? Inequitable treatment of workers can cause dissatisfaction and low morale and ultimately low output. Workers whose professional ethos will not permit a lowering of standards of their work may nevertheless lower their work rate, for example see fewer patients, to register their displeasure.

Expectancy theory (Porter and Lawler, 1968) takes this process one step further by asking two questions. First, if I work harder, what is the chance of my being able to achieve the standard of performance required? If there are problems with personal confidence, experience, training or availability of equipment, working harder will not mean that I achieve the right standard, so I may decide against the extra effort. Second, if I can surmount these hurdles, what is the likelihood of my receiving my reward, intrinsic and/or extrinsic, recognition and/or treasure?

Process theories are about cognition, how people experience and perceive their working environment and respond to it. Indeed, Handy (1993) has described it as a calculus – the effort needed to achieve the required work performance and reward needed to perform. These processes depend in part on the confidence each worker has in their leader's ability to deliver a working environment that allows them to do their best work.

Motivation, according to Herzberg (1966), comes from the satisfaction of a person's intrinsic needs, not payment. Once again, the leader is crucial in providing a supportive environment that enables self-development. In considering both content and process theories of motivation, then, management/leadership is the key, particularly when so many health service employees are professionals and expect to be treated as such.

Example 9.2

JOB DESIGN

Where Taylor sought to impose rigidity of operation and to inhibit each worker's scope for innovation, current approaches involve the introduction of variety, autonomy and task defragmentation. Variety of task not only helps to reduce monotony at work, but calls on a wide repertoire of skills and experience. Autonomy increases personal control, and responsibility for a complete task serves to enhance meaningfulness and satisfaction.

The trend to develop jobs in this way depends on three moderators (Hackman and Oldham, 1980):

- The ability and skill of the worker – related to training, qualification and experience
- The strength of the employee's growth needs (at work) – their 'comfort zone' on Maslow's hierarchy or Alderfer's continuum
- The employee's satisfaction with the context of the work – the psychological contract, which may include issues such as pay and conditions, organizational policy and rules, ethics and intrinsic rewards such as recognition. This third factor appears to relate as much to the process

theories of motivation as to Herzberg's hygiene factors.

While horizontal job loading, where all tasks are of a roughly similar level of skill and responsibility, can increase variety, it can also increase stress if imposed to an unreasonable level for a particular individual. Vertical job loading, where greater responsibility for the task is given, such as planning, financial control, management of others, is usually accompanied by higher grading and extrinsic rewards.

One further important finding by Katz (1978) and cited by Schein (1988) was that for those workers remaining in the same job for over 15–20 years, contextual factors such as pay and benefits, co-worker relations and compatibility with supervisors were of equal importance. Contextual factors therefore became relatively more important as job longevity increased. When this occurs, job redesign may be less motivating than better pay or working conditions. Alternatively, a step change of job function or a change of occupation may reinvigorate some employees.

Systems theory and the sociotechnical system approach

Health and social care services comprise a plethora of systems, each aimed at delivering one or more elements of care – prevention, diagnosis, treatment, rehabilitation and long-term care. Systems theory proposes that the whole is greater than the sum of its parts. This means that each component subsystem acquires a greater significance when part of a superordinate system than when on its own. Indeed, the significance of subsystems depends upon their inclusion. Ludwig von Bertalanffy (1951), a biologist who first wrote about systems theory, made the connection between biological systems, for example the homeostatic system, and organizational systems.

 CONNECTIONS

Chapter 1 describes the basis of homeostasis as a system in balance.

Figure 9.2 illustrates very well the relationship between organizational components and the organization and its environment. Changes in organizational arrangements will effect changes in every other subsystem and thus moderate the rate of change occurring within the organization.

The Nadler and Tushman congruency model of organizational behaviour examines the relationship between the main components of the organization. The extent to which they are congruent with each other is an indicator of the likely efficiency of the organization and, therefore, its survival and effectiveness. Put simply, the greater the congruence, the more efficient will be the organization, given its environmental constraints. Are there sufficient numbers of trained employees? Are they deployed in the most efficient manner? For example, if the government's policy is to encourage patient choice, including giving birth at home, will there be enough appropriately trained midwives, together with appropriate back-up facilities, in time to meet the introduction of the policy?

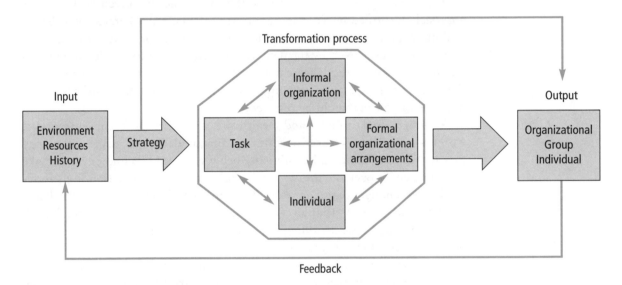

Figure 9.2 A congruency model of organizational behaviour
Source: Nadler and Tushman, 1979

Nadler and Tushman (1979) suggest that four organizational components need to be optimized in order to achieve effective operations:

- The formal organizational structure: relationships, responsibilities (job descriptions)

- The tasks to be performed: caring and curing, educating and researching

- The individual employees: sufficient, trained, qualified, experienced and competent

- The informal structure: the way the organization works, its behavioural norms, its 'culture'.

The model specifically does not include groups or technology, both of which can have an important bearing on organizational efficiency. But neither does it necessarily exclude them.

Changes made to a single element in one part of the system inevitably have repercussions for many other systems and subsystems. For example, efforts in health education, such as smoking cessation or obesity prevention, will result in longer healthy lives and less demand on curative services over the long term. And when changes are made within the healthcare organization itself, similar effects occur. For example, changes made to increase the autonomy and responsibility of frontline workers may increase anxiety within the organization with regard to budgetary control. On the other hand, withdrawal of financial control to the centre to ensure savings may well lower the morale and motivation of those same frontline workers.

A particular variant of systems theory is the sociotechnical systems approach, identified by Trist and Bamforth (1951). Their context was that of coal mining following the introduction of mechanization. The social patterns of work were destroyed by the new technology, leading to a reduction in coal output. The new methods were potentially more efficient but, after investigation, further changes were required to take account of the workers' social needs before output could be restored.

Although coal mining and healthcare are very different enterprises, workers in both workplaces operate in teams, under stress, using technology that is still developing and continually being replaced. Technology can make a significant impact on the way we work and its introduction constitutes significant change that can extend to the psychological contract being compromised, even though job designations may remain unaltered. Technology can cause deskilling but also lead to reskilling. Not everyone will be able to accept either outcome.

There are, however, occasions when change brings unexpected consequences, or shifts in behaviour or performance arise for no apparent reason. The models described so far do not help in such circumstances: so what might do so?

Chaos (or complexity) theory

This chapter has addressed a number of theories aimed at imposing order on otherwise potentially unstable organizations. The bureaucratic approach seeks to limit discretion and impose rigidity, while the management techniques associated with motivation and leadership appear to be more flexible levers of control. But are these approaches effective in every case? If they were, then once mastered, all organizations would run like well-oiled machines, optimizing effectiveness and efficiency. Clearly this is not the case. So what is happening to cause such variation in performance in output and outcomes between similar organizations and between different operational periods within the same organization?

In the 1960s, two researchers, Henri Poincaré and Edward Lorenz, identified chaos theory by discovering non-repeating patterns of behaviour in complex systems, which nevertheless remained contained within a broad framework of predictability. Lorenz's work applied to weather forecasting, a highly complex problem, but more recently, the theory has been used to explain unpredictable and non-repeating patterns in biological behaviour and in complex organizations.

Some NHS organizations appear to have greater competence in treating patients than others. Some improve both their clinical and financial performance while others underperform. Many experience variation over time in these and other parameters and appear to go in and out of control inexplicably. According to Tiplady (2003, p. 2):

> Chaos theory is based on the recognition that real world systems never settle down into a steady state. All systems go through continual patterns of order and disorder, always changing, never repeating. Chaos ... exhibits a kind of stability within instability.

The source of this disorder comes from the complexity within the system, the effects of which are unpredictable. For example, the emergence of HIV/AIDS in the 1980s placed considerable demands on healthcare services and ring-fenced money. New forms of treatment in the 1990s that meant people were living with the disease (rather than dying from it) required new, more integrated forms of service delivery. Very small changes in policy and managerial adjustments can often effect very significant changes over time and this fact gives us a clue as to the manner in which change might best be achieved within organizations. Tiplady likens the initiation of change to sowing seeds in people's minds, which will bear considerable and unforeseen fruit in the future. He believes that successful change is best seen as an iterative process of small steps, rather than a heavy-handed imposition from above. Whatever the approach, however, outcomes may vary considerably from those predicted. Moreover, while the performance of the organization as a whole may be unpredictable, the same is found to apply within its component parts.

It is clear that from the earliest attempts to identify a workable management hypothesis, managers and researchers alike have seen the necessity to exercise control over workers and organizations in order to achieve planned output. While chaos theory may help us to understand why some targets are missed and others unexpectedly exceeded, there is an unremitting requirement for better management of all types of organization. We attempt to illustrate some of these points in the following case study on the formulation and implementation of a local obesity strategy.

CASE STUDY Formulating an obesity strategy

Organization and management skills are vital for both the planning and the implementation of a PCT's obesity strategy. All organization and management activity takes place within a policy context. The obesity strategy required goals and targets to be set, partnership working to be operational and effective, resources to be available, and monitoring and evaluation to demonstrate its effectiveness. The following case study uses these categories to discuss Central PCT's obesity strategy.

The policy context for the obesity strategy was positive and proactive. In 2004, the government set a public service agreement (PSA) target to halt the year-on-year rise of obesity in children aged under 11 by 2010, and to reduce obesity across the population as a whole. This target was owned by three different governmental departments: the Department of Health, the Department for Education and Skills, and the Department for Culture, Media and Sport. Following this PSA, in 2006, the National Institute for Health and Clinical Excellence (NICE) published its guidelines for the prevention and treatment of obesity (NICE, 2006), and the National Heart Forum, in association with the Faculty of Public Health and the Department of Health, also published *Lightening the Load*, a toolkit on tackling obesity. The Department of Health's White Paper *Choosing Health* (DoH, 2004) set out to demonstrate how people can be encouraged and empowered to make healthier choices, including choosing a healthy diet and increased physical activity. This was followed by the White Paper delivery plan *Delivering Choosing Health: Making Healthier Choices Easier* (DoH, 2005), which sets out how the White Paper commitments will be delivered.

In addition, the government has set targets relating to obesity for local authorities and PCTs. These include:

- Local public sector agreement target to increase levels of sport and active leisure activities to over 50-year-olds and 15–19-year-olds
- Public sector agreement target to increase breastfeeding initiation rates by 2% per annum, focusing particularly on women from disadvantaged groups
- Healthy schools target that schoolchildren should do a minimum of two hours' physical activity at school each week.

An obesity and healthy eating strategy needs to provide a framework that integrates an organization's major goals, policies and actions. In other words, a strategy should result from a process of formal planning based on extensive data collection and analysis. On the one hand, a strategy can be cutting edge, offering innovative approaches, but in the public sector, they may become permeated by cumbersome, slow and change-resistant personnel and procedures. As we have seen in this chapter, however, all organizations operate in an environment and a strategy merely articulates an approach used by military strategists – how to ensure a fit between goals, resources (including staff capacity and capability) and environment.

Figure 9.3 illustrates the factors that need to be taken into account.

Following a period of consultation with practitioners and the public, an obesity strategy must select a range of goals and targets. One goal is the creation of an

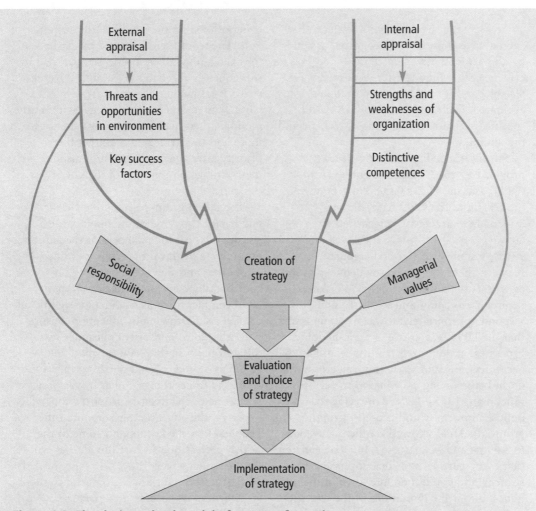

Figure 9.3 The design school model of strategy formation
Source: Mintzberg et al., 1998, p. 26

ongoing data set measuring the local population's BMI especially all reception year and year 6 schoolchildren as well as adults. This data set could be used to evaluate the impact of the strategy on the population's body weight. Other targets included those aimed at early years' interventions (such as Sure Start) and schools, encompassing the provision of healthy meals, educating staff and children on what a healthy diet consists of, supporting the National School Fruit and Vegetable Scheme, and providing healthy tuck shops and cookery lessons. The physical activity targets include the provision of healthy transport plans, showers and secure cycle parking for workplaces. For schools, targets include timetabling more physical activity sessions for schoolchildren, promoting walk to school and cycle to school schemes and improving playground facilities. For the general public, targets include extending the provision of leisure facilities to all age groups and socioeconomic classes and the provision of dedicated cycle lanes.

The key requirements for a target to be agreed were that: it was recognized as valid by all partners; it was based on sound evidence regarding its effectiveness; it was feasible; and it could be monitored and evaluated. Each target had to be SMART – specific, measurable, achievable, realistic and time limited.

Strong leadership and support was provided by the Director of Public Health (DPH) and the PCT's CEO. Between them, the DPH and the CEO have all the leadership characteristics identified by Stewart (1989) – vision, values, valour, virtue, visibility, vigour and vigilance. Between them, this duo provided inspiration as well as the all-important people skills – the ability to communicate, listen and respond appropriately. It was also important that the DPH was aware of team-building processes, and ensured that the team had the necessary time and space to form, storm and norm before being called upon to perform (Tuckman, 1965). Instead of trying to impose uniformity and consensus on the group, the DPH allowed conflicting agendas to emerge and be discussed, but also ensured that every partner had some input into the strategy and could therefore 'own' it. Being honest about the limitations of the strategy was also important, so that partners did not develop unrealistic expectations of what the strategy could deliver.

While the DPH focused on team-building, the CEO focused more on the motivations of the different individuals involved in the team. Using theoretical frameworks such as Maslow's (1943) hierarchy of needs and Alderfer's (1972) motivation theories, the CEO has consciously tried to reinforce people's engagement with the team. For example, after finding out that a team member was interested in the media, the CEO provided funding for this team member to participate in a training programme on using the mass media effectively, which was being offered by the local health promotion unit. The team then delegated media liaison to this team member, and were rewarded by subsequently receiving favourable coverage in the local media. Nevertheless, while the CEO wanted an obesity strategy 'within nine months', there were other things she wanted more and the strategy did not get the priority after the initial few months and maintaining commitment of members was difficult.

The initial group formulating the strategy had been led by one of the public health consultants. All the members of the planning group were health professionals of one sort or another and they were focusing on coordinating care for people once obesity had been identified as a source of significant clinical risk. Drawing in education, leisure and other local authority colleagues was difficult because they saw the planning group as a 'doctors and nurses' group and it was hard to get things going. It was only when one of the doctors proposed that other experts – the education, leisure and other people – join the group, and some of the health professionals stand down, that work on the strategy took off.

Partnership working was crucial to the strategy and its success. Key partners were identified as those working in the health, social care, education and leisure sectors as well as workplaces in general, the media and commercial sectors, and the general public. The public was accessed via community, neighbourhood and voluntary organizations. The local strategic partnership was tasked with ensuring that the impact on health would be routinely considered when applications for new communities and transport planning were received. In this way, it is anticipated that the obesity strategy will become embedded within everyone's agenda, with a knock-on serendipitous effect.

In order to be implemented, the strategy required funding and resources. While some of the resources (for example people's expertise, time and energy) were available as part of normal working patterns, other items (for example healthy cooking lessons in schools, exercise facilities in workplaces) required dedicated funding. It was important therefore that the PCT could ring-fence funding for the implementation of the strategy, even if at the outset this was secured for only three years. Some funding was also obtained from the Big Lottery Fund programme.

Monitoring and evaluation was necessary to demonstrate the strategy's effectiveness and secure long-term sustainable funding. The BMI measurements for schoolchildren and adults will provide ongoing data that can be used to assess the effectiveness of the obesity strategy. Specific initiatives will include monitoring of uptake, for example the number of children using supervised walk to school and cycle to school schemes will be logged by supervisors. Different partners will also be conducting their own routine audit and monitoring activities that will shed light on the strategy's impact. However, one of the challenges of the strategy is to devise a means of collating and

combining these diverse forms of monitoring and evaluation in order to provide an overall evaluation of the strategy. A second challenge is to identify what changes (if any) can be attributed to the strategy, and what changes would have happened anyway, as part of secular shifts and movements, regardless of any additional local input. These challenges pose significant dilemmas that require specialist expertise and funding to address. Central PCT has been fortunate in obtaining some research funding enabling it to employ a part-time researcher to evaluate the first 18 months of the strategy.

Taking an overview, it appears that the PCT's obesity strategy has been carefully planned and should prove effective in tackling obesity. The various elements of a successful strategy – a positive policy environment, setting appropriate goals and targets, strong leadership and partnership working, adequate resourcing, and ongoing monitoring and evaluation are all in place to varying degrees. Many challenges remain, not least to secure sustainable funding and establish that the strategy is effective, but the basic requirements of an effective strategy have all been addressed.

Summary

- Theoretical and empirical work can help us to understand why organizations and the people that comprise them behave as they do

- An organization's goals, strategies, structure, technology and external environment all relate to each other and this relationship is critical to its performance and effectiveness

- Managers face many challenges in managing internal dynamic processes in an organization, including the role of culture, managing change, decision-making processes, managing work in groups and teams, and power and politics

Questions for further discussion

1. You will find a doctor leading healthcare organizations in the USA and many European countries. Why are there so few who do this in the UK?

2. Can members of the public have any real say in decision-making about healthcare and health services?

3. What experience, skills and competences does a manager of a healthcare service need? Are these different from those required to manage another sort of organization?

4. Could a professionally cross-trained (generic) worker such as a children's worker replace many of the current well-differentiated professions? Would this help or hinder the development of a teamwork ethos in healthcare?

Further reading

Buchanan, D. and Huczinsky, A. (2000) *Organizational Behaviour*. New York: Prentice Hall.
A multidisciplinary text that enables students to study the behaviour of organizations and the role of management. It explores core concepts and debates in a readable and accessible manner.

Hatch, M.J. (1997) *Organization Theory: Modern, Symbolic and Postmodern Perspectives*. Oxford: Oxford University Press.
An interesting analysis of different perspectives on organizations. It discusses the ways in which organizations can be analysed including as social structures or cultures and looks at key concepts such as decision-making, power and change.

Iles, V. (2005) *Really Managing Healthcare* (2nd edn). Maidenhead: Open University Press.
Deals with practical issues in healthcare management.

Klein, R. (2004) *The New Politics of the NHS: From Creation to Reinvention* (5th edn). London: Longman.
Concentrates on those issues that seem to best illuminate the analytic themes and to provide the most insight into political processes.

Levitt, R., Wall, A. and Appleby, J. (2004) *The Reorganised National Health Service* (6th edn). Cheltenham: Stanley Thornes.
Deals with the structure of the NHS and the many changes that have occurred since 1948.

Mullins, L.J. (2005) *Management and Organizational Behaviour* (7th edn). London: Pitman.
This is a major text dealing with all the management theories and thinking, both historic and current. It does not deal specifically with the health services.

Senior, B. and Fleming, J. (2006) *Organizational Change* (3rd edn). Harlow: Pearson Educational.
Excellent accessible treatment of organizational change, highly applicable to health services and to a wide range of public and private sector organizations.

Developing Change Management Skills; a resource for healthcare professionals and managers can be downloaded at www.sdo.lshtm.ac.uk/publications.

References

Adams, J.S. (1965) Inequity in social exchange, in L. Berkowitz (ed.) *Advances in Experimental Social Psychology*, vol. 2. New York: Academic Press.

Alderfer, C.P. (1972) *Existence, Relatedness and Growth*. New York: Free Press.

Alimo-Metcalfe, B. and Alban-Metcalfe, R. (2000) 'Heaven can wait'. *Health Service Journal* 12 October: 26–9.

Ansoff, I.H. and McDonell, E.J. (1990) *Implanting Strategic Management*. Engelwood Cliffs, NJ: Prentice Hall.

Bertalanffy, L. von (1951) 'Problems of general systems theory: a new approach to the unity of science'. *Human Biology* **23**(4): 302–12.

Deal, T. and Kennedy, A. (1982) *Corporate Cultures: The Rites and Rituals of Corporate Life*. Reading, MA: Addison-Wesley.

DHSS (Department for Health and Social Security) (1983) *NHS Management Inquiry: Report to the Secretary of State for Social Services* (the Griffiths Report). London: DHSS.

DoH (Department of Health) (2004) *Choosing Health: Making Healthier Choices Easier*, White Paper. London: DoH.

DoH (Department of Health) (2005) *Delivering Choosing Health: Making Healthier Choices Easier*, White Paper. London: DoH.

Fayol, H. (1949) *General and Industrial Management*. London: Pitman.

Fiedler, F.E. (1967) *A Theory of Leadership Effectiveness*. New York: McGraw-Hill.

Fincham, R. and Rhodes, P (1999) *Principles of Organisational Behaviour* (3rd edn). Oxford: OUP.

French, J.R.P and Raven, B. (1968) The bases of social power, in D. Cartwright and A.F. Zander (eds) *Group Dynamics: Research and Theory* (3rd edn). London: Harper & Row.

Gleicher, D., Beckhard, R. and Harris, R. (1987) The change equation, www.valuebasedmanagement.net.

Hackman, J.R. and Oldham, G.R. (1980) *Work Redesign*. Reading, MA: Addison-Wesley.

Handy, C.B. (1993) *Understanding Organisations* (4th edn). London: Penguin.

Handy, C.B. (1995) *Gods of Management*. Oxford: OUP.

Herzberg, F. (1966) *Work and the Nature of Man*. New York: World Publishing.

Kakabadse, A., Ludlow, R. and Vinnicombe, S. (1988) *Working in Organizations*. London: Penguin

Katz, R. (1978) 'Job longevity as a situational factor in job satisfaction'. *Administrative Science Quarterly* **23**: 204–23.

Lewin, K. (1951) *Field Theory in Social Science*. London: Harper & Row.

Maslow, A.H. (1943) 'A theory of human motivation'. *Psychological Review* **50**: 370–96.

McGregor, D. (1987) *The Human Side of Enterprise*. London: Penguin.

Mintzberg, H., Ahlstrand, B. and Lampel, J. (1998) *Strategy Safari: A Guided Tour Through the Wilds of Strategic Management*. New York: Free Press.

Moss Kanter, R. (1989) *When Giants Learn to Dance*. New York: Simon & Schuster.

Mullins, L.J. (2005) *Management and Organisational Behaviour* (7th edn). Harlow: FT/Prentice Hall.

Nadler, D.A. and Tushman, M.L. (1979) A congruence model for diagnosing organisational behaviour, in D. Kolb, I. Rubin and J. McIntyre (eds) *Organisational Psychology: A Book of Readings* (3rd edn). Englewood Cliffs, NJ: Prentice Hall.

National Heart Forum (2006) *Lightening the Load: Tackling Overweight and Obesity*, www.heartforum.org.uk/Publications, accessed 31/8/07.

NICE (2006) *Obesity: the Prevention, Identification, Assessment and Management of Overweight and Obesity in Adults and Children*. London: NICE/DH.

Porter, L.W. and Lawler, E.E. (1968) *Managerial Attitudes and Performance*. Homewood, IL: Dorsey Press.

Pugh, D.S. and Hickson, D.J. (1996) *Writers on Organisations* (5th edn). London: Penguin.

Roethlisberger, F.J. and Dixon, W.J. (1943) *Management and the Worker*. Cambridge, MA: Harvard University Press.

Rose, M. (1978) *Industrial Behaviour: Theoretical Developments since Taylor*. Harmondsworth: Penguin.

Schein, E.H. (1988) *Organisational Psychology* (3rd edn). Englewood Cliffs, NJ: Prentice Hall.

Stewart, R. (1989) *Leading in the NHS: A Practical Guide*. Basingstoke: Macmillan – now Palgrave Macmillan.

Tannenbaum, R. and Schmidt, W.H. (1973) 'How to choose a leadership pattern'. *Harvard Business Review* 51(3): 162–75, 178–80.

Taylor, F.W. (2003) *Scientific Management*. London: Routledge.

Tiplady, R. (2003) 'Letting go: chaos theory and the management of organisations', www.tiplady/org.uk.

Trist, E. and Bamforth, K.W. (1951) 'Some social and psychological consequences of the longwall method of coal-getting'. *Human Relations* 4(1): 37–8.

Tuckman, B.W. (1965) 'Development sequence in small groups'. *Psychological Bulletin* 63: 384–99.

Watson, C.M. (1983) 'Leadership, management and the seven keys'. *Business Horizons* March–April: 8–13.

Weber, M. (1964) *The Theory of Social and Economic Organisations*. London: Collier Macmillan.

DAVID COHEN

Health economics

Outline of chapter

LEARNING OUTCOMES

This chapter will enable readers to:

- Appreciate why economics exists
- Understand the basic principles of economics
- Understand how these principles can be applied to health
- Be familiar with and describe the different types of economic appraisal
- Understand the contribution that health economics can make to health studies

Overview

There is a growing awareness worldwide that the resources available to maintain and improve health are finite, whereas the demands made on these resources appear to be virtually infinite. Consequently, many are looking to economics – the science of making choices in situations of scarcity – for assistance. This chapter explains what economics is and, equally importantly, what it is not. The emphasis throughout is on how economics does not deal with problems that are uniquely economic but instead addresses common issues through different eyes. Economics is about the allocation of resources to production and the distribution of those outputs to society. The way in which this is done in unregulated markets is explained in the first part of the chapter, followed by a discussion of what might make healthcare differ from other market goods. Problems in the allocation and distribution of services in non-market situations, such as with the UK NHS, are examined, with particular emphasis on the difficulties that arise when healthcare is given according to people's 'needs' rather than their ability to pay. The second part explains the cost–benefit approach, this being defended through a return to the basic economic principle of scarcity, the fact that choice always involves sacrifice and the importance of being explicit about the criteria on which inescapable choices are made. Efficiency is defended as a criterion for choice on the basis that it seeks to maximize the health that can be achieved from whatever level of resources are available. There is an explanation of the three key techniques of economic appraisal: cost–benefit, cost-effectiveness and cost–utility analyses. It is emphasized that these tools ought to be employed only with a firm understanding of the principles upon which they are based. The chapter ends with a case study exploring how economic evidence was used to inform a policy decision for the treatment of obesity.

Introduction

The past few decades have witnessed an unprecedented growth in healthcare expenditure worldwide. An example of the magnitude of this rise can be seen in the case of the UK, where, in 1973, £3,364 million was spent on healthcare, both public and private. This was equivalent to £60 per person, representing 4.6% of GDP. By 2005, this had increased to £109,226 million, equivalent to £1,820 per person and 7.7% of GDP (OHE, 2006). This increase has occurred under both Labour and Conservative governments.

With overall economic growth during this period, an increase in healthcare spending is to be expected and indeed ought to be regarded as a good thing. After all, more spending on healthcare should mean more health for the population. Yet the increased spending on healthcare does not appear to have been accompanied by a corresponding fall in the demands being made on the healthcare systems.

Given these trends, it is not surprising that there is a growing recognition that resources for healthcare are unlikely ever to be sufficient to meet all health needs. This, in turn, means an increasing acceptance that not everything that can be done will be done and that choices are inescapable. Economics is the science of making choices.

> **? ** What do you understand by 'economics'? What insights into health and healthcare provision might its study offer?

Economics has been defined as:

> the study of how men and society end up choosing, with or without the use of money, to employ scarce productive resources to produce various commodities over time and distribute them for consumption, now and in the future, among various groups and people in society. It analyses the costs and benefits of improving patterns of resource allocation. (Samuelson, 1976, p. 5)

The discipline exists because the resources (inputs) available to produce goods and services (outputs) are finite, whereas humankind's desire to consume these goods and services appears to be virtually infinite. Economics concerns how society makes a choice about how much of its scarce resources are allocated to the production of what, and how these outputs of production are then distributed to members of society.

Economics is a discipline – a recognized body of thought – and health economics is the application of this body of thought to the topic 'health'. Thus it deals with questions such as:

● How much of society's scarce resources should be devoted to the production of health?

● How should health outputs be distributed?

These are couched in words that make them recognizable as 'economic' questions, but what about the following?

● What is the best way of treating people with disease X?

● Should we introduce a programme to screen for disease Y?

These may appear to be clinical and policy issues respectively rather than economic ones. Indeed, decisions of this sort are regularly made without seeking the assistance of economists. Yet from the perspective of economics, both can also be viewed as legitimate economic questions since both involve the use of scarce resources (inputs) and both are concerned with making people healthier (outputs). Health economics is first and foremost a 'way of thinking' based on a defined set of principles. It does not address a unique set of problems but puts a different perspective on the issues and problems that others would address from their own perspectives.

The two questions above could be rephrased by asking 'What is the most cost-effective way of treating people with disease X?' and 'Do the benefits of introducing a programme to screen for disease Y outweigh the costs?'

? **What knowledge would a health economist need to answer these questions?**

Health economics can be viewed as having a 'toolkit' containing a number of different appraisal techniques. All are concerned with examining policies and interventions by comparing the resources needed (costs) with the effects produced (benefits). The broad umbrella of the cost–benefit approach also includes cost-effectiveness analysis and cost–utility analysis which are discussed later in this chapter.

If health economics is concerned with the production of health, it must clearly be concerned with more than just interventions provided by health professionals. Road safety and environmental measures also affect people's health. Macroeconomic issues, such as the effect of unemployment on health, and policy issues, such as increasing taxes to reduce the demand for unhealthy goods, are also within the remit of health economics.

The contribution of economics to health studies

Economics deals with two basic problems:

- the allocation of resources to production
- the distribution of the outputs of that production.

One way of dealing with these is for government to eschew any role at all, leaving everything to 'market forces' – essentially the interaction of supply and demand. How much of a country's resources to allocate to the production of shoes, for example, and what mechanism to employ to distribute shoes are rarely issues to which governments pay much heed. If left alone, market forces do the job perfectly well. If any government feels that it is somehow wrong when poor people cannot afford the shoes they need, the response is normally one of income redistribution rather than any direct interference in the workings of the market for shoes.

Market forces and healthcare

The principle of market forces and the relationship between supply and demand are key concepts in economics. Demand is defined as that quantity of a good for which consumers are willing and able to pay at any given price.

Economic theory says that consumers will demand more at a lower price than they will at a higher price, as shown by the line dd in Figure 10.1. Similarly, supply is defined as that quantity which producers are willing to offer for sale at a given price. The theory states that they will wish to supply smaller quantities when prices are low than when prices are high, as shown by the line ss in Figure 10.1. There are textbooks full of theories to explain why this is the case, but for present purposes we will simply assume that such supply and demand behaviour makes intuitive sense.

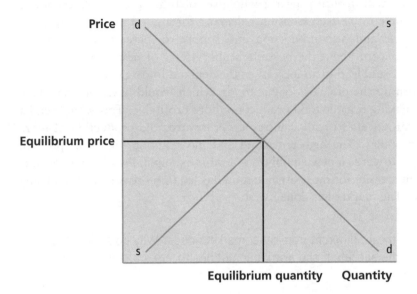

Figure 10.1 Supply, demand and market equilibrium

A market is where the exchange takes place, the price determining how much money changes hands for every unit of the good bought and sold. If at any price the quantity that producers supply exceeds the quantity that consumers demand, there will be a pressure on prices to fall. The opposite occurs when demand exceeds supply – there will be a pressure on prices to rise. There is one price, the 'equilibrium price', at which supply and demand are equal and there is no pressure from within the market for the price to change. The quantity that is both supplied and demanded at the equilibrium price is the 'equilibrium quantity'.

This simple analysis shows how market forces have solved the first economic problem – the allocation of resources. Some level of resources is required to produce the equilibrium quantity, but no one has told producers how many resources to allocate to the production of this good, it just happened. The market has also dealt with the second economic problem – the distribution of output – since, by definition, only those consumers willing and able to pay the equilibrium price can consume the good. Price can therefore be seen as a rationing mechanism limiting the distribution of the good only to those who demand it at the equilibrium price.

Of course, markets do not settle down at an equilibrium and stay there for all time. Changes are occurring outside the market that cause supply and demand to change. On the demand side, people's incomes, tastes and preferences, as well as the prices of other goods, are constantly changing. On the supply side, production techniques and the cost of labour and materials are also constantly altering. Equilibrium is thus rarely reached, but that hardly matters. What does matter is that if demand and supply are not in equilibrium at any moment, economic theory can predict what will happen to the price, which will in turn trigger a whole set of other predictable economic forces to come into effect. Consumer demand for a good may initially cause prices to rise and also production and supply to increase. For example, increased concern about the possible health effects of pesticide use in food production could lead to an increase in the demand for organic produce. This would push up the price of organic foods, which would have the immediate effect of making organic food production more profitable. This would send a signal to producers to reallocate resources towards the production of more organic products. The higher demand and the resulting higher supply will push prices towards a new equilibrium. In this example, the ultimate result is that people's desire for more organic food has led to more organic food being produced. The market has done its job.

? **Is healthcare different from other market goods? Why do so few countries leave the allocation and distribution of healthcare entirely to market forces?**

Although not stated explicitly, a number of assumptions have to hold for the free market to work in the way described. Donaldson et al. (2005) outline these as:

● consumers making their own choices (consumer sovereignty)

● consumers being well informed

● consumers' choices affecting only themselves

● competition between suppliers.

In a free market, no elite with some 'preferred' set of values tells consumers what they should or should not demand. Individuals are assumed to be the best judges of their own welfare, and economic theory shows how, subject to certain assumptions, perfectly competitive and unregulated markets produce socially optimum results. In the case of healthcare, however, the appropriateness of consumer sovereignty can be challenged. Is the patient necessarily the best judge of his or her own welfare? Does the patient necessarily want to be the judge? Many may prefer to be left out of the decision process altogether and leave it to the doctor, who 'knows best what's good for me'.

Market theory assumes that consumers are well informed and can judge how much utility (satisfaction) they get from consuming a good. In the case of healthcare, however, individuals will rarely be able to diagnose themselves, are unlikely to be aware of the range of available treatments and cannot judge how much utility they will get from a treatment even after consuming it since they do not know what would have happened in the absence of any treatment. They have to rely on the doctor's superior knowledge so there is an 'asymmetry of information' between supplier and consumer, with the doctor deciding both the treatment that the patient will demand and supplying it.

A consumer considering buying a new car may, of course, be no more knowledgeable about cars than she is about healthcare, yet she is unlikely to leave the decision about which car to buy totally to the salesman. Why not? The difference between these two cases is simply that she trusts the doctor – at least more than she trusts the salesman. Doctors are expected to act according to a code of medical ethics; car salesmen are not. But it is debatable whether an ethical code means that doctors will end up making the same consumption decisions that fully informed consumers would make if they had the medical knowledge. Factors such as attitudes to risk, aversion to pain, or personal circumstances (who will mind the children if I go into hospital?) can affect consumption decisions. Doctors are unlikely to have all this information and possibly would not take it into account even if they did.

Also implicit in the theory of how unregulated markets produce socially optimal results is the assumption that individuals' consumption decisions affect them and them alone. This may not, however, always be the case. Someone's decision to buy a guard dog that barks all night may well provide their neighbour with a great deal of negative utility. Where such 'externalities' (positive or negative) exist, it can be easily shown that unregulated markets will not produce socially optimal solutions. Healthcare arguably has externalities, both positive and negative. The decision to seek treatment for a communicable disease affects not only the treated individual, but also others, in that their risk of catching the disease is reduced. It has also been argued that a 'humanitarian externality' may exist in healthcare if people derive positive utility from the knowledge that others are receiving the healthcare they need.

CONNECTIONS

Chapter 11 discusses how codes of practice influence the work of health professionals and how philosophical activity can help to understand the balance of actions and effects.

For the market to work as described earlier, a number of assumptions are also needed on the supply side, chief among these being assumptions concerning the competitive behaviour of firms. In reality, private healthcare markets are rarely if ever characterized by many small hospitals competing with each other on the grounds of price. Elements of monopoly powers normally exist together with many other features, which suggest that the free-market model does not describe what happens in the market for healthcare.

Healthcare is thus arguably very different from other goods or services in the marketplace. Various forms of regulation could be introduced, however, to overcome specific problems without taking the step of removing healthcare from the marketplace. In the end, the issue can only be settled by resorting to philosophy and ideology. Most countries intervene in some measure in the provision of healthcare. In the UK, the decision to take healthcare (almost) completely 'off the market' by setting up the NHS was taken mainly because of a social consensus that access to healthcare should be regarded as a 'funda-mental human right' – like access to the courts of justice – rather than as part of society's reward system. Unsurprisingly, in the US, where political ideology favours rewards rather than rights, a far greater proportion of healthcare is delivered through private firms.

The allocation and distribution of healthcare 'off the market'

If healthcare is taken off the market, some alternative means of allocation and distribution have to be found. On the allocation side, this is normally done by a committee deciding what proportion of total public expenditure will be spent each year on healthcare. On the distribution side, healthcare is provided to those who need it.

In 1948, healthcare was taken 'off the market' in the UK by the creation of the NHS. It was assumed that doctors would determine how much need there was and government would simply allocate the appropriate volume of resources to ensure that all needs would be met. This clearly has not happened. To explain why requires a deeper examination of what is meant by need.

THINKING ABOUT

In your view, should a person with a crooked nose be able to have NHS surgery to correct it? What criteria should you use to decide whether that person should have treatment?

To an economist, need means 'capacity to benefit' from treatment. Economists use the terms 'wants' and 'demands' to refer to consumer-based judgements and 'need' to refer to judgements made by some third party. In a private healthcare system, the consumer will be given a nose-straightening operation if he or she is willing to pay the money price. In a zero-priced public healthcare system, the doctor will judge whether or not the individual needs the operation – perhaps because of breathing difficulties. If there is no clinical need, the operation will be denied.

Defined in terms of capacity to benefit from treatment, need is clearly a dynamic concept. Every new medical development that allows the previously untreatable to be treated is increasing need. Similarly, any development that allows the previously treatable to be better treated is also increasing need. It was not long ago, for example, that there was nothing that could be done to prevent very premature, low birth weight babies from dying. Today, thanks to new technology and skills, those same babies have a need for neonatal intensive care.

There can, of course, be developments that actually free up resources for other uses, but in most cases, new interventions involve an increase in resource use. Given the pace of new technological development, it is hardly surprising that year-on-year increases in expenditure on healthcare are not hitting the target of meeting total need. It is possible to argue, however, that whereas need may grow with time, it is still finite at any given point in time. This would be true but for the fact that need is also both relative and subjective.

Relativity can be shown by the fact that many of today's needs would not have been considered to be needs 60 years ago when diseases such as smallpox, diphtheria and polio were the pressing problems of the day. Similarly, the current pressure on resources is raising questions about whether some needs ought to be considered needs at all. In some parts of the UK, interventions such as tattoo removal, gender reorientation and fertility treatment are currently being withdrawn from the needs-based NHS.

Subjectivity of need can be demonstrated by the wide variation in treatments given to similar populations that cannot be explained by a difference in disease prevalence. Moreover, it is not only a judgement of whether or not a patient needs treatment, but also one of how much they need. All may agree on a patient's need for physiotherapy, but how often and for how long are subjective judgements.

CONNECTIONS

To an economist, need means 'capacity to benefit' from treatment. Chapter 11 discusses how the values we hold about health may influence views about entitlement to treatment.

Example 10.1

THE RELATIVITY OF NEED: THE CASE OF VIAGRA

Until the introduction of Viagra (sildenafil), erectile dysfunction in men had always been considered to represent a clinical need. Available treatments included:

- psychological management
- vacuum constriction devices
- intracavernosal injection therapy
- transurethral drug delivery (MUSE)
- a penile prosthesis
- surgery.

All were provided free on the UK NHS apart from vacuum pumps, which patients in some parts of the country had to purchase privately. The cost of meeting erectile dysfunction need was not an issue.

In 1997, Viagra was licensed by the US Federal Drug Administration. Prior to its launch, the sexual function disorder market in the US had total sales of $157 million (£78 million), mainly on MUSE. Within four weeks of Viagra being launched, the market increased to over 10 times its previous size, Viagra capturing a staggering 97.5% of the total market (IMS America, 1998). In the UK, with its publicly funded, zero-priced healthcare system, it was estimated that Viagra could add £1 billion per annum to the NHS drugs bill (*Daily Mail*, 8 July 1998). The government quickly stepped in, setting specific criteria for who could and could not be prescribed Viagra on the NHS. Those who did not meet the criteria obviously did not 'need' Viagra. Moreover, the decision of whether or not there was a need was no longer to be left to doctors.

In a world of infinite resources, all men who could benefit from treatment would be prescribed Viagra. In the real world of scarcity and choice, those at the less severe end of the sexual dysfunction continuum are judged not to need it.

Why will resources for healthcare always be scarce?

Economists argue that, even if health needs were finite, it would still not be in society's interest to allocate sufficient resources to meet all health needs. This somewhat provocative statement can be justified by focusing on the fact that society clearly has needs other than those relating to health (education, defence, transport and law and order, for example). However, since the total amount available to spend on all these is finite, spending in one area means having less to spend in another. Similarly, more public expenditure means higher taxes and thus less to spend on private consumption.

Both the balance between private and public expenditure and the distribution of the latter between the different public sector areas are driven by a fundamental economic principle known as 'diminishing marginal benefit'. This states that as any activity expands, the extra benefit produced by each extra unit of input gets progressively smaller. For example, a single nurse working in a community will focus her efforts on where the need is greatest. A second nurse will also produce benefits, but as the most pressing needs are already being met by the first nurse, the marginal (extra) benefit produced by the second will be less than that of the first. And so on.

Increased spending on health produces positive marginal health benefits, but at the cost of foregoing the benefits that the spending could have achieved elsewhere in the economy. If healthcare's relative share of total spending is increased, then that of another area must be reduced. According to the above economic principle, the extra spending on health will produce decreasing marginal benefits, while reduced spending in the other area will incur increasing marginal sacrifices. If the marginal gain exceeds the marginal sacrifice, the total benefit from the shift in expenditure will increase, but this can only go on for so long. Eventually, the continually decreasing marginal benefits in health will no longer exceed the marginal losses elsewhere.

If society has a multiplicity of needs, the socially optimal balance of expenditure will be at that point at which any further shifts will begin to make total benefit fall, that is, society will begin to be made worse off, and this will not be at the point at which all health needs are being met. Put another way, since the share of total societal resources devoted to health will always be less than the level at which all needs can be met, some form of rationing is inevitable.

Theoretical and methodological approaches

Resources and money

Anything being considered – from the level of broad policies down to individual interventions – involves the use of resources. Given scarcity, choices in how those resources should be used are inescapable.

Resources are defined as those things which contribute to the production of an output. Producing corn requires resources such as land, seeds, workers and tractors. No amount of money will produce corn unless it is used to buy land, hire workers and so on. Resources in healthcare include doctors, nurses, hospital buildings, bandages and drugs. Again, money pays for these resources, but, by the above definition, volunteers and informal carers are also resources even though they do not receive monetary reward. The distinction between money and resources is thus important. More money normally means control over more resources, but this is not always the case. A shortage of nurses trained in intensive care will constrain activity in an intensive care unit, regardless of the cash available.

For present purposes, money also has a second function in that it provides a common measure of value. Expressing resources in terms of a common measure allows them to be added together and compared with other combinations of resources. The same is true for outputs. By definition, all the outputs of healthcare are of value, and expressing each in terms of its monetary value allows different outputs to be added and compared.

THINKING ABOUT

Do you think a monetary value can be put on health? Can you compare the life of a premature baby (whose life depends on intensive care) with the pain relief of thousands of older people achieved through simple hip replacements?

The output of healthcare

Economists have long argued that, while not necessarily its only output, the principal output of the healthcare industry is 'health'. The inverted commas reflect the fact that many health services, for example palliative care of the terminally ill, are not intended to raise health status as such. However, if 'health' is perceived in the broad sense of wellbeing, all effective interventions will make people better off than they would otherwise have been.

The practical difficulties of viewing output in this way stem from the fact that health is notoriously difficult to define, measure and value. Broad definitions, such as that by the World Health Organization of health as a 'state of complete physical, mental and social well-being' (WHO, 1946), are unhelpful when trying to compare the output of alternative therapies.

In practice, therefore, intermediate measures are often used as proxies for the final (health) outputs. This is acceptable as long as the link between the proxy measure and health is well established. Thus, evidence that a reduction in smoking prevalence will result in a reduction in smoking-related morbidity and mortality means that the 'number of quitters' is an acceptable proxy for the output of a smoking cessation programme, even though smoking is not a disease and quitting is not in itself a health gain. The less well established the link between the proxy and health, the less useful the proxy.

CONNECTIONS

Chapter 3 discusses some of the problems of identifying outcomes from health interventions.

The economic notion of cost

To an economist, cost means sacrifice: an accountant will measure cost as the amount of money spent; an economist will look at what has been forgone. The term 'opportunity cost' is used in economics to emphasize this notion of an opportunity forgone. Within economics, 'cost' is used as shorthand for 'opportunity cost'.

A cost can thus be incurred without money changing hands. A new clinic that takes a nurse off a ward for one hour a week will not affect the nursing wages bill, but it will involve the sacrifice of the benefit that the nurse could have achieved in one hour on the ward. Similarly, freeing an hour of nurse time provides the opportunity to use that hour to produce benefits that could not otherwise be produced. The freed-up hour is valued, regardless of the fact that no money will be saved.

 On what basis should resource allocation choices be made?

The principal criterion used in economics is **efficiency**, which maximizes the benefits from the available resources. It concerns the relationship between inputs and outputs, that is, most benefit being available at least cost. Being efficient means getting as much health as is possible from the available resources; being inefficient means getting less.

It is important to note, however, that whereas efficiency is a good rule to be guided by, it is never a substitute for decision-making (Drummond, 1981). Demonstrating that A is more efficient than B suggests that A should be pursued unless alternative criteria can be identified to argue otherwise. B may be justified, for example, on equity, public relations or political expediency grounds, and no economist would argue that these are not relevant alternative criteria. However, it becomes difficult to argue for the pursuit of inefficient B over efficient A on grounds such as the political power of the doctors involved, historical precedent or who can get most public support by waving a shroud in front of a television camera – factors which at least in part explain the current pattern of resource allocation.

The cost–benefit approach

Figure 10.2 illustrates the cost–benefit way of thinking. The principle of weighing gains against sacrifices is the cost–benefit approach. In each situation, there are costs, which means that an alternative must be forgone. There will also be particular benefits that result.

Something will fail the cost–benefit test if the benefits achieved are judged to be of lower value than the benefits forgone by not using the resources in other ways. In this case, the gains and sacrifices are both couched in terms of health. Failing the cost–benefit test does not mean that these health gains are not worth some amount of money.

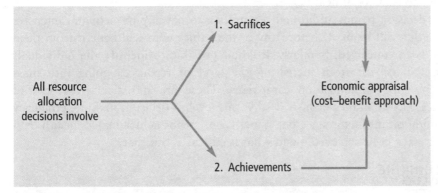

Figure 10.2 The cost–benefit framework

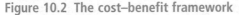 **Is it ethical to make healthcare decisions on the basis of efficiency?**

It is important to stress that the cost–benefit approach is not being advocated at the level of decision-making relating to the individual patient; it is natural for doctors and other health professionals to want to do what is best for their patients. Doctors have always practised under a system of medical ethics that has conventionally focused on the two ethical theories of 'virtue' and 'duty' (Jonsen and Hellegers, 1987). These are individualistic ethics based on the doctor's responsibility for the individual patient, a guiding principle of which has long been that it is unethical to do anything that does more harm than good.

Chapter 11 discusses the guiding principles of beneficence and non-maleficence, which, in medical ethics, means that health workers should not take any action that does more harm than good.

Given that a doctor's first duty will inevitably be to his or her patient, a doctor's preference for making clinical decisions on the basis of clinical effectiveness rather than efficiency is understandable. It is still legitimate to take the costs that others will have to bear into account, but the patient in front of the doctor is a person with a name, a face, a family, a history. Efficiency is still relevant, but in this situation is relatively unimportant.

More recently, and due to an increasing awareness of the scarcity of resources, ethicists have begun focusing on a third ethical theory, that of the 'common good' (Mooney, 1992). This is a social ethic based on responsibility for the health of populations. In this, the guiding principle of only doing those things which do more good than harm still applies, but the terms now reflect a social perspective. On this basis, any intervention that yields only a small benefit to the patient but will mean a large sacrifice to other patients will, from a social perspective, be doing more harm than good. Those responsible for health policy-making and broad resource allocation decisions have to see their duty as being to the whole population – including the potential future consumers of healthcare.

A decision to put additional resources into developing neonatal intensive care units will be made before any of the babies who will benefit from them have been conceived. Similarly, it is not possible to identify the individuals who will benefit from increasing the level of resources going into mass screening or immunization campaigns. These are statistical lives without names, faces, families or histories. At this level of decision-making, efficiency is an important factor since being inefficient means achieving less health than could have been achieved – and what is ethical about that?

THINKING ABOUT

Think about some health policy decisions that benefit populations but may adversely affect individuals.

Example 10.2

THE CASE OF CHILD B

In 1995, a 10-year-old girl referred to as Child B suffered a relapse of acute myeloid leukaemia. Having previously undergone two courses of chemotherapy and a bone marrow transplant, her doctors considered that further active treatment would not be in her best interests. The chances of remission following further chemotherapy were put at between 10 and 20%, with a similar chance of survival following further bone marrow transplantation. The treatments would cost £15,000 and £60,000 respectively.

Child B was denied further active treatment by her local health authority on two grounds: first, because of the suffering involved, further treatment would not be in her best interest, and second, the resources available were finite and the needs of other patients had to be borne in mind. Her father took the case to court.

The judge ruled in the father's favour, claiming that the health authority had not adequately explained their funding priorities. This decision was, however, overturned by the Court of Appeal on the same day (*Times*, 15 March 1995). The Master of the Rolls rejected the original judge's criticism of the health authority, claiming that it was common knowledge that health resources were scarce and therefore the health authority had not exceeded its powers or acted unreasonably. Child B was subsequently admitted to a private hospital after an anonymous donor provided £75,000 for her treatment. Sadly, she died soon afterwards.

It could perhaps be argued that, ethically speaking, the duty of the health authority was to endeavour to preserve life. However, in economic terms, the treatment of this individual would have incurred a high sacrifice elsewhere. In other words, the opportunity costs far outweighed the benefit to the individual patient.

Economics is often given a bad press when it comes to healthcare because of a mistaken belief that it is all about saving money, but that is not what economics is trying to do. In the above example, the issue was how to spend a finite budget given the competing needs of those to whom the budget holders were responsible. The need to choose is a reality; the question is whether or not choices are made on the basis of rational and defensible criteria. Economic thinking and the techniques of economic appraisal are aids to decision-making that can lead to greater efficiency and hence a greater overall level of health.

Techniques of economic appraisal

All the techniques of economic appraisal fall under the broad umbrella of the cost–benefit approach. All are concerned with examining one or more interventions by comparing the resources needed against the effects produced. How they differ depends essentially on how these effects (benefits) are perceived, which in turn depends on the objective of the appraisal.

Cost–benefit analysis

The most comprehensive technique of economic appraisal is **cost–benefit analysis**. Its objective is to assess whether – or to what extent – something is worth doing. Cost–benefit analysis thus addresses *allocative* efficiency, in that it tells us whether or not (or how much) resources should be allocated to this programme. This involves weighing all the benefits of the programme (or the extra benefit from an expansion of the programme) against the total (or extra) cost of achieving them. This can only be done if all the costs and benefits are expressed in common units. Although similar to a financial appraisal, cost–benefit analysis is concerned with the value of gains and losses rather than the money spent and money received, which is the basis of financial appraisal.

In economics, costs are all the resources directly or indirectly used by the programme that have alternative uses, that is, which incur opportunity costs. Benefits are everything of value that results. Cost–benefit analysis normally adopts a 'social welfare' perspective, in that all costs are considered regardless of who bears them, and all benefits are included regardless of to whom they accrue. Cost and benefit variables are identified, measured in appropriate physical or other relevant units and finally valued.

Where they exist, market prices are normally used to express the money value of costs and benefits. Where market prices do not exist, 'shadow prices' can be used. For example, the time of volunteers does not command a market price, but it is possible to impute a price to volunteers' time using the wages of paid workers who do roughly the same work as a proxy.

THINKING ABOUT

Do you think a monetary value can be put on health?

The valuation of health and other intangible benefits and costs is, however, clearly no easy task. A variety of methods are available to do this, which will not be detailed here (see, for example, Drummond et al., 2005). Nevertheless, many people find the very act of placing a monetary value on such things as pain relief or the extension of life to be at best distasteful and at worst immoral. According to the economic way of thinking, the values are always there – the only issue is whether they are to be explicit or implicit. Economic appraisal attempts to make valuations explicit in order to assist the pursuit of efficiency. For example, if an economic evaluation shows some new intervention to have a cost per life saved of £100,000 and a decision is taken not to introduce that intervention, then it is implied that those lives are valued at less than £100,000. The rejection of a programme with a low implied value of a life would be difficult to defend if another programme is currently running with a much higher implied value of a life. Efficiency in terms of maximizing the number of lives saved from any given level of expenditure will be improved by making a marginal reduction in the latter programme in order to support the former.

Many people feel an understandable distaste at the idea on putting a money value on intangible health benefits: such things ought somehow to be above considerations of cost. Yet if cost is perceived in terms of sacrifice, it is evident from both individual behaviour and collective decision-making that this is clearly not the case. For example, the decision to reject a proposal to build a flyover at a dangerous intersection on grounds of costs implies that the value of the anticipated lives saved and injuries avoided is less than the cost of building the flyover. The fact that preventable road deaths are tolerated shows that society does not put an infinite value on the lives that could be saved.

Cost-effectiveness analysis

Often the issue is not whether or not to do something but more simply how to do it. For example, if the question is one of deciding how to treat people with raised blood pressure – given that a decision has already been taken to treat them – **cost-effectiveness analysis** can compare alternative blood pressure-reducing interventions in terms of their cost per unit reduction. Cost-effectiveness analysis addresses *technical* efficiency in the sense that it can tell us the best way to do something but not whether or not that something is worth doing. That is an allocative efficiency issue that can only be dealt with by cost–benefit analysis.

Cost-effectiveness analysis is a simpler technique than cost–benefit analysis. By perceiving benefits more narrowly and measuring them only in physical units, it avoids the difficult task of benefit valuation. At the same time, it provides information that is much more limited, since it can only compare alternative ways of pursuing the given objective – in this case to reduce blood pressure. It says nothing about how efficient any blood pressure reduction programme is compared with other programmes of healthcare.

Cost-effectiveness analysis can, however, be broadened by using more general benefit measures that are not unique to the programme in question. For example, since reducing blood pressure is expected to reduce mortality, the objective of a blood pressure reduction programme can be expressed in broader life-saving terms. By comparing alternative ways of reducing blood pressure in terms of cost per life year saved, the most cost-effective way of reducing blood pressure can then be compared with the cost effectiveness of any other life-saving programme.

> **?** Why might it be difficult to assess the effectiveness of blood pressure reduction using broad measures?

Assessing cost per life year involves a more complex appraisal than assessing cost per unit reduction in blood pressure. Whereas blood pressure can be accurately measured, translating today's reduced blood pressure into tomorrow's lives saved involves a greater use of assumptions and estimations. Moreover, this broader cost-effectiveness analysis will still be limited because it is restricted to comparing interventions that extend life and many health-care interventions, for example hernia repair, do not affect length of life. It also has to assume that each year of life is of equal value, regardless of the quality of that life.

This problem can be overcome by broadening the object to take in both life extension and **quality of life** improvements, or, stated more generally, to produce 'health'. The advantage of so doing is that the cost-effectiveness of all the interventions, whether preventive, curative or caring, can then be compared in terms of cost per unit of 'health' produced.

If 'health' is the output of healthcare, some means of measuring health is needed. Perfect measures of health will, however, never exist because health is both multidimensional and value laden. People who are in pain, who suffer depression or who have impaired vision or restricted mobility are all in a state of health that is less than perfect. Although each of the dimensions of ill health can be measured independently (more versus less pain, greater versus lesser visual impairment and so on), a measure of 'health' will have to combine all these into a unidimensional index. Who will have worse health, the person with depression or the person in pain? Such a decision obviously involves a value judgement, but who should be the judge? The depressed person will quite rightly feel that depression is the worse state and will value an improvement from depression to perfect health more highly than an improvement from a state of pain to perfect health. The person in pain may, not surprisingly, disagree. A 'perfect' health status measure therefore cannot exist until such problems are reconciled.

Nevertheless, economists have made considerable progress in measuring health by focusing on the idea that all interventions must either extend life, improve the quality of life or achieve some combination of the two. Therefore, in principle, all effective interventions produce quality adjusted life years (**QALYs**). If the effectiveness of any programme is measured in terms of QALYs, a comparison of cost per QALY can indicate the most technically efficient ways of producing health. Economic evaluations that use QALYs (or similar utility-based health measures) are often called cost–utility analyses. They are often, however, regarded as just a special form of cost-effectiveness analysis and not given a different name.

Priority-setting in healthcare

In a perfect world of infinite resources, priority-setting would not be necessary: everyone would receive whatever healthcare they needed fully and immediately. Sadly, we do not live in such a perfect world. In the real world of scarce resources, not everything that can be done will be done, so some means of prioritizing is necessary if what does and what does not get done is to be at all rationally based.

Prioritizing is needed at all levels of decision-making from broad policies to decisions about treating individual patients. An illustration of how economic thinking can help at both levels is provided in Example 10.3.

Example 10.3

PRIORITY-SETTING IN HEALTHCARE

In the early 1970s, Grogono and Woodgate (1971) attempted to prioritize patients in need of non-urgent surgery using an index based on 10 dimensions of ill health. The thinking behind this was that while treating people purely on a first come, first served basis may have its attractions, surgeons are unlikely to ignore factors such as how much pain patients are in, or whether or not their condition is preventing them going out to work, when deciding priorities for treatment.

If surgeons are therefore implicitly making judgements of need on the basis of undeclared criteria, would it not be possible, and more ethical, to make these criteria explicit? Grogono and Woodgate came up with the following list:

● ability to work
● ability to enjoy hobbies and recreation
● malaise, pain or suffering

- worry or unhappiness
- ability to communicate
- ability to sleep
- independence of others
- ability to eat/enjoy food
- bladder and bowel control
- sex life.

The idea was that, in the course of a normal consultation, it ought to be possible to give patients a score of 0, 0.5 or 1 according to whether they were normal, impaired or incapacitated on each of the dimensions. These figures could be added together: the higher the Grogono–Woodgate index score, the higher the patient's priority.

The problem with the Grogono–Woodgate index is that the dimensions are not weighted to reflect their relative importance. The absence of weighting implies that all are valued equally, which is clearly unrealistic. Most people would probably agree that someone with a score of 1 as a result of double incontinence is worse off than someone with a score of 1 resulting from an inability to participate in hobbies and recreation. If so, and assuming that effective interventions exist for both, the former has a greater need. But this is a value judgement rather than a clinical judgement.

Note that this approach did not prioritize patients according to diagnosis, for example hernias versus ingrown toenails, but according to how the condition was affecting them in terms of pain or their ability to get out and about. The sought-after valuations occur between the dimensions of ill health rather than between diagnosed conditions.

In an early attempt to see whether there were such things as 'social values', Rosser and Kind (1978) used a matrix of eight rows representing different degrees of 'disability' and four columns representing different degrees of 'distress' in order to produce the grid shown in Figure 10.3. Everyone will agree that a cell representing less pain and less disability is valued more highly than one representing more pain and more disability, but what about a cell representing less pain and more disability? Each of us can have our own view depending on our own values, but if 90% of a representative sample of the population preferred one cell to the other, would such a consensus not allow us to say that 'society' puts a higher value on one state than the other?

Rosser and Kind (1978) took a sample of people representing doctors, nurses, patients and healthy individuals and asked them to rank each health state in the matrix and then give a score of 1 to the top-ranked state (which would inevitably be no disability and no distress) and a score of 0 to the state judged to be equivalent to death. All other states were to be scored cardinally (0.8, for example, being 'twice as good' as 0.4), negative scores being permitted for states judged to be worse than death.

Although this exercise can be criticized on a number of grounds, for example that the sample was small and possibly unrepresentative, the fact that reasonably consistent scores were produced suggests that there can be such a thing as 'social values'. Health gains could now be measured directly, the difference in score between the pretreatment cell and the post-treatment cell representing the extent of the health gain. More recently, and using other means, social valuations of health states from much larger and more representative samples have been obtained (see, for example, EuroQol Group, 1990).

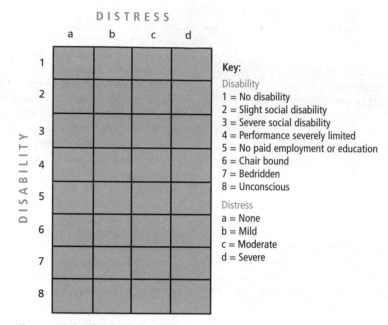

DISTRESS

a   b   c   d

DISABILITY

1
2
3
4
5
6
7
8

Key:

Disability
1 = No disability
2 = Slight social disability
3 = Severe social disability
4 = Performance severely limited
5 = No paid employment or education
6 = Chair bound
7 = Bedridden
8 = Unconscious

Distress
a = None
b = Mild
c = Moderate
d = Severe

Figure 10.3 The Rosser grid
Source: Rosser and Kind, 1978

CASE STUDY The use of economic evaluation in the treatment of obesity

The direct cost to the NHS of treating obesity was estimated to be £50 million in 1998, with an additional £1,800–£1,900 million to treat obesity-related illnesses.

A range of interventions are available for the management of overweight and obesity. These include work/school/community programmes (for primary prevention), dietary modification, exercise programmes, behaviour modification programmes, pharmacological agents, commercial programmes (for example WeightWatchers), and alternative therapies (NHS Centre for Reviews and Dissemination, 1996; SIGN, 1997; HDA, 2003). Surgery is occasionally used as a last resort for those with very severe obesity and for whom other treatments have failed. In 1998, a newly developed drug, orlistat (Xenical), which prevents the absorption of fat in the intestine, was licensed for the treatment of

obesity. At issue was whether or not treatment with orlistat should be available free on the NHS.

The treatment of obesity has an ethical dimension and is not simply a matter of most effective or most cost-effective management. Notwithstanding biological explanations (see Chapter 1), many people regard obesity as a self-induced condition with a simple solution – eat less and exercise more. It can thus be argued that it would be inappropriate for the NHS to pay for drug treatment since 'more deserving' patients would have to bear the opportunity costs.

The National Institute for Clinical Excellence (NICE, www.nice.org.uk) was created in 1999 as an independent organization responsible for producing national (England and Wales) guidance on treatments. Its remit was later broadened to include guidance on promoting good health as well as preventing and treating ill health (and the word 'health' was added to its title). The thinking behind the creation of NICE was that guidance on which treatments to provide should be *evidence based*. One important – and controversial – decision was that NICE guidance would be based not only on evidence of clinical effectiveness but also on evidence of cost-effectiveness. NICE decided early on that, where possible, evidence should be presented in the form of a cost–utility analysis with outcomes measured in QALYs (see above). This would allow comparisons to be made across a wide range of different ways of producing health.

Universities in the UK and the Netherlands were jointly commissioned to conduct a systematic review of the evidence of the clinical and cost-effectiveness of orlistat in the management of obesity (O'Meara et al., 2001). In addition, NICE considered evidence provided by the drug's manufacturer as well as from a number of professional, patient/carer and other groups.

Interestingly, if not surprisingly, there was a significant difference in the evidence from the systematic review and that from the manufacturer. In the former case, the cost per QALY gained was £46,000 (range, £19,000–£55,000) compared with the manufacturer's estimate of £10,400 (range, £8,400–£16,000). The difference between the two was due mainly to differences in key assumptions, for example with regard to the effect of short-term weight loss on longer term illnesses. The NICE committee felt that the manufacturer's assumptions were overly optimistic and this had the effect of underestimating the true cost per QALY.

As stated earlier, cost-effectiveness analyses address technical rather than allocative efficiency, that is, they show the relative cost-effectiveness of different ways of producing an output (in this case QALYs) but do not directly address the issue of how much society should be willing to pay for additional QALYs. NICE has been dealing with this by applying a broad rule of thumb that interventions with extra cost per QALY gained above £30,000 are unlikely to be recommended for implementation on the NHS.

The analysis of orlistat showed that a cost per QALY below £30,000 would only be achieved if patients achieved a significant weight loss; specifically, if they lost about 5% of their body mass for each three months of treatment or showed a cumulative loss of at least 10% of body weight from the start of treatment over the first six months.

NICE guidance on the use of orlistat was issued in March 2001 and reviewed in 2004. It recommended prescribing orlistat only to people who had demonstrated they were able to lose weight (had lost at least 2.5kg by dietary control and increased physical activity alone in the month prior to the first prescription) and to continue maintaining them on orlistat only if they met the weight loss conditions above (NICE, 2004). A recent summary in *Bandolier*, the guide to evidence-based healthcare, concludes: 'The bottom line is that weight reducing drugs are of value in a few, with significant adverse events in many', basing this on a recent review (Padwal et al., 2003). In the UK, France and Canada, the drug is available on prescription. In Australia and the US, certain formulations can be obtained over the counter.

Conclusion

Economics is the study of trade-offs. It explicitly recognizes that health improvements are achieved at a cost, that is, by foregoing (trading off) the benefits of something else in exchange. Although this has been discussed above in terms of choices regarding the distribution of healthcare, the same way of thinking can be applied to decisions made by individuals regarding their own behaviour. This may at first sight seem odd, and indeed one of the reasons why health issues were ignored by economists for so long was the belief that health was so important that no individual would be willing to trade it off for anything else (Fuchs, 1972). It is, however, easy to show that this is not in fact the case.

Smokers who are aware of the associated health risks are trading off the risk of future illness or death against the present satisfaction and pleasure they get from smoking. Careful driving reduces risk but can mean longer journeys. As Cullis and West (1979) stated:

> Few people, if any, seek to maximize their health and life expectancy per se. To do so, involves sacrificing opportunities to eat,

drink, play games, drive and so on that at the margin may be a greater source of utility than any additional (expected) minute or so of life.

Of all the disciplines that examine health, economics is perhaps unique by its focus on *optimum* health as opposed to *maximum* health. Optimum health is achieved when the marginal benefits of improved health (or the reduced risk of future ill health) are outweighed by the marginal opportunity cost. Optimum health is thus likely to be lower than maximum health. While maximum health is something that everyone wants, it is clearly not something that everyone demands (in the sense that demand equals willingness to pay for).

Summary

- The focus of health economics is on finding rational ways to allocate scarce resources to healthcare services

- In a period of scarce resources, priority-setting is important. Economics provides a framework for this to take place at a broad policy level and in individual treatment decisions. Various techniques have been used to assess what type of value can be put on aspects of health

- Health economics uses different types of economic appraisal technique to help to make more effective decisions: cost–benefit analysis is the process of weighing gains against sacrifices. Benefits need to be set against the costs, which means that an alternative is foregone. Economics is not concerned with optimum health. The health improvements need to outweigh the benefits from doing something else

Questions for further discussion

???

1. Why is it important that health services operate efficiently?

2. Is it unethical to put a monetary value on human life and suffering?

3. Can there be any justification in disinvesting in programmes known to be effective?

Further reading

Donaldson, C., Gerard, K., Mitton, C. et al. (2005) *The Economics of Healthcare Financing* (2nd edn). Basingstoke: Palgrave Macmillan.
Covers the theoretical issues in an applied way, giving examples of how these economic issues are being addressed in different healthcare systems.

Drummond, M., Sculpher, M., Torrance, G. et al. (2005) *Methods for the Economic Evaluation of Programmes in Healthcare* (3rd edn). Oxford: Oxford University Press.
Jefferson, T., Demicheli, V. and Mugford, M. (1996) *Elementary Economic Evaluation in Healthcare*. London: BMJ Publishing.
These two books explain the 'how' of economics. Both offer guidance to those wishing to undertake economic evaluations.

Edgar, A., Salek, S., Shickle, D. and Cohen, D. (1998) *The Ethical QALY: Ethical Issues in Healthcare Resource Allocations*. Surrey: Euromed Publications.
Assesses the role that quality of life measures can play in the allocation of healthcare resources, with an emphasis on the ethics of doing so.

Mooney, G. (2003) *Economics Medicine and Healthcare* (3rd edn). London: Harvester Wheatsheaf.
Mooney, G. (1994) *Key Issues in Health Economics*. London: Harvester Wheatsheaf.
Together these two volumes provide a good overview of the economic way of thinking and the range of issues addressed by the discipline. They deal with conceptual issues such the nature of the commodity of healthcare and whose values ought to be used in deciding how to use scarce healthcare resources.

Phillips, C.J. (2005) *Health Economics: An Introduction for Health Professionals*. Oxford: Blackwell.
Covers basic principles in the context of decision-making in the British NHS.

References

Cullis, J.G. and West, P.A. (1979) *The Economics of Health: An Introduction*. London: Martin Robertson.

Donaldson, C., Gerard, K., Mitton, C. et al. (2005) *The Economics of Healthcare Financing: The Visible Hand* (2nd edn). Basingstoke: Palgrave Macmillan.

Drummond, M.F. (1981) *Principles of Economic Appraisal in Healthcare*. Oxford: Oxford Medical Publications.

Drummond, M., Sculpher, M., Torrance, G. et al. (2005) *Methods for the Economic Evaluation of Programmes in Healthcare* (3rd edn). Oxford: Oxford University Press.

EuroQol Group (1990) 'EuroQol – a new facility for the measurement of health related quality of life'. *Health Policy* **16**: 199–208.

Fuchs, V.R. (1972) 'Healthcare and the US economic system'. *Milbank Memorial Fund Quarterly* **50**: 211–37.

Grogono, A.W. and Woodgate, D.J. (1971) 'Index for measuring health'. *Lancet* **2**(7732): 1024–6.

HDA (Health Development Agency) (2003) *The Management of Obesity and Overweight: An Analysis of Reviews of Diet, Physical Activity and Behavioural Approaches. Evidence briefing*. London: HDA.

IMS America (1998) Viagra prescriptions continue to climb. IMS America Health Facts press release, 4 May.

Jonsen, A.R. and Hellegers, A.E. (1987) Conceptual foundations for an ethics of medical care, in L.R. Tancredi (ed.) *Ethics of Healthcare*. Washington: National Academy of Sciences.

Mooney, G. (1992) *Economics Medicine and Healthcare* (2nd edn). London: Harvester Wheatsheaf.

NHS Centre for Reviews and Dissemination (1997) *A Systematic Review of the Interventions for the Prevention and Treatment of Obesity, and the Maintenance of Weight Loss*. CRD Report (10). York: NHS Centre for Reviews and Dissemination.

NICE (2004) *Guidance on the Use of Orlistat for the Treatment of Obesity in Adults*. London: NICE/DoH.

O'Meara, S., Riemsma, R., Shirran, L. et al. (2001) *A Systematic Review of the Clinical Effectiveness and Cost Effectiveness of Orlistat in the Management of Obesity*. University of York/University of Maastricht: NHS Centre for Reviews and Dissemination.

OHE (Office of Health Economics) (2006) *Compendium of Health Statistics*. London: OHE.

Padwal, R., Li, S.K. and Lau, D.C. (2003) Long-term pharmacotherapy for overweight and obesity: a systematic review and meta-analysis of randomized controlled trials. *International Journal of Obesity* 27: 1437–46.

Rosser, R. and Kind, P. (1978) 'A scale of valuations of states of illness: Is there a social consensus?' *International Journal of Epidemiology* 7: 347–58.

Samuelson, P.A. (1976) *Economics*. Tokyo: McGraw-Hill.

SIGN (Scottish Intercollegiate Guidelines Network) (2006) *Obesity in Scotland: Integrating Prevention with Weight Management*. Edinburgh: SIGN.

WHO (World Health Organization) (1946) *Preamble of the Constitution of the World Health Organization*. Geneva: WHO.

Ethics and law and health

LEARNING OUTCOMES

This chapter will enable readers to:

- Understand the key concerns and principles of ethics and law
- Understand and describe how the theory and methodology of ethics inform and illuminate policy and practice in healthcare
- Understand and describe how the law and its methods inform and illuminate healthcare policy and practice
- Understand and describe how and why ethical judgements on the dilemmas posed by healthcare may differ substantially from legal judgements

Overview

This chapter explores the central relevance of ethics and law to health studies. It exposes a range of dilemmas facing those involved in healthcare provision in developed countries. These dilemmas relate to issues such as the nature and value of life (at both its beginning and its end), the rationing of scarce resources and the accountability of health professionals to the public whom they are supposed to serve. In the UK recently, there have been legal cases investigating whether a doctor is right to hasten or assist patients towards their deaths, whether economic priorities can determine treatment and whether a health authority was negligent in not investigating the standards of consultant cardiac surgeons. These are dilemmas that can only be fully understood by a consideration of the disciplines of ethics and law. Furthermore, dilemmas are not confined simply to 'life and death' situations but cover the whole span of healthcare activity, from prevention and health promotion through treatment to rehabilitation. In the first part of the chapter, ethical theory is discussed and related to practical health and healthcare examples; then the law, its nature and application to health and healthcare are explored. The second part exposes difficulties in the relationship between ethics and law, and poses the essential question: is what we must do (our legal obligation) always the same, in healthcare, as what we ought to do (our ethical or moral duty)? The chapter closes with an extended example of the dilemma posed by policy-makers' attempts to intervene in the food choices of children and young people and in so doing it draws out both the problems and possibilities attached to the consideration of healthcare through the lenses of the law and, especially, ethics.

Introduction

Those involved in and planning healthcare are faced by major decisions concerning:

● life and death

● the power held by professions and the point at which the level of power becomes unacceptable

● priorities for the way in which we spend public money.

In addition, such decisions and issues are not only relevant when we are talking about 'acute' treatment and care: for those concerned with the prevention of disease and the promotion of health, they are of equal relevance. In the area of healthcare rationing, for example, to what extent should we devote resources to population health promotion when this might result in some individuals being deprived of the treatment and care they acutely need?

CONNECTIONS
CONNECTIONS

Chapter 10 considers how economic principles can be applied to decisions concerning spending on public health and healthcare services.

To what extent should a health professional use his or her power to 'persuade' someone to give up what the professional believes to be an 'unhealthy' behaviour? Given medicine's increased ability to 'decide', in a technical sense, when life can end, does killing or assisting people towards death become acceptable in certain circumstances? Equally, from developments in the field of reproductive technology, and the so-called genetic revolution (Kitcher, 1994), should we be concerned about the implications of medicine's technical capacity to decide whether and when life should begin, or even what kinds of lives are created in the first place? As the expectations of the health services rise, and as more people are helped to live longer, the burden on the NHS is increased. Recent reforms have stressed the importance of both clinical excellence and limits to public expenditure. To what extent should economic priorities determine treatment (or the lack of it)?

Such dilemmas can of course be helpfully investigated by disciplines such as sociology (in relation to, say, the understanding of professional power) and economics (considering, for example, the financial cost of particular healthcare decisions). Doubtless pathology, genetics, pharmacology and other medical disciplines would also have a lot to say about aspects of 'life' and 'death' dilemmas. But none of the dilemmas can be thought about simply in these 'nuts and bolts' ways. They concern **values** (for example the value of 'health for its own sake' as against the value of economic efficiency).

We often expect others to hold the same kinds of values as ourselves, for example that killing is wrong. Such values can be thought of as normative, that is, we believe the value concerned should be assumed and accepted without argument. We often believe that a certain value – such as 'killing is wrong' – is so important that we establish prescriptive rules to prevent action contrary to the value, or to punish those who do act in such a way. Such issues become the subject of laws, which society as a whole upholds and enforces. This is the territory of ethics and law, making a consideration of these two disciplines vital to the study and understanding of health.

The contribution of ethics to health studies

There are three main branches of philosophy, of which ethics forms a part:

- **epistemology** (enquiry into the nature and grounds of belief, experience and knowledge)
- metaphysics (the study of the nature of being)
- ethics (enquiry into how we ought to act and conduct ourselves).

Ethics is the branch of philosophy that has traditionally concerned itself with examining the worth or value of conduct, with developing and defending views on what might be meant by a 'worthwhile life' and with how such a life could be led. Different ethical traditions have developed separate – and conflicting – views on the purpose of ethics and the kind of conduct in which we should actually engage. In particular, Western philosophy has been profoundly shaped by three theories of ethics: Aristotelianism, deontology and utilitarianism. Each of these three theories can in turn be seen as essentially a product of the times in which it was originally born. These theories are based on trying to determine:

● what is meant by leading a good or virtuous life – the focus particularly of Aristotelianism

● what kinds of duties or obligations we owe each other – the focus especially of deontology

● how we might take account of consequences when deciding a particular course of action – the focus particularly of utilitarianism.

Aristotelianism

Aristotle was a Greek philosopher who lived from 384–322 BC. His *Ethics* is representative of those ethical theories that aim to work out what a good (moral) life might mean and how the development of such a life can be encouraged. Aristotle attempted to do this by looking at the nature of the world and the individuals within it in order to assess what being virtuous might mean. For this reason, Aristotle is frequently thought of as an empiricist, that is, his theory is based on observation and experience. In observing the world, he argued that we become virtuous by performing virtuous actions.

For Aristotle, the virtuous lies in the moderate action, leading him to the famous 'doctrine of the golden mean' (Russell, 1979). Every virtue is a mean between two extremes (or vices). For Aristotle, what is most important is not simply the identification of the mean (the virtuous) in all aspects of human action. It is the idea that, through reflection and contemplation, we should develop our lives so that we know how to act according to the mean – in other words, how to act virtuously (or morally). We thus become more morally expert, reflection and the consequent performance of virtuous action determining what it means to lead 'the worthwhile (good) life'.

THINKING ABOUT

Can you think what a virtuous action might be?

Example 11.1

THE DILEMMA OF LIFE

In August 2005, retired GP Dr Michael Irwin travelled to Zurich in Switzerland with terminally ill widow Mrs May Murphy, who intended to kill herself. In an apartment owned by the Swiss organization Dignitas, which offers support to people with grave medical conditions who wish to take their own lives, Mrs Murphy committed suicide. Dr Irwin was in the room as she took a lethal dose of barbiturates:

> He recalls her saying, 'I want to die, my body has gone'. 'She could hardly move her arms. She had to use both hands in order to hold this little glass', he said. (Dyer, 2006)

The issue of assisted suicide is deeply contentious and controversial. It is legal in Switzerland, but against the law in the UK, which is why Dr Irwin and Mrs Murphy travelled to Zurich. In May 2006, peers blocked a bill introduced to the House of Lords by Lord Joffe to legalize assisted suicide in certain circumstances. Although not entirely clear, the distinction between assisted suicide and euthanasia lies in the former involving doctors giving patients the means to kill themselves, while the latter involves medical practitioners directly administering fatal doses of medication themselves (Harding, 2005). In January 2006, the Crown Prosecution Service (CPS) was actively considering charges against Dr Irwin after he admitted helping a number of people, including Mrs Murphy, to receive support from Dignitas.

? In your view, did Dr Irwin carry out a virtuous act?

Whether Dr Irwin did the right thing and acted morally may depend on our conception of caring. It could be argued that Dr Irwin was acting virtuously and caring for Mrs Murphy because the requirement in this situation was to relieve the distress, pain and anguish she was suffering as she faced her death.

Much depends here on the intention of Dr Irwin's action. While under current UK law, the doctor would have been culpable whether he had given Mrs Murphy the means for suicide or actually killed her himself, if his motive was to care, then arguably he was acting morally. In Aristotelian terms, his action was virtuous. It is necessary to emphasize the word 'arguably' because of the extremity of the situation and the related action. If the virtuous is the mean between two extremes, the virtue of caring lies somewhere in the middle between excessive 'caring' leading to dependency and loss of autonomy and not caring at all (or not caring in the 'right' way). Given that we do not usually understand caring as killing or even helping people to die, Dr Irwin's action could only be seen as a 'mean' within a situation of enormous and distorted extremes. The guidance offered by Aristotelianism in this particular situation might therefore be somewhat limited, although it does allow for an interpretation of the action. That interpretation is likely to become more substantial if we look beyond the particular situation involving Mrs Murphy, consider a range of others in which Dr Irwin had been involved and from that try to determine whether he demonstrated 'caring' according to more usual means. If this was possible, it could be suggested that Dr Irwin was leading the 'worthwhile (good) life'.

Immanuel Kant and deontology

Immanuel Kant (1724–1804) was a German philosopher who developed ideas representative of deontology – thinking based on the notion that we owe each other particular **duties** or obligations.

Kant claimed the existence of a reality independent of our experience. Part of his justification for this claim lay in his analysis of our experience as humans. We live in a world subject to scientific laws of causation, yet we retain freedom of will, having the capacity to act morally or otherwise. Our moral choices must therefore be framed within an independent reality. Kant argued that reason exists independently of experience and that the right use of reason is directed towards moral ends. Reason moves us to act out of duty for its own sake and independently of any thought about the consequences. This leads to Kant's famous statement of the categorical imperative: 'I ought never to act in such a way *that I cannot also will that my maxim should become a universal law*' (Paton, 1948).

Example 11.2

KANT AND THE DILEMMA OF LIFE

? In your view, was Dr Irwin carrying out his duty?

At first glance, Kant's view that we hold certain moral obligations independent of ideas about consequences seems to hold the possibility of a definitive judgement in the case of Dr Irwin. We might say that helping people to die is always wrong; therefore we should judge the doctor to have committed an act of which we morally disapprove even if it is a legal act. There is, however, a major difficulty at this point. We seldom act with regard to only one moral imperative: we usually have multiple ethical considerations. Dr Irwin would have known that in the UK helping people to die is legally wrong and that many people believe it to be morally so as well. But he would also have known that allowing suffering is wrong (or, framed more positively, that he had a duty to care for Mrs Murphy). If Dr Irwin had not helped her to die, Mrs Murphy would have continued with her terrible suffering. The deontologist faces a problem at this point. There is either agreement that conflicting duties exist, in which case helping people to die may not always be wrong, or there is a persistence in the belief that the overriding duty is to preserve life. We need to be clear, though, that not acting will result in continued suffering.

How, then, is the difficulty overcome? One way (which of course the strict deontologist could not accept) is to allow that the consideration of consequences plays an important part in making moral decisions. This leads to the third ethical tradition to be considered – utilitarianism.

J.S. Mill and utilitarianism

John Stuart Mill (1806–73) was a Scottish philosopher and probably the most famous advocate of the ethical theory known as **utilitarianism**. In this view, careful thought needs to be given to the consequences of any action, and if those consequences are likely to be adverse for some, the reason for the action must be robust.

Put simply, the theory of utilitarianism seems appealing:

Utility, or the greatest happiness principle, holds that actions are right in proportion as they tend to promote happiness, wrong as they tend to produce the reverse of happiness. By happiness is intended pleasure, and the absence of pain; by unhappiness, pain, and the privation of pleasure. (Mill, 1962, p. 257)

Utilitarianism – and consequentialist ethical theory in general – corresponds with a belief held by many that whereas there are important moral duties, action simply for the sake of duty, whatever the consequences, is problematic. In addition, a deliberation about consequences may well include thoughts about the level of 'happiness' or 'unhappiness' likely to accrue from a particular course of action.

Example 11.3

J.S. MILL AND THE DILEMMA OF LIFE

? In your view, were the consequences of Dr Irwin's action beneficial?

Dr Irwin's view might have been that helping Mrs Murphy to die would have been a merciful release for the patient herself and the end of much anguish for her family. But there are at least two difficulties in relying too heavily on consequences to determine moral decision-making:

1. How is it ever possible fully to know the consequences of any particular action? Mrs Murphy's self-administration of the lethal barbiturates might have resulted in considerable distress before her death. The choice may not have been a clear-cut one between intolerable pain and a peaceful death. Introducing a chance of the existence of a complex set of possible consequences may make some likely to see Dr Irwin less as someone acting in the patient's best interests and more as someone toying with a person's fate.

2. What if Dr Irwin's actions had resulted in members of Mrs Murphy's family being terribly distressed by her death, far more so than if her passing had been different?

Dr Irwin may not have intended this to be the case, but if either or both of these had been the consequences of his actions, the end result could be argued to have been more misery than if he had not acted. Utilitarianism contains the paradoxical possibility that someone can intend an action to be ethical but for it to become unethical as it is mediated by circumstances (even more problematic of course is the notion that someone can intend an unethical action but circumstances render it unexpectedly ethical). These difficulties all contribute to the view that a reliance solely on consequences as the measure of moral judgement makes ethics a somewhat haphazard business.

Creating 'worthwhile lives': perspectives from ethics on 'the genetic revolution'

Historically, the concern of ethics has been with understanding how lives already in existence can be 'worthwhile'. But the huge leaps in scientific understanding about the nature of life itself that have taken place since the discovery by Crick and Watson of the structure of DNA in the 1950s have led ethics into completely new territories. The so-called genetic revolution has made it possible for science to create and shape certain kinds of lives. These technological possibilities lead us immediately towards profound ethical problems. Glover (2006) suggests that we need to consider the justifiability of genetic and reproductive technologies used to minimize or eliminate the possibility of babies being born with disabilities or disorders. At first sight, such projects seem eminently justifiable – how could we not want fewer babies who will suffer the pain and distress of being disabled or suffering from chronic ill health being born into the world? But the issue is not as clear-cut as this. At its heart, it is an issue about the nature of 'the worthwhile life'. What causes us to believe that lives of disability and chronic ill health are less worthwhile than lives free of these things? We know that many people who are disabled or are living with a chronic disorder lead lives that are purposeful and worthwhile. Why should we deny the possibility of such lives? Where do we draw the line? If we agree that it might be reasonable to prevent the birth of people with a disability such as Down syndrome, why might we disagree that we should also prevent the birth of people with a sensory handicap such as deafness? As Glover (2006, p. 2) argues, if we are engaged in projects about limiting or eliminating lives of disability and disorder, what does this say about societal attitudes towards people currently living with these things? Surely they are entitled to 'equality of respect', a notion that does not seem very evident within projects designed to make everyone 'normal' (whatever that means). For many, this idea (contained within genetic engineering projects designed to reduce or eliminate disability and disorder or, even more contentiously perhaps, to create the kinds of lives desired by some parents, so-called designer babies) smacks of Nazi eugenics (Glover, 2006, p. 1). The horrors of this particular project have reverberated through the second half of the twentieth century and into the present one (Burleigh, 2001), and for this reason alone it is hardly surprising that we have significant ethical worries about medicine's capacity to create and alter particular kinds of lives.

Example 11.4

NORMALITY AND ABNORMALITY

While the ethical focus on genetic and reproductive technologies often centres on issues around the creation of 'normal lives' (and the prevention or elimination of 'abnormal' ones), there are also questions related to their use in creating certain kinds of lives we might consider likely to be 'problematic':

In 2002 a lesbian couple, Sharon Duchesneau and Candy McCullough, who are both deaf, used sperm donated by a friend with hereditary deafness to have a deaf baby. They took the view that deafness is not a disability but a difference. During her pregnancy, Sharon Duchesneau said, 'It would be nice to have a deaf child who is the same as us ... A hearing baby would be a blessing. A deaf baby would be a special blessing. (Glover, 2006, p. 5)

? Would you agree with the couple's course of action? If so, why? If not, why not? Do you think your reactions and thoughts might be different here than in the case of a couple who were trying to use genetic and reproductive technologies to avoid giving birth to a baby who was deaf? If so, think about why this might be the case.

The contribution of law to health studies

? How would you define 'law' and what is its contribution to the study of health?

A straightforward definition of 'law' might be 'the development and study of a society's prescriptive laws and rules'. Given this, it is likely that the law will (either actually or potentially) have a view on many healthcare dilemmas. In the example of Dr Irwin, he was facing charges because his actions may have broken laws relating to the protection of life, in this case that of the terminally ill Mrs Murphy. At the other end of life, the law makes certain prescriptions with regard to the status and protection of foetuses and in what types of circumstance that protection could be legitimately neglected. There are laws relating to the provision of health services, which could inform or influence debates and dilemmas connected to healthcare rationing (although, as will be seen, this is a very vague area).

In addition, the study of law helps us to recognize the value placed by society on health and the expectations we have about the ways in which health workers conduct themselves. In the 'Bristol heart babies' case, for example, two surgeons were found guilty of professional misconduct by the General Medical Council (GMC) in 1998 (Hill, 1999). This highlights the matter of rules and the capacity for self-regulation that a particular professional cabal (medicine) has been allowed to develop. The high number of deaths in paediatric cardiac surgery at Bristol Royal Infirmary was known about by the hospital, the Royal College of Surgeons and the Department of Health for three years before action was finally taken. For some, the Bristol case demonstrates the fundamental weakness in allowing the self-governance of professions.

The sources of law

The laws governing all those who live in England and Wales (general laws) have historically had two sources: legislation or statute; and law decided through the courts, that is, case law. In Scotland, there are both different statutes and a different system of courts. Since 1999, much law applicable to Scotland has been decided by the Scottish Parliament in Edinburgh, which also has some independent power to raise revenue through taxation, a fundamental support to its legislative capacity (Ham, 2004).

Legislation (statute law)

Notwithstanding recent changes in legislative power related to devolution, the source of law has traditionally been developed and enacted by Parliament at Westminster. In recent times, 1999 also saw the creation of separate assemblies for Wales and Northern Ireland, both with less legislative power than the Scottish Parliament. During the twentieth century and into the twenty-first, **statute law** has assumed great significance, partly because of a more active national legislature (including, latterly, the bodies created by devolution) and the emergence of supranational (for example European) legislative bodies. Acts of Parliament (statutes) are primary legislation and become law after both Houses of Parliament have passed them and royal assent has been received. Recent examples of primary legislation directly affecting healthcare provision include the various Acts and amendments to Acts following on from the new Labour government's reform for the NHS, embodied in *The NHS Plan* and *Delivering the NHS Plan* (Ham, 2004). This included the Health and Social Care (Community Health and Standards) Act 2003, which provided the legal grounds for the establishment of NHS foundation trusts.

As well as enacting primary legislation, Parliament has the ability to delegate the right to the relevant secretary of state (in the case of the legislation above, for health) to draw up regulations or orders dealing with details or future situations that cannot be included in the main Act. This is known as 'delegated legislation'.

Case law

Case law emerges from decisions made in the courts of England and Wales. Court decisions may be the only authority with regard to a particular issue, or they may be the authority charged with interpreting a particular piece of legislation. If, however, there is a conflict between case and statute, the latter must always be followed. If the outcome of this is not acceptable, it is the responsibility of legislators to consider changing the statute. Case law's essential ingredient is legal precedent, judges referring back to similar cases in order to make consistent decisions. Not all decisions made by the courts are binding on later cases. The English court system is hierarchical, a decision made by a higher court becoming binding on lower ones. Cases creating precedent have generally been heard in the Court of Appeal or the House of Lords. The House of Lords is the highest court in the land and can therefore overturn any decision made in lower courts and, in some circumstances, decide not to follow a decision that it might have made previously.

A striking example of healthcare-related case law is that of Anthony Bland. Mr Bland was a young football supporter who fell into a persistent vegetative state following massive injury at the Hillsborough football stadium disaster in April 1989. Mr Bland's parents petitioned the courts to declare that it would be lawful for doctors to remove life support and allow him to die. In a highly distinctive judgement *(Airedale NHS Trust (Respondents)* v. *Bland*, 4 February 1993), the Law Lords ruled that, on the basis of opinions given by Mr Bland's loved ones about his character before being injured, he would, given his state at the time of judgement, have chosen to die rather than live. The principle of self-determination was allowed over that of the sanctity of life, although in their judgement, the Law Lords emphasized continuing treatment as not being in the patient's best interests, rather than Anthony Bland's right to choose death (Dworkin, 1995).

While statute decided by Parliament, together with case law, has historically been the source of law for England and Wales, recent years have seen European law become a further crucial influence over its development.

European law

The European Communities Act 1972 allowed for the application of European Community law within the UK. The essential purpose of applying European law to member states of what is now the European Union (EU) is to effect harmonization, frequently to support economic aims (for example the free movement of goods and labour). There is, however, a different kind of impact on our domestic law emerging from Europe. The Human Rights Act 1998 incorporated the European Convention on Human Rights into domestic law for the first time, meaning that courts have a duty to take into account case law decided by the European Court of Human Rights (ECHR) in Strasbourg (Outhwaite, 1999). Key articles that actually or potentially affect the health service include:

- the right to life (Article 2)

- the right not to be subjected to inhuman or degrading treatment (Article 3)

- the right to liberty (Article 5)

- the right to marry and have a family (Article 12).

Criminal law and civil law

Most criminal law derives from statute law (although murder is defined through common law). Such laws create offences, which can be prosecuted. Usually it is the CPS that decides on and undertakes the prosecution of offences against the criminal law, as was mentioned in the case of Dr Irwin above. In some specific areas, however, other bodies have the power to engage in criminal prosecutions: local authorities can, for example, prosecute environmental health-related offences.

Civil law, on the other hand, enables individual citizens to make legal claims against others (either individuals or organizations) where a civil wrong has been committed. Such wrongs include negligence and breach of statutory duty (part of a group of wrongs sometimes referred to as torts).

Although it is necessary to make the distinction between criminal and civil law, it should be noted that some actions can be pursued both as criminal offences and civil wrongs.

As expectations of health services rise and more people are helped to live longer, the burden on the NHS is increased. Recent organizational reform (embodied, for example, in *The NHS Plan*) has emphasized the importance of clinical excellence, individual choice and the finite nature of public expenditure on health.

The resource decisions that inevitably underpin these strategic directions can, in part, be understood as being made on the basis of empirical evidence (cost–benefit, cost-effectiveness, a knowledge of the total financial package available to the NHS and so on). There sometimes comes a point, however, at which decisions are whittled down to being about competing values, for example economics versus health and wellbeing. The theoretical and methodological perspectives adopted in both ethics and law support our analysis of the range of values related to health and represented within healthcare.

Theoretical and methodological perspectives in ethics

The territory of ethics – the examination and discussion of the values underpinning conduct – is largely conceptual, and in the case of many of the concepts discussed in ethics, there is a large degree of dispute, or contestedness.

Some philosophers have attempted to suggest that value ('ought') judgements have a status roughly equivalent to those concerning empirical fact, for example that asserting 'killing is wrong' is stating an undeniable truth. Aristotle, Kant and Mill are all philosophers attempting such normative moral projects. More recently, contemporary philosophers have suggested that there are important principles that should underlie healthcare provision. Beauchamp and Childress (2001) and Gillon (1994) have suggested that the following principles are particularly important for healthcare workers:

- respect for **autonomy**: the obligation to respect the autonomy of others, for example patients or clients, to the extent that this is compatible with the autonomy of all who are likely to be affected by the action being considered

- **beneficence**: the ethical commitment in healthcare to produce benefit for patients or clients

- **non-maleficence**: the obligation not to harm patients or clients, closely linked to the previous principle, because any given action has the potential to result in both benefit and harm. The obligation on healthcare professionals is to ensure that the balance is always in favour of benefit in any given situation

- **justice**: the obligation to act fairly when dealing with competing claims to do with, for example, resources or rights.

Importantly, the four principles are prima facie binding (literally, 'at first sight'), which is interpreted as meaning that each is binding unless it conflicts with another. In this case, a choice must be made between the competing principles as to which one should be followed. Those who support the four principles argue that whereas they cannot yield a definitive ethical judgement in all healthcare situations, they do provide a framework for considering, and reasoning about, obligations.

The study of ethics cannot provide us with ready-made answers to difficult situations (these simply do not exist), but it does give us the 'tools' to enable reflection on the dilemmas we confront and thus helps us to make greater sense of them. Arguably, actively attempting to understand ethical dilemmas through reflection will help us to become more moral individuals, a return to the Aristotelian idea that the purpose of ethics is to help us to lead the good (worthwhile) life.

If we are to become 'better' at dealing with the ethical difficulties facing us in healthcare, we need at least three things:

● an awareness of moral theory

● an awareness of the kinds of principles, duties and obligations to which everyone working in this field might agree to abide by

● a capacity to reflect on how theory and principles connect with our own intuition, thus developing the ability to think coherently, in a moral sense, by and for ourselves.

> **Example 11.5**

SOME TECHNIQUES FOR THE DEVELOPMENT OF MORAL REFLECTION AND INTUITION

Sue Hunt is a health visitor who is concerned about the nature of smoking advice being given by her colleagues in the multipartner general practice where she is based. Her anxiety centres on whether she and her colleagues – including the GPs – are being too directive, possibly even coercive, in the advice they give. Sue has recently studied ethical problems in healthcare. She has recognized the ease with which healthcare workers may assume control and think that their advice should be directive in tone and be readily accepted by patients.

Sue decides to explore further whether the smoking cessation advice work she and her colleagues undertake poses ethical problems. She arranges to discuss the issue with her mentor. Together, they talk through her concerns and agree the following plan of action:

● Sue will undertake a short 'self-audit' of her own advice-giving on smoking cessation. She will make notes in a diary after each relevant session with patients for a week. She will then describe the advice she gave, how she dealt with questions, the reaction of patients and how she dealt with that reaction.

● At the end of the week, she will use the notes actively to reflect on her advice-giving practice. To what extent did she feel she was respecting patients' autonomy and listening to what they said? If it was hard to do so, why was this? For example, were listening difficulties related to pressure of time or a feeling that you 'had to do something'?

● Following the audit and reflection, Sue will seek the views of her health visitor colleagues in the practice and see whether they have similar perceptions and experiences in this area.

● She will use her experience, and hopefully that of her colleagues, to frame a presentation to other colleagues in the practice on the difficulties with and possibilities for giving advice that is patient centred.

● Sue will review progress with her mentor in a month's time.

From this example, it is possible to identify processes such as understanding moral theory through reading, mentoring, reflective diary-keeping and discussion as all potentially contributing to the development of moral reflection and intuition (Duncan, 2007).

Theoretical and methodological perspectives in law

The methodology of law is analytic and frequently engages with written statutes and recorded cases. Such engagement often occurs with the purpose of discovering whether legislation or existing precedent is sufficient to apply to a new case or whether a new precedent will have to be set. To this extent, there will always be – actually or potentially – a particular legal perspective (a judgement) on a situation. Analysis in law yields more absolute conclusions than analysis in ethics, although, as will be discussed in the following section, this does not mean that we cannot question some of the conclusions that the law makes.

The provision of a healthcare service exposes some of the limitations of the law and its relative weakness. The UK is said to have committed itself – through the NHS – to the provision of a comprehensive healthcare service equally available to all according to need and free of charge at the point of delivery (McHale et al., 1997). This commitment has been expressed by all recent governments despite their different attitudes to the socioeconomic context within which healthcare services are delivered.

This continuing political commitment can be seen as representing the value placed by our society on health and healthcare. A legal framework – expressed through the NHS Act 1977, together with subsequent amendments and related legislation – seeks to ensure this commitment. The 1977 Act states that the secretary of state has a general duty to:

> Continue the promotion in England and Wales of a comprehensive health service designed to secure improvement:
>
> a. in the physical and mental health of the people of those countries
> b. in the prevention, diagnosis and treatment of illness, and for that purpose to provide or secure the effective provision of services in accordance with this act.

Section 3(1) of the Act requires the secretary of state to provide health services to the extent considered necessary to 'meet all reasonable requirements'. The secretary of state's power is, with certain exceptions, discretionary. There is very frequently no legal right to insist that particular services are available, and the courts are reluctant to scrutinize decisions made by health service organizations that have denied patients access to the services they want.

In this area, the law's position is difficult. It might be generally accepted that individuals have a right to healthcare, but statute allows the nature of that right to be decided by those controlling healthcare. In addition, unless a right can be acted on, it is hardly a right at all. There are two main ways in which individuals can attempt to enforce their **rights** to healthcare, both with their roots in the civil law. These are:

- the public law action for judicial review, which allows a challenge to be made to the decisions of public bodies on the basis that they have been irrational, illegal or procedurally improper

- claims for compensation on the basis of the right to healthcare having been breached.

Example 11.6

CHILD B

The case of Child B in 1995 provides an example of a judicial review (R. v. Cambridge DHA, ex p. B). The father of a 10-year-old girl (referred to at the time as Child B) brought a review of the decision by Cambridge Health Authority not to fund further treatment of her leukaemia. Her doctors made the clinical judgement that she would not benefit from further chemotherapy or a second bone marrow transplant. A second opinion sought by the child's father disputed this, but the health authority declined to pay for the treatment proposed. The case was taken to the High Court, where Mr Justice Laws judged that the authority had not adequately explained the priorities that had led to its decision in this case. He required it to be re-examined, although he did not order the treatment to be funded. The health authority took the case to the Court of Appeal. Sir Thomas Bingham, Master of the Rolls, began his judgement by commenting on the very high value placed by society on human life but concluded that the courts could neither make judgements on healthcare resource allocation nor require a health authority to be explicit about its decision-making. Child B died in May 1996.

The case of Child B underlines the reluctance of the law to interfere in both clinical judgements and decisions on resource allocation (rationing). As a society we place a high value on health and healthcare, but as individuals we are extremely limited in our capacity to pursue that right. Although the introduction of the Human Rights Act in 1998 was thought likely to strengthen individual rights to particular forms of health-related care and treatment, its effects have not been clear-cut. For example, Dianne Pretty was a woman in the late stages of motor neurone disease. The terrible and painful nature of her condition caused her to seek to commit suicide. Physically, however, she was unable to take her own life. If her husband helped her to do so, as she wanted, he would be guilty of assistance and face legal repercussions. With the help of Liberty, the human rights organization, Mrs Pretty began a legal challenge against the application of the Suicide Act using certain Articles of the Human Rights Act (Liberty, 2001). She was given leave to appeal for a judicial review against the Director of Public Prosecutions by the High Court in August 2001. This appeal was dismissed in the House of Lords in November 2001. Mrs Pretty then took her case to the ECHR, but again the case was rejected. The ECHR ruled that the fact that assisted suicide was a crime was not a breach of Mrs Pretty's human rights (*Guardian*, 2002). Dianne Pretty died in May 2002, having failed in her attempts to be allowed to be assisted towards death. Despite human rights legislation, there appear to be limits to our pursuit of what we might perceive to be health-related rights.

The law also expresses societal expectations of how healthcare professionals should conduct themselves and the obligations they have to clients or patients. Professionals owe those whom they serve a general duty of care. If this is breached, the professional has acted not only unprofessionally, but also negligently. If patients' or clients' expectations of the duty of care are not met, they may wish to seek redress in civil law through a negligence action – from patients' perspectives, to achieve compensation in some way for the wrong believed to have been done. This reinforces the point that legal mechanisms serve both of the following closely connected purposes of law applied to healthcare:

● the expression of societal values

● the expectations we have of professionals.

It appears quite right, then, in terms of the law, to talk about individual expectations of healthcare professionals. There is an expectation that they hold a duty of care, and if there is a failure in this respect, there is an equal expectation that they should be subject to redress. This is perhaps optimistic because the legal system is, in practice, so complex, and its use so costly, that individuals very often have little chance of fulfilling the complete 'expectation equation'.

The basis of the duty of care was laid in a judgement in 1932 by Lord Atkin *(Donoghue* v. *Stevenson)*. He judged that someone must take reasonable care to avoid actions or omissions in action that could be reasonably foreseen to cause injury to someone directly affected by those acts. (Note that this is quite different from an obligation to act for the benefit of another, which generally does not exist in English law.) Breaching this duty and causing harm is negligence, and a civil liability has thus been created, so compensation can be claimed. If a negligence action is to be successful, three things must, on the balance of probability, be established:

● The plaintiff (the person pursuing redress) must establish that the defendant (the person defending the action) owes her or him a duty of care

● This duty has been breached

● The result of the breach has been that the plaintiff suffered foreseeable harm.

If healthcare professionals consider the duty of care, it is likely that they will want to ask a number of questions. First, to whom do they owe a duty? The law would usually deem that they have a duty to their patients and probably their patients' relatives, as well as to their colleagues.

Second, when would a duty be regarded as having been breached? The law would probably take the view that the duty has been breached if the required standard of care has not been met. The 'Bolam test' (based on the judgement resulting from *Bolam* v. *Friern Hospital Management Committee*, 1957) indicates that healthcare professionals would breach the standard of care if they failed to meet the standards of their peers. This, however, is not a simple test, at least in part because the law is less likely to take a judgement on 'acceptable care' provided by some professional groups in healthcare than others.

Third, what is the extent of proof required that the damage or harm done was actually caused by negligent professional behaviour? In the case described in *Barnett* v. *Chelsea and Kensington Hospital Management Committee* (1968), a night watchman was turned away from a hospital A&E department, later to die of arsenic poisoning. It was judged in this case that there is an obligation to provide care to someone presenting at an A&E department. However, it was also judged that the factors causing death in the case were not within the capacity of a medical practitioner to treat, and therefore the doctor who turned the patient away could not be held liable for his death.

The relationship between ethics and law: is what we *must* do the same as what we *ought* to do?

When we approach healthcare professionals, we generally do so because we need help and have an expectation and confidence that those whom we approach can offer us such assistance. We believe – or hope we can believe – that they will take their duty of care towards us seriously, respect our confidentiality, inform us of what they intend to do on our behalf and why, and only go ahead and do it if we consent to their proposed actions.

Yet healthcare practices, and the relationships between professionals and patients, are frequently messy and difficult. We are right to expect the possibility of redress when things go wrong. And the law might to some extent be able to provide this as part of its role in 'formally' expressing societal expectations of both the healthcare systems operating on our behalf and the individual professionals working within them. But when we go to healthcare professionals, our expectations are not simply that they will operate within relatively narrow and legalistic conceptions such as those of 'negligence' and 'duty of care'. It has been argued, for example, that in law, the duty of care centres on the requirement to avoid actions or omissions that are likely to result in injury or harm. Would we seek the help of a practitioner simply because we knew that he or she had an excellent reputation for avoiding harm, which is largely all the general law requires him or her to do?

This is moving towards the view that there is a difference between what we *must* do (that which the law requires us to do) and what we *ought* to do (that which – for want of better words – our personal and professional moral character obliges us to do). In addition, it may be that it is the healthcare professional who does what he or she ought to do (rather than simply what must be done) whom we would regard as a 'good' or 'moral' practitioner (Lesser, 2002; Duncan et al., 2003).

In the case described above of Dr Irwin, who was facing legal charges associated with the death of Mrs Murphy, it could be argued that he did what he felt he ought to do in supporting the relief of her pain and suffering. There are cases, for example that of the Northumbrian GP Dr David Moor, where the law seems to agree that the relief of pain and suffering is paramount, even though it might lead to a patient's death. In this case, Dr Moor was cleared of the murder of his patient Mr George Liddell, to whom he had administered a huge dose of diamorphine (Dyer, 1999). In other cases in which there is arguably a similar motivation, the conclusion of a jury might, however, be different. In 1992, Dr Nigel Cox was tried for the attempted murder of one of his patients, Mrs Lillian Boyes. She was dying from a crippling and agonisingly painful form of rheumatoid arthritis and begged Dr Cox to kill her, which he did with a lethal injection of potassium chloride (Dworkin, 1995). He was convicted and received a suspended jail sentence. Both Dr Moor and Dr Cox wanted to relieve their patients of terrible suffering. The roots of the different outcomes of the legal cases lie in the decision of the jurors and the direction of the judges, but the law itself remains the same: killing is wrong. Yet we might want to argue that both doctors *ought* to have performed the action they did. (Or, equally, we might want to argue that both actions were wrong.)

The law was reluctant to intervene in the judgement made by Cambridge Health Authority about the extent to which the priority of treatment for Child B superseded the many other priorities it believed itself to have. Sir Thomas Bingham, in the Court of Appeal, effectively ruled that the authority had no legal obligation to fund treatment for Child B. Yet while there might not have been a legal obligation (as in, this treatment *must* be funded), at least some would argue that it *ought* to have been paid for. Here was a young girl with a life-threatening condition whose prognosis was to some degree disputed by doctors who knew her case. The problem of rationing and priority-setting is made more acute by the undoubted fact that the health authority had to make choices about what to fund across a whole range of possible health promotion, prevention, treatment and care activities, given the duties delegated to it by the secretary of state. Would it have been better, for example, if the authority had funded treatment for Child B at the expense of a smoking prevention programme, which, if effective, might ultimately – in 20 or 30 years' time – have saved or prolonged several hundred lives?

The death of 29 babies and toddlers at Bristol Royal Infirmary following heart surgery performed by two cardiac surgeons raises a complex set of issues centred around professional competence. One of the surgeons and the infirmary chief executive were eventually found guilty of serious professional misconduct by the GMC and banned from practising medicine. The other surgeon was banned from operating on children for three years and later sacked. A public inquiry into children's heart surgery at Bristol Royal Infirmary, chaired by Sir Ian Kennedy, led to the Kennedy Report (2001). This concluded that much more effective safeguards were needed to protect patients; the Bristol failures had occurred, the report said, because it had been the surgeons who themselves had been operating on the children who were responsible for the quality of care provided. So the report endorsed measures that were already being taken by the Labour government to strengthen the audit of health services, including the establishment of the Commission for Health Improvement and the National Patient Safety Agency. The government also accepted a number of recommendations made by Kennedy, including the need for a Council for the Regulation of Healthcare Professionals, to strengthen systems for professional self-regulation (Ham, 2004). This was established in 2003, but has since changed its name to the Council for Healthcare Regulatory Excellence (CHRE). It needs to be distinguished from the Health Professions Council, which is the body responsible for the day-to-day regulation of many professions allied to medicine, including occupational therapy and physiotherapy.

We could reasonably argue in relation to Bristol that what *must* be done and what *ought* to be done should be indistinguishable from one another, in a way that is indisputable and unlike the other situations we have reviewed. We *must* have protection to ensure that those who are charged with our fundamental wellbeing are competent to undertake the task. And those who perform the task (and others who regulate them) *ought* to ensure that this is the case. Yet despite this indisputability, 29 children died in Bristol Royal Infirmary before action was taken, and even when cases were proved against the professionals concerned, varying degrees of sanctions against them were applied (and were objected to). This state of affairs seems to suggest that what we might consider to be the moral duty to professional competence held by those working in healthcare might not be matched by equally rigorous laws. Even with the regulatory strengthening that has been one of the fundamental health-related projects of the Labour government, we might be doubtful about its ultimate effect on individual practice. After all, Bristol has not proved to be the end of professional scandals. For example, in 2006, the *Observer* alleged that there were at least 175 nurses accused of serious misconduct who were still working in British hospitals (Revill, 2006a).

Part of the difficulty in the Bristol case lay in the fact that monitoring of the surgeons concerned was essentially a process of self-regulation (or at best regulation by peers). This applied even when the case entered the wider professional domain; the professional body to which it would have been referred was the then completely self-regulating GMC. This concept of self-regulation is highly problematic because it might lead to a climate in which it becomes hard for professionals to do what they might feel they *ought*. In 1990, a young consultant anaesthetist working at Bristol Royal Infirmary wrote to the local health authority raising his concerns about what seemed to be a higher than average death rate among babies undergoing cardiac surgery. These allegations were dismissed, the anaesthetist later claiming that the main surgeon had threatened to ruin his career prospects if he pursued the matter (Hill, 1999).

That professionals should find 'whistle-blowing' so threatening is another disturbing feature of the Bristol case. This – and other instances – have contributed to the GMC strengthening its mechanisms for self-regulation and to the CHRE overseeing doctors' regulation (Bradshaw and Bradshaw, 2004).

Indeed, as this chapter was being written, a further effect of Bristol (and related 'medical scandals' such as the case of mass-murdering GP Dr Harold Shipman) was being played out through the implementation of another raft of reforms to the GMC. These involved the requirement for it to move, at least to some extent, away from self-regulation towards greater involvement of people other than doctors in decisions about medical conduct. The threat to potential 'whistle-blowers' from their managers or other employees is also a concern of the Public Interest Disclosure Act 1998, which provides certain protections for those genuinely 'blowing the whistle' from victimization and dismissal (RCN, 2001).

 What are the advantages and disadvantages of a professional group regulating itself?

It could be argued that it is professionals themselves – by virtue of their technical expertise and moral commitment – who stand the best chance of closing the *must–ought* 'gap'. After all, cases such as Bristol are relatively rare, even though we may naturally be concerned that they exist at all. One of the ways in which professional groups have attempted to close the gap is through the development of codes of conduct.

Closing the 'gap' between what we must do and what we ought to do: consent and professional conduct

Nurses, midwives and specialist community public health nurses are bound to practise according to the duties set out in the Nursing and Midwifery Council's **code of conduct** (NMC, 2004). A commitment to the code of conduct seems to bind these professionals to do certain things that they *ought* to do (the code being an expression of moral commitments) and what they *must* do (the professional being likely to be sanctioned if the commitments are neglected or breached).

Article 3 of the code declares that the practitioner must: 'Obtain consent before you give any treatment or care' (NMC, 2004). This is a rather broad statement, although slightly more specific and directive advice supplement it. However, if we accept what has just been said, it is clear that the professional both *ought* to and *must* engage in processes aimed at achieving informed consent on the part of his or her patients.

What difficulties do you think there might be with the concept of informed consent?

Informed consent is a very reasonable obligation and expectation. The difficulty comes when we start going beyond generality and think about what it might mean in practice. Informed consent involves two processes – informing and consenting (Gorovitz, 1985). The end result of informing should be understanding, yet there are many possible barriers to understanding, particularly in the healthcare context:

● Patients or clients are frequently in a critical state in which their ability to understand is limited

● Individuals have different capacities with regard to understanding

● Informing has a cost in that it is time-consuming and demanding of skills that health professionals have in different measures.

Moreover, some people do not want to be informed and understandably dread 'bad news'. Consenting should also be regarded not simply as one instance of a patient or client acquiescing but an ongoing process, with a healthcare practitioner's duty perhaps being continually to nurture and confirm understanding and awareness.

Teasing out the complexities of informed consent both as a moral obligation and professional duty for the health worker raises at least two problems for the NMC code of conduct. (Of course, these problems also apply to other professional codes.) First, the complexity of informed consent exposes the generality of the code, which makes it more difficult to decide when it is being breached. There will be many circumstances in which professionals are 'pushed' to achieve informed consent; at what point is it possible to step in and suggest that duty has been breached? This problem relates particularly to the *must* side of the gap. Professionals generally know what they must do, but is it possible to blame them when they cannot do it? The second problem is that by pushing deeper into this article of the code, we are made aware of how much commitment a health worker must have to practise according to its general requirements. This problem relates especially to the *ought* side of the gap. The health worker must be involved in a continuous process of self-deliberation, and possibly of negotiation and agreement with clients or patients. Is it reasonable to expect this sort of commitment from nurses and other professionals?

It appears, then, that regarding codes of conduct as devices to close the gap between *must* and *ought* in the actions of healthcare professionals is simplistic. Codes by themselves are at once too general and too intimidating. We can probably expect health workers broadly to work according to their code, and it is right to demand sanctions for those who grossly offend against it. But these are by and large exceptional cases and do not help most practitioners who are involved in the messy and complicated everyday context of healthcare. We outlined above a range of 'techniques' that might help people to develop their capacity to determine what they *ought* to do (as well as what they *must* do).

CASE STUDY Banning 'junk food' advertising

Recent years have seen an increasing concern in the UK (as in other developed countries) with rising levels of obesity in childhood and the risk that this poses to the future health of the nation (DoH, 2004).

This concern has led to experts and politicians pursuing a range of strategies to address the problem. In November 2006, Ofcom announced a ban on so-called junk food being advertised during children's TV programmes, on dedicated children's channels and around all programmes that have a 'particular appeal' to under-16s (Campbell, 2006; Sweney, 2007). This ban was likely to be the first control on media advertising of junk food. The Advertising Standards Authority was planning a scheme, at the end of 2006, to ban such advertising in children's magazines and the Department of Health was considering similar restrictions related to billboards, radio and the internet (Campbell, 2006).

For some politicians, however, this was not enough. The *Observer* reported that supporters of a complete pre-9 pm watershed ban on TV advertising of junk food were gathering behind a private members' bill from the Labour peer, Baroness Thornton (Campbell, 2006). If this was successful and enacted, TV companies would be prevented by law from advertising unhealthy foods before 9 o'clock in the evening. Television advertising of junk food would simply be illegal within specified times. But the ethical question remains; should we be trying to restrict this kind of advertising? What is the moral justification for such action?

To some, this question might seem strange. There is a growing incidence (some experts have referred to it as an epidemic) of childhood obesity. There is also strong evidence that obesity is connected to problems of health and wellbeing in childhood and in later life. It would not be unreasonable to suggest that obesity trails behind it a huge burden of morbidity and premature mortality. The widespread availability of junk food, that is, food characteristically high in salt, fat and sugar and with little nutritional value, and consequent changes in dietary behaviour have been linked to the increased incidence of obesity (NHS Centre for Reviews and Dissemination, 2002). So if junk food leads to obesity and obesity leads to health problems (even death), then surely those concerned about health and its protection and promotion should be unequivocal in their support for any measure likely to reduce the consumption of unhealthy foods?

Perhaps this is true. But we have argued throughout this chapter that issues and questions of healthcare centrally involve values. As a consequence, there is a need for us to develop our skills of moral reflection, and our ethical intuition. If our arguments are accepted, we cannot take for granted the position on the banning of junk food advertising to children outlined above. We need to subject it to further examination and critique. One way of undertaking this is to examine the action of banning advertising in relation to the four principles of healthcare ethics described earlier: beneficence, non-maleficence, respect for autonomy and justice.

Banning junk food advertising and the principle of beneficence

At first sight, the case here seems clear. After all, the 'common-sense' position that has just been outlined on the matter (ban advertising, reduce obesity and prevent suffering through ill health and early death) is one that resonates with many. How can bans not produce benefit and do good? This position depends, though, on at least two further things being the case:

● There is a causal relationship between the advertising ban, reduction in junk food consumption and lowering of obesity levels
● The ban, and in particular what is included and excluded from it, is carefully constructed.

With regard to the first point, while we might be able to claim some relationship between the ban, food consumption and obesity levels, we cannot claim that it is causal. There are two reasons for this. First, childhood obesity is causally complex and involves broader aspects of lifestyle beyond simply eating behaviour (NHS Centre for Reviews and Dissemination, 2002). We not only eat in different ways than we have done previously; we also work and play and generally live our lives in different ways, too. So while we could say that banning junk food advertising might play a part in the eventual reduction of childhood obesity (and of course this in itself might be enough to convince us of the worth of such a ban), the nature and extent of this role is relatively unclear.

In relation to the second point, some interest groups have claimed that the model used to decide which foods Ofcom should ban from advertising is a very imprecise tool. According to the model (supplied by the Food Standards Agency), it is claimed, raisins and All-Bran would be banned but not chicken nuggets and white bread (Sweney, 2007). Perhaps this does no more than highlight the question of the complexity and disputability of nutritional information, but it adds to the view that the relationship between any ban and eventual health benefit is not as clear-cut as some might have thought. There is thus a need to analyse this

case against the other principles of healthcare ethics.

Banning junk food advertising and the principle of non-maleficence

If benefit emerging from the action could be contested, this underlines the importance of assessing it in terms of not producing harm. (We may be less prepared to concede harm, even of a limited nature, if we are less clear about benefit.) It might be possible to construct an argument for the ban causing harm in terms of the social context to which it is applied. If we ban advertising of junk food, some might believe that those who continue to buy it are engaging in harmful behaviour. The child buying a McDonald's Happy Meal, say, becomes demonized, an object of ridicule and fun. (This might be exacerbated by the fact that they are already overweight and subject to potential difficulties of self-image.) In this demonization of junk food, its consumers also become vilified, and so harm is caused to them.

The other side of this coin is the economic effect of the ban on both junk food producers and advertisers. The Ofcom ban has already been recognized as contributing to a fall-off in sales of some junk food (especially takeaway fast foods) (Sweney, 2007) and a wider legislative ban may well hasten this decline. Moreover, some pundits have suggested that bans would starve some TV networks of cash and possibly cause closures, with a resulting loss of jobs (Brook, 2004). While we might be less inclined to have sympathy for supermarket and takeaway overlords and TV moguls, there is a need to recognize the effect of changing patterns of consumption on the employees who work for them.

Banning junk food advertising and the principle of respect for autonomy

For many considering the ethics of this case study, the principle of respect for autonomy is of crucial importance. Why should the nanny state (albeit indirectly through advertising restrictions) try and direct the preferences and wishes of individuals? Can't we allow children and young people (and their parents) to make up their own minds about junk food and its consumption? Here there are important questions of vulnerability and capacity. In the UK, we have strong traditions of legislative and other protection for children and young people, including protection from harms to health. Smoking and drinking are banned for children and young people because we believe they do not necessarily have the awareness of harm and capacity for self-protection from it that most adults possess. This vulnerability might make us more inclined to believe that in this kind of case, restrictions on autonomy could be justified. Moral philosophers often refer to such restrictions as paternalistic, with some finding it relatively easy to defend 'soft' or 'weak' paternalism (Wikler, 1978).

On the other hand, a cherished goal of health promoters is the empowerment of those with whom they work (Tones and Green, 2004), because this is likely to lead to more authentic action, including action for health. If we deliberately coerce and restrict (even if only very weakly), to what extent are we providing children and young people with models of how we would like them to behave as they become adults, that is, as individuals in charge of their own destinies and carefully deliberating on the choices available to them?

Banning junk food advertising and the principle of justice

As has been suggested, there are a number of justice-related areas that are potentially relevant for healthcare-related ethical thought. The most obvious in this case is distributive justice; the fair adjudication of competing claims to the scarce resource of healthcare. We know that there is a

relationship between childhood obesity and morbidity. Treating illness costs the NHS money, so we need to do what we can to reduce the incidence of obesity and banning junk food advertising might contribute to this. NICE has recently recommended that teenagers should be allowed access to the 'last resort' treatment of bariatric (stomach-stapling) surgery if the condition cannot be dealt with by any other means. Such an operation can cost in the region of £8,000 (Revill, 2006b). This is not considering the economic burden that the adult consequences of childhood obesity (chronic heart disease, cancers and so on) might result in. So an analysis of banning junk food advertising using the principle of distributive justice might reasonably come to the conclusion that the economic burden presented by unchecked obesity is unfair for those who have to bear it (taxpayers). It would also be unfair to those with other conditions who might be denied treatment as a result of scarce resources being devoted to dealing with severely overweight people.

However, this conclusion again depends on a strong relationship between banning junk food advertising and the reduction in obesity incidence. We have argued that it is not possible to claim such a relationship in an unproblematic way. So any argument for the ethical worth of the intervention based on distributive justice needs to be carefully balanced with arguments both for and against its worth in relation to the other principles.

This short analysis of the ethics of banning advertising of junk food does not necessarily lead us to definitive conclusions. As we have already argued, principles alone cannot support our ethical reasoning and decision-making; we also need an awareness of theory and a capacity to reflect on how both theory and principles connect with our own ethical intuition and 'moral sense'. However, this kind of analytical exercise can begin, in a very real way, to expose the complexity and difficulty inherent within health-related interventions and actions that appear, on the surface, to cause little problem. Together with the rest of this chapter, we hope that it has begun to feed your own ideas about the significance of work in health and healthcare in terms of ethical and legal perspectives.

Summary

- The study of ethics is conceptual enquiry, largely concerned with trying to understand how people ought to behave towards one another. It involves clarifying the meaning of concepts such as 'benefit' or 'duty'

- The study of law is an analytical enquiry into the development of society's prescriptive rules or laws, and into establishing whether legal statute or precedent applies in a particular situation

- Ethics tries to describe what we *ought* to do. The law prescribes what we *must* do

- The study of ethics and law can help to identify the value placed on health over and above other values, the guides or limits to professional conduct and the scope of the obligations of health workers

- Neither ethics nor law can provide a definitive 'solution' to contemporary health dilemmas (for these do not exist), but their study can provide a framework for considering key questions. Reflecting on ethical and legal principles and dilemmas may help in forming consistent judgements and in the search for a moral life

Questions for further discussion

1. Does the law's concern with prescription and attempts to establish definitive judgements help or hinder those striving to be good (moral) health workers?

2. Consider a health dilemma that you are personally aware of or have become aware of through the media. Can the application of ethical principles clarify what should be done in this situation?

Further reading

Beauchamp, T. and Childress, J. (2001) *Principles of Biomedical Ethics* (5th edn). Oxford: Oxford University Press.
Beauchamp and Childress developed the idea of the 'famous four principles' of healthcare ethics, and here their ideas are most completely expressed. It is detailed and technical but offers many helpful points of reference, including extensive signposts to further literature.

Cribb, A. and Duncan, P. (2002) *Health Promotion and Professional Ethics*. Oxford: Blackwell.
An extended consideration of the ethical challenges facing those involved in promoting health, an area of healthcare often – and wrongly, it is argued – assumed to be morally unproblematic.

Dworkin, R. (1995) *Life's Dominion: An Argument about Abortion and Euthanasia*. London: HarperCollins.
An elegantly written attempt to make sense, from a legal/philosophical perspective, of the ways in which we think about the beginning and ending of human life. This well-constructed and closely argued book provides a model for thinking about how we might employ ethics and law in consideration of other areas of health and healthcare.

Gillon, R. (1990) *Philosophical Medical Ethics*. Chichester: John Wiley & Sons.
Writing for a mainly British audience, Gillon has 'translated' Beauchamp and Childress's ideas and arguments from the North American context in which they were originally framed.

Glover, J. (2006) *Choosing Children: The Ethical Dilemmas of Genetic Intervention*. Oxford: Clarendon Press.
A beautifully written book by a leading moral philosopher, based on a series of lectures in which he explores the dilemmas faced by a society in which genetic and reproductive technology is radically changing the nature of life's beginnings.

Tingle, J. and Cribb, A. (eds) (2002) *Nursing Law and Ethics* (2nd edn). Oxford: Blackwell.
An accessible introduction to issues of law and ethics facing those involved in nursing practice.

References

Beauchamp, T. and Childress, J. (2001) *Principles of Biomedical Ethics* (5th edn). Oxford: Oxford University Press.

Bradshaw, P.L. and Bradshaw, G. (2004) *Health Policy for Healthcare Professionals*. London: Sage.

Brook, S. (2004) Junk food ban would starve TV networks. *Guardian*, 14 October.

Burleigh, M. (2001) *The Third Reich: A New History*. London: Pan Macmillan.

Campbell, D. (2006) Junk food ads face ban in youth magazines. *Observer*, 19 November.

DoH (Department of Health) (2004) *Choosing Health*. London: Stationery Office.

Duncan, P. (2007) *Critical Perspectives on Health*. Basingstoke: Palgrave Macmillan.

Duncan, P., Cribb, A. and Stephenson, A. (2003) 'Developing the good healthcare practitioner: clues from a study in medical education'. *Learning in Health and Social Care* 2(4): 181–90.

Dworkin, R. (1995) *Life's Dominion*. London: HarperCollins.

Dyer, C. (1999) Doctor cleared of murdering patient. *Guardian*, 12 May.

Dyer, C. (2006) GP questioned over journey to suicide clinic. *Guardian*, 31 January.

Gillon, R. (1994) 'Medical ethics: four principles plus attention to scope'. *British Medical Journal* 309: 184–8.

Glover, J. (2006) *Choosing Children: The Ethical Dilemmas of Genetic Intervention*. Oxford: Clarendon Press.

Gorovitz, S. (1985) *Doctor's Dilemmas: Moral Conflict and Medical Care*. New York: Oxford University Press.

Guardian (2002) Dianne Pretty loses right to die case, *Guardian*, 29 April.

Ham, C. (2004) *Health Policy in Britain* (5th edn). Basingstoke: Palgrave Macmillan.

Harding, L. (2005) Swiss hospital will be the first to allow assisted suicide. *Guardian* Weekly, 23 December.

Hill, M. (1999) Uncovering the Bristol scandal. BBC Online News, 15 March, www.bbc.co.uk/news.

Kennedy Report (2001) *The Report of the Public Inquiry into Children's Heart Surgery at the Bristol Royal Infirmary 1984–1995*, Cm 5207(1). London: Stationery Office.

Kitcher, P. (1994) *The Lives to Come: The Genetic Revolution and Human Possibilities*. London: Penguin.

Lesser, H. (2002) An ethical perspective: negligence and moral obligations, in J. Tingle and A. Cribb (eds) *Nursing Law and Ethics*. Oxford: Blackwell, pp. 90–8.

Liberty (2001) Dianne Pretty's right to die case: High Court clears way for judicial review, www.liberty-human-rights-org.uk, accessed 13/2/2007.

McHale, J., Fox, M., with Murphy, J. (1997) *Healthcare Law: Text and Materials*. London: Sweet & Maxwell.

Mill, J.S. (1962) *Utilitarianism and Other Writings*. Glasgow: Fontana.

NHS Centre for Reviews and Dissemination (2002) *The Prevention and Treatment of Childhood Obesity*. York: NHS Centre for Reviews and Dissemination.

NMC (Nursing and Midwifery Council) (2004) *Code of Professional Conduct*. London: Nursing and Midwifery Council.

Outhwaite, W. (1999) 'Indefinite articles'. *Health Service Journal* Special Report, 27 May: 9–11.

Paton, H.J. (1948) *The Moral Law*. London: Hutchinson.

Revill, J. (2006a) Patients' lives being left at mercy of abusive nurses. *Observer*, 25 June.

Revill, J. (2006b) NHS must pay for fat children to get surgery. *Observer*, 19 November.

RCN (Royal College of Nursing) (2001) *Blowing the Whistle*. London: RCN.

Russell, B. (1979) *A History of Western Philosophy*. London: Unwin.

Sweney, M. (2007) MPs seek tougher junk food ad ban. *Guardian*, 6 February.

Tones, K. and Green, J. (2004) *Health Promotion: Planning and Strategies*. London: Sage.

Wikler, D. (1978) 'Persuasion and coercion for health: ethical issues in government efforts to change lifestyles'. *Millbank Memorial Fund Quarterly* 56(3): 303–38.

Glossary

Administration	the practice of being accountable for carrying out the decisions of others. Involves initiating action within defined limits of authority, and monitoring and recording progress, outcomes and events. It is an essential component of, particularly, a bureaucratic organization
Aetiology	concerns assigning a cause to a given outcome. For example, the aetiology of coronary heart disease might involve smoking, a high cholesterol level, obesity and a stressful lifestyle
Association	an identifiable relationship between exposure to a risk factor and disease. Causation implies there is a mechanism that leads from exposure to disease
Attitude	the feelings an individual has about an object or action. There are three aspects to a person's attitudes to an issue – cognitive (knowledge and information), affective (their emotions, likes and dislikes) and behavioural (their skills and competences)
Attribution	the perceived or reported reason given for an action, event or feelings
Attribution theory	attributions are perceived or reported causes of actions, events or feelings. Attribution theory concerns the beliefs that individuals possess about the causes of events
Autonomy	the capacity to be in charge of your own actions and your own destiny. The principle of respect for autonomy asserts that we have a moral obligation to allow this capacity to individuals to the extent that it does not infringe on the equal rights of others
Beneficence	the production of good, or benefit. This is frequently regarded as a moral obligation that ought to be held by healthcare workers
Bias	the result of any process that causes observations to differ from their true values in a systematic way (as opposed to chance, which is defined as random variation). Bias may be introduced into a study at its inception (for example when selecting the sample), during its course or during the analysis
Biomedicine	the application of the principles of natural science (biology and physiology) to the human body. Focuses on the biological causes and treatment of ill health and disease

Body	the physical body, a concept encompassing not only the experience of living within our bodies, but also the meanings we attach to the body
Bureaucracy	a term describing particular features of organizations in which structure, role relationships and procedures are specified in writing and are followed impartially and without deviation over long time periods, irrespective of the individual's personality or the personal preferences of the role occupants
Cells	the smallest self-contained living units in the body. Some, like those in the blood, are separate; others are connected to each other to form tissues
Citizenship	the possession of civil, political and legal rights (for example free speech and voting). In social policy, the possession of social rights (for example to economic security) is also regarded as a precondition to citizenship
Class	the division and ranking of groups of people according to occupational role, which arose during the growth and development of capitalism. Social class refers to status and power as well as to income
Cloning	involves the transfer of a nucleus from a body cell to a denucleated egg. No fertilization by sperm is involved
Code of conduct	an attempt to prescribe the ways in which members of an occupational or professional group ought to behave. Such attempts are frequently made by representatives of that occupational or professional group itself
Cohort	a group that can be followed or tracked over time
Collectivism	the general responsibility of all members of society to meet the needs of individuals, for example services funded through taxation
Community	a contested term that is usually taken to refer to a group of people living in a defined geographic area, but may also refer to those sharing a common culture or values
Compliance	behaving in line with that which has been suggested, such as taking medication, eating more healthily or attending a health check. Also known as adherence
Consumption	the way in which cultural artefacts are used or purchased, and the way in which we take meaning from them
Cost–benefit analysis	a technique of economic appraisal that assesses allocative efficiency by comparing the money value of all the costs of a policy, programme or intervention against the money value of all the benefits

Cost-effectiveness analysis	a technique of economic appraisal that assesses technical efficiency by comparing the money value of the costs of a policy, programme or intervention against a single, non-monetary measure of its effectiveness (for example number of life years gained)
Culture	may be portrayed as monolithic, implying that all members of society share a common language, religion, traditions and customs. Culture is, however, increasingly pluralistic, different cultures interacting and influencing each other
Deduction	the converse of induction, whereby a specific inference or prediction is made from a generalization
Discipline	a field of study with a bounded area of knowledge and agreed areas of interest and methods of inquiry
Discourse	can be used in the sense of language to refer to talk or writing. It can also be used to describe a set of ideas and norms about a topic
Disease	a biological definition sees disease as an alteration in the state of the body or some of its organs that changes it from its 'normal' state, interrupting or disturbing the performance of the vital functions. It can be used to refer to a specific, medically diagnosed condition with distinctive, recognized symptoms, which may cause pain or sickness. The concept of disease can also be seen as relative and has been differently defined historically and culturally
Duties	things that we morally or legally ought to do. Duty is usually distinguished from obligation. We incur obligations because of specific circumstances, but duty is something of longer standing and primarily connected with role. A nurse, for example, has a duty to care in a long-standing and general sense because he or she is a nurse. Nurses also incur obligations to care in a much more short-term sense and with regard to particular people (patients) by virtue of placing themselves in situations in which caring is required
Efficiency	achieving outcomes in the most economic manner possible
Empiricism	the view that knowledge is based on experience, not theory. Knowledge can therefore be proven to exist, because it is tested in real-life experiences. Empiricism is the basis of scientific knowledge
Empowerment	a process through which individuals and groups are able to recognize and express their needs and take appropriate action to meet them

Epistemology	the philosophical study of the nature of knowledge and its production
Equity	being fair and just. This may involve targeting specific services for those most in need rather than providing the same blanket service for everyone
Ethnicity	characteristics of social life, such as culture, religion, language and history, which are shared by groups of people and passed on to the next generation. Often used instead of 'race', which focuses on physical differences and thus has been largely discredited
Eugenics	the process of using selective breeding for the goal of improving the human race
Evidence	that which tends to prove or disprove something. Used legally, data presented to a court or jury in proof of the facts in issue
Evidence-based healthcare practice	the conscientious, explicit and judicious use of current best evidence in decision-making
Experiment	characteristic of science as a way of testing a hypothesis. The aim is to reduce the number of factors that may affect the results so that the procedures are reproduceable
Feminism	the theoretical perspective focusing on gender inequality and the role of women in society. This theory stresses the social and historical origins of women's inferior position in society
Functionalism	the theoretical perspective that sees institutions and processes as having specific social functions, which may differ from their overt function and which contribute to social continuity and consensus
Gender	the social role that is attached to being biologically male or female
Genes	a section of genetic material (DNA) that codes for a protein, that is, instructs the cell how to assemble amino acids into proteins. As there are thought to be about 100,000 proteins in humans, there are about 100,000 genes
Globalization	the increasingly interdependent social and economic relationships that span different countries around the world
Health	a contested concept that is variously defined according to place and time. Health is defined by the WHO (1946) as 'a state of complete physical, mental, and social wellbeing, not merely the absence of disease or infirmity' and more recently as [the extent to which] an individual or group [is] able ... to realize aspirations, to satisfy needs, and to change or cope with the environment.

Health is, therefore, seen as a resource for everyday life, not the objective of living. Health is a positive concept emphasizing social and personal resources, as well as physical capacities.' (WHO, 1986)

Health behaviours	acts that relate to health, such as eating, drinking or wearing a seat belt
Health beliefs	the opinions or thoughts that a person has concerning an object or action, for example the belief that potatoes are fattening
Health indicator	a characteristic that is used to describe an aspect of a population, for example quality of life or life expectancy
Hegemony	domination of one group or set of ideas over others through political means
Holism	from the Greek *holos* (whole), it is a theory that the parts of any whole cannot exist and cannot be understood except in relation to the whole. In health terms, holism refers to the view that the body cannot be separated from the emotions or mind
Homeostasis	the relatively constant and optimal internal environment, or conditions within organizations or cells, or the physiological processes that maintain these conditions
Hypothesis	a proposed explanation for a phenomenon
Identity	can be signified by the way in which we consume culture in order to convey a certain image
Ideology	a framework of concepts and values, similar to an intellectual paradigm, that shapes a view of the world, for example liberalism, feminism
Illness	commonly understood as the subjective experience of ill health or disease. Illness perceptions are constructed by the social, cultural, historical and geographical contexts which we inhabit
Incidence	the number of newly diagnosed cases during a specific time period
Induction	in science is the process of reaching a generalization or law from many individual specific observations
Interactionism	the theoretical perspective that emphasizes the meaning of social life. Meanings emerge from social interaction and interpretation and are conveyed via language, labels and signs
Interdisciplinary	the relationships both between and among disciplines that enable different perspectives on an issue
Internal market	the introduction of a commercial culture into health services in which different agencies (for example GP

practices, hospitals and health authorities) seek to provide or purchase services in managed competition with the intention of increased efficiency

Justice — fairness in terms of one or other (or more) of: resource allocation (distributive justice), meeting natural rights (rights-based justice) and the law (legal justice)

Lay health beliefs — non-professional interpretations of what causes health and illness. Lay beliefs may contrast with biomedical interpretations of cause

Lifestyle (conducive to health) — a way of living based on identifiable patterns of behaviour. Lifestyle is often presumed to be a matter of personal choice. However lifestyles are determined by the interplay between an individual's personal characteristics, social interactions, and socioeconomic and environmental living conditions

Locus of control — refers to an individual's generalized expectations concerning where control over subsequent events resides – internal locus of control being the belief that control over future events resides primarily in oneself, while external locus of control is the expectancy that control is outside oneself – either in the hands of powerful others or due to fate/chance

Marxist and political economy perspectives — see medicine as a tool of capitalism and economic growth, stressing the conflict inherent in capitalism, characterized by opposing classes with different interests

Materialism — the theoretical perspective that emphasizes the importance of material resources and access to resources such as income and education. This theory focuses on social inequality

Medicalization — the process by which medicine has increased its power in society. This includes the use of medical technology and the professional power of doctors to make decisions about social and ethical problems

Methodology — the theoretical analysis of methods belonging to a specific discipline or branch of knowledge, for example 'the methodology used in this psychosocial research project is qualitative and social constructionist'. Also used to refer to a body of practices or the overall orientation of a piece of research, for example 'the study's methodology employed qualitative methods including questionnaires and observation'

Methods — the means to achieve something. In research, methods refers to specific means of collecting and analysing data, for example interviews and content analysis of interview scripts

Mixed economy of welfare	the provision of welfare through a mixture of state, private, voluntary and informal services. Sometimes referred to as welfare pluralism
Model	an abstract construction presenting possible relationships between phenomena, for example health belief model
Morbidity	the state of being diseased, usually measured by the number of cases of people with a medical condition in a given population at a given time
Mortality rate	the number of deaths in a population. Thus, the crude mortality rate is the total number of deaths in the population divided by the total population size. Specific mortality rates refer to particular subpopulations, for example the rate of deaths in males of social class I
Multidisciplinary	the study of a subject that applies the methods and approaches of several disciplines. It may also be used to describe a planning approach that includes professionals from different disciplines
Need	a socially constructed and highly contested concept related to want. It may be publicly expressed by individuals or groups, or be professionally defined (normative needs)
Neoliberalism	a political movement of the 1980s espousing the free market and resisting state interference as a means of promoting economic development and securing political liberty. Critics see it as a means of sustaining inequalities
Non-maleficence	doing no harm. This is frequently regarded as a moral obligation that ought to be held by healthcare workers and is closely connected with beneficence
Null hypothesis	a prediction that there is no causal relationship between two factors. This hypothesis is then tested, by examining the likelihood that any observed relationship between the factors could have arisen by chance. Disproving the null hypothesis means that there is a strong possibility that a cause and effect relationship between two variables (which is very unlikely to happen by chance) has been discovered
Organizational culture	a set of collectively held, relevant, distinctive and shared meanings, values and assumptions, which operate unconsciously and define an organization's (unchallenged) view of itself, its environment and its mission. It also defines and governs the expected behaviour of its members
Organs	are composed of tissues that form a structure such as the heart, stomach, liver or skin tending to restore the status quo (in this case, raising the body temperature again)

P value	the probability that the data under consideration would have occurred by chance (that is, just due to sampling variation). The p value is crucial in deciding whether or not two variables are likely to be causally related. Quantitative research commonly tests a null hypothesis, that is, a statement that there is no relationship between two variables. If the p value is small, then the null hypothesis is more likely to be rejected, because the data under consideration are unlikely to have occurred by chance. A common threshold p value is less than 0.05, which means that the data could have arisen by chance (that is, without a causal relationship) in only 1 in 20 instances. When the p value is 0.05 or less, it is commonly accepted that a causal relationship between the two variables being considered exists
Paradigm	in an intellectual discipline, this refers to a framework comprising the assumptions, concepts, theories and values within which the search for knowledge is conducted, for example a scientific paradigm
Paradigm shift	a term first used by Kuhn to describe the process by which one way of thinking is replaced by another through a series of 'revolutions', for example Keynesian economics replaced by monetarism
Partnership	two or more individuals, teams or organizations working collaboratively towards the achievement of agreed goals and targets. A partnership for health is a voluntary agreement between two or more partners to work cooperatively towards a set of shared health outcomes
Pathogenic	the presence of disease caused by a pathogen (a disease-causing agent such as a virus or bacteria)
Policy	goals, decisions and purposeful actions generally associated with governments but also with a range of other organizations
Postmodernism	an umbrella term referring to the rejection of modernism, linear progress and essential truths in favour of fragmentation, plural discourses and relativism
Prevalence	refers to disease rates in populations. The prevalence of disease X refers to the number of people with disease X alive on a certain date
Primary care or primary healthcare	healthcare that is located in communities and is the first point of call
Proteins	large (macro) molecules made of smaller subunits called amino acids. In living organisms, there are about 20 amino acids that can join together in a number of combinations to make many different proteins. Amino

acids are formed from groups of chemicals similar in structure and composition to ammonia. The breakdown product of amino acids is ammonia, which gives urine its particular characteristic. The proteins formed from amino acids have a variety of functions, such as structural products (for example collagen), enzymatic products (for example the enzymes catalase, amylase) or transport products (for example albumin, haemoglobin)

Quality of life   an individual's perception of his or her position in life. May include an assessment of physical health, psychological state, level of independence, social relationships, physical environment and personal beliefs

QALY   quality adjusted life year. A measure of health output that captures both length of life and quality of life

Randomized controlled trial   an experimental study in which subjects are randomly allocated to receive or not receive an intervention

Rationing   a mechanism to reconcile an excess of demand over supply. In competitive markets, consumption is rationed by price; that is, only those willing and able to pay the market price can consume the goods. With public provision, consumption is rationed using more explicit methods such as waiting lists, limited prescribing lists and so on. Often euphemistically referred to as prioritization

Reductionist   a scientific approach of seeking explanation and understanding by focusing on smaller and smaller units, for example seeking to understand disease processes by focusing on cellular changes

Representation   how cultural artefacts are portrayed, discussed and given symbolic meanings

Rights   inalienable properties of all human beings, as in the right to independence and autonomy. Rights are often derived from moral and ethical frameworks, and may be protected by national or international legal frameworks

Risk factors   are those that make an individual or population susceptible to a disease or illness. They may be environmental (for example exposure to asbestos), related to lifestyle (for example drinking alcohol) or genetic (for example a familial history of breast cancer)

Risk groups   used in epidemiology to describe groups vulnerable to certain diseases or conditions, whether because of their behaviour or their economic, environmental or social characteristics

Science   from the Latin *scientia* (knowledge), science comprises two main fields – the natural sciences, which study natural phenomena such as the human body, and the social sciences, which study human behaviour and societies

Scientific method
a systematic way of gathering data through observation and experimentation, and the formulation and testing of hypotheses. The scientific method, and resulting knowledge, is often viewed as more rigorous and dependable than alternative forms of gathering knowledge, for example reflection

Screening
the presumptive identification of a disease or condition through the use of tests (for example blood tests in newborns to detect phenylketonuria) or examinations (for example the use of chest X-rays to detect tuberculosis)

Self-efficacy
the belief relating to the degree of confidence an individual has in whether a behaviour can be performed

Sick role
Parsons' theory that ill people enter into the sick role, which confers both rights and obligations. The sick role legitimates and regulates illness and hence minimizes the disruption caused by illness

Social capital
the degree of cohesion that exists in communities, characterized by networks of belonging and trust, linked to social participation and access to resources

Social constructionism
the theoretical perspective suggesting that all knowledge and discourse (as well as ideology and representations) are socially constructed within a context in which different groups of people have differing interests and priorities, and therefore represent only a partial truth

Social inequalities
inequalities in income, access to resources, power and status that are produced, reproduced and maintained by social processes and institutions

Social justice
the concepts of rights and fairness in the distribution of resources

Statute law
a law made by a sovereign or legislative authority

Structuralism
a term covering theoretical perspectives arguing that the social world is shaped by underlying forces such as economic structure and the role of language

Target
a formalized goal set by an individual, team or organization. Health targets state, for a given population, the amount of change (using a health indicator) that could be reasonably expected within a defined time period. Targets are generally based on specific and measurable changes in health outcomes, or intermediate health outcomes

Team-building	an essential component of organizational development, whereby the needs and roles of individual group members and team objectives are identified and clarified, and responsibilities are negotiated and assigned. Team-building can take place both 'off the job' through facilitated training exercises and also through work-related activity, innovation and feedback on work performance
Theory	a logical and plausible explanation of why systems or people behave in observed ways, for example why people adopt protective health behaviours. A theory is capable of predicting future occurrences and being tested through experiment or otherwise falsified through empirical observation, for example theory of planned behaviour
Universalism	benefits and services available to all within a society, regardless of ability to pay
Utilitarianism	the moral theory asserting that we always ought to do what will produce the greatest good
Values	things which are valuable. Value may be subjective (something is valued simply because it is wanted), instrumental (something is valued because it has a useful function) or intrinsic (something is valued because it has fundamental and irreducible importance). It is of course possible for something to be valuable in more than just one of these separate senses
Welfare	the conditions necessary to secure the wellbeing of individuals in any society

Index

Page numbers printed in **bold** type refer to figures; those in *italic* to tables. An asterisk (*) before a page number indicates a glossary entry